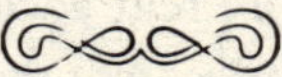

In the book *Mastering Yoga*, all the aspects of yoga have been described precisely. The specialty of this book is that the *yogasanas* have been presented clearly with illustrations, for the reader. I hope that this book will be a guide to students, researchers and all those who seek knowledge of yoga.

Prof. Ganesh Shankar Giri
Head, Department of Yogic Science,
Dr Harisingh Gaur University, Sagar

The strength of this knowledge-enhancing book is that by reading it, any reader can develop their internal and external self and make their personalities, complementing the present times. They can also bring about the desired changes in their physical, mental, educational, spiritual and cultural aspects of life.

Dr Shailendra Parashar
Professor and Director,
Ambedkar Peetha, Vikram University, Ujjain

The book *Mastering Yoga* written by Mr Rajeev Jain 'Trilok' is like a bouquet in the garden of this world. Just as a gardener chooses the most beautiful flowers of his garden to make a bouquet, similarly Mr Trilok has picked various yoga *kriyas* and written them down in the form of a book, which is very useful for students, yoga practitioners and those who have interest in yoga.

Shri M. P. Yadav
Trainer, State Yoga In-charge – M.P.
Govt. Yoga Training Centre, Bhopal

This effort by Shri Rajeev Jain 'Trilok' is really a novel one. He has comprehensively described Yoga in context to the Indian philosophy. This is indeed a great accomplishment in the field of Yoga. I congratulate him and expect that the readers would benefit from this.

Dr Mahesh Jain
Director,
Maharshi Patanjali Sanskrit Sansthan, Bhopal

The efforts of Shri Rajeev Jain 'Trilok' cannot be expressed in words. His efforts have given the world the encyclopedia of yoga. In present time, where everyone is stressed and have fast dynamic lifestyle and environment is pollutted, each and every person needs peaceful, stressfree and healthy life. And I think this book is the ultimate solution for all your problems.

Dr Subhash Atre, IPS, Chief Secretary, Home Chhattisgarh/ **Dr Ramesh Tevani,** Bhopal,/**Dr H. Malvi,** MD, Bhopal;/ **Dr Mohan,** Canada;/**Dr Pooja Rai,** Melbourne, Australia/ **Sakina Husain Malvi,** Auckland, New Zealand/**Rachna Jain,** Jabalpur/**Vivek Tantray,** Damoh/**Vijay Kukreja,** Badalapur/ **Dr Manoj Sharma,** Bhopal/**Harish saxena MD (AIECCE)** New Delhi

MASTERING YOGA

MASTERING YOGA

Yogasanas, Pranayama, Mudra, Body-locks (Bandha), Purification of the Body (Shatkarma), Meditation and Kundalini Yoga

With scientific explanations

Yogacharya
RAJEEV JAIN 'Trilok'

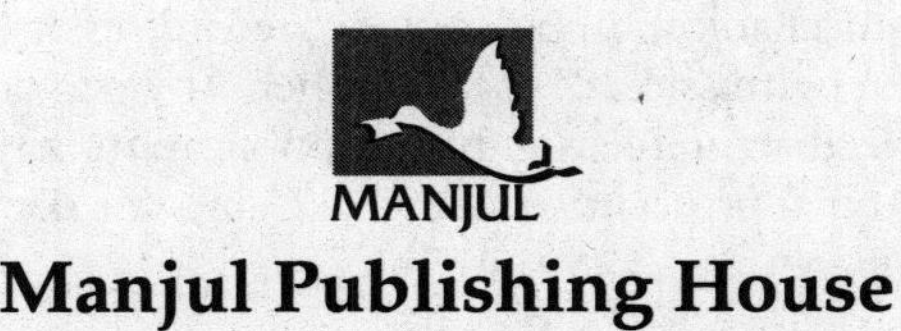

Manjul Publishing House

First published in India by

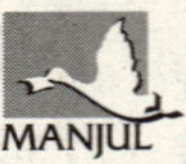

Manjul Publishing House
• C-16, Sector 3, Noida, Uttar Pradesh 201301, India
Website: www.manjulindia.com

Registered Office:
• 2nd Floor, Usha Preet Complex, 42 Malviya Nagar,
Bhopal 462 003 – India

Distribution Centres:
Ahmedabad, Bengaluru, Chennai, Kochi, Kolkata,
Hyderabad, Mumbai, New Delhi, Pune

Mastering Yoga
Yogasanas, Pranayama, Mudra, Body-locks (Bandha), Purification of the Body (Shatkarma), Meditation and Kundalini Yoga
With scientific explanations

This edition first published in 2021
Fourth impression 2025

ISBN 978-93-91242-45-9

Printed and bound in India by Saurabh Printers Pvt. Ltd.

The publisher or the author do not intend to provide any professional advice or service through this book. The ideas, procedures, and suggestions given in the book are in no way alternative to any medical assistance. Therefore, in any matter related to health, only medical advice should be taken and given priority. The publisher and the author shall not be liable for any loss or damage caused to any reader by the use of any information contained in the book.

Contents

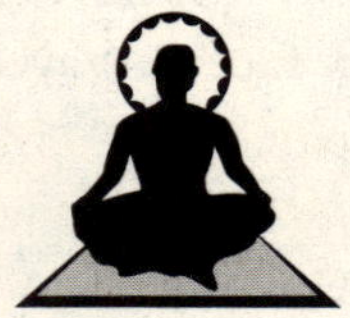

Tribute

I pay my respect to my Gurudev Acharya Shri 108 Vimalsagar Ji Maharaj. I pay homage to my respected father, late Mr Vijay Kumar Jain (Keolari M.P.) and mother, late Mrs Kamala Jain. I pay my respect to late Shri Krishnachandra Rakheja and Mrs Manjul Devi Rakheja, who have played the roles of a father and a mother to me. Their guidance and inspiration has made me who I am today.

At the tender age of two, when I lost my mother, the one gentle hand that held me, was that of late Mrs Uma Devi Jain. Now she is on her way to her journey towards salvation. I bow to her in reverence.

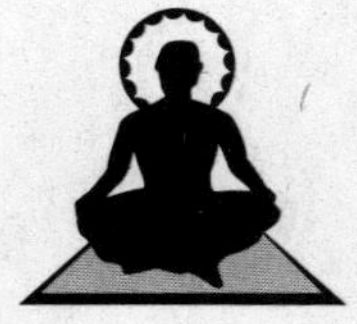

Dedication

This book is dedicated to:

- The Almighty, all pervading God, who has made me a capable medium of transmitting my knowledge about good health to people.
- To all those who wish to be healthy and those who aim to maintain their good health.
- To all those who wish to see everyone happy, disease free and prosperous by walking on this path.

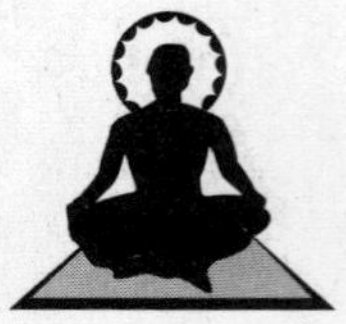

Acknowledgement

At the very outset, I would like to express my heartfelt thanks to the Director of Manjul Publications, Mr Vikas Rakheja and his wife Mrs Anu Rakheja, who not only encouraged me to write this book, but also showered their affection on me.

I owe the presentability of this book to Mr Vijay Gulsundare and Mr Abraham G. Varghese, who did their job of typesetting and designing with diligence and creativity.

I am grateful to all my well wishers and to my wife Asha Jain, daughter Anushree Jain and son Aadish Jain, who stood by me throughout this endeavour.

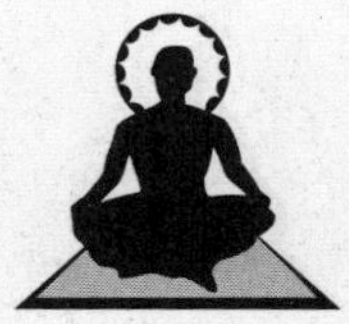

Words of Encouragement

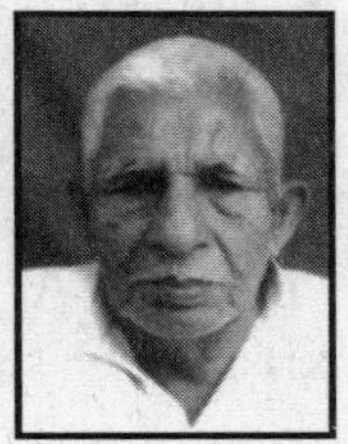

There have been many enlightened people in the Indian civilization. They have always nurtured the earth with their profound knowledge, and motivated people to move towards wellness by spreading the light of their wisdom. One such ray of light, that is emitted through this wisdom, has been instrumental in keeping our bodies healthy. My disciple, Rajeev Jain 'Trilok' has humbly received this tradition and knowledge and has written it down in the form of this book *Mastering Yoga*, so that everyone can attain physical and mental happiness, thereby achieving welfare of the self. This book has been written keeping in mind the requirements of a modern life. Though there are thousands of books available on yoga in the market, there has always been some aspect or the other lacking in them. Hence, this endeavour of Rajeev Jain 'Trilok' to make up for all these shortcomings is certainly praiseworthy. Since it includes many topics in one volume, it justifies the name *Mastering Yoga*. Hence, this book is worth reading from many perspectives. I extend my blessings and abundant good wishes to him.

Govind Prasad Gupta
Founder
Indian Council for Yoga Research

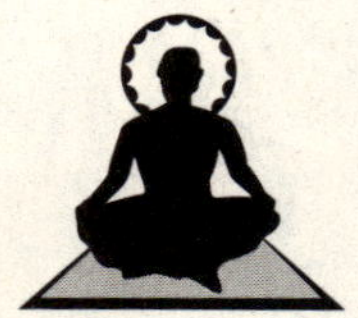

Blessings

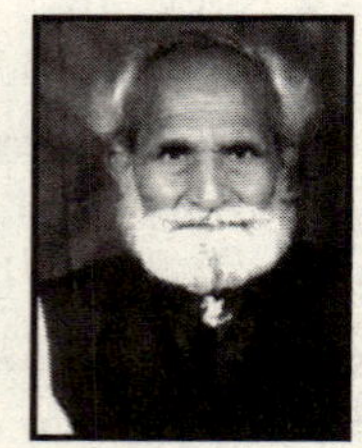

I am very pleased to know that just as I have tried to imbibe and disseminate with commitment and dedication, the knowledge and skills acquired from my gurus – Acharya 108 Shri Vimal Sagarji Maharaj, Aryikaratn Gyanmati Mataji, Shri Krishna Dasji Paramhans Maharaj 'Nepalibaba', Swami Satyanand Saraswati Ji Maharaj, Munger (Bihar), Swami Sachchidanand Saraswatiji, Munger (Bihar), who addressed me as 'Swami Pranavanand Saraswati' in Harda (M.P.), Swami Dheerendra Bramhachari Ji, Director, Antarashtreey Vishvayatan Yogashram, Katra (Jammu & Kashmir) – to all the people and continue to do so. Similarly my worthy disciple dear Rajeev Jain 'Trilok' has written and dedicated such a book to the society which will be helpful in bringing happiness, peace, health and self-development in the lives of all people worldwide. This book incorporates almost all the topics which are important to make life worthwhile, and are beneficial for the humankind.

For about last 50 years, I have been selflessly disseminating this knowledge (of yoga) obtained from my gurus, for the health of the people along with their spiritual and emotional progress, so that they may live worthy lives and reach great spiritual heights.

Here, I would like to mention that my Yoga guru, Swami Satyanand Saraswatiji and Swami Dheerendra Bramhachariji always used to say, 'Just as we have taught these skills to you, similarly you too should pass them on to your disciples and to everyone else.' Keeping these words in mind, I told my disciple Rajeev Jain 'Trilok', who had been practicing and learning Yoga for the last 20 years, that 'whether you take Yoga classes, or write books on Yoga, you must try to write exactly as you have been taught, so that the art and science of Yoga does not become obsolete. It should remain immortal. Simultaneously, you too must reach great spiritual heights.' With these good wishes and blessings, may you continue to do the good job of disseminating the knowledge of Yoga, which has been brought down from generations through the guru disciple tradition and which has been imparted to you by me.

God bless you

Yogacharya Dr Phoolchand 'Yogiraj'
'Ayog Mitra' (M.P. Human Rights Commission)
Dy Chairman – Madhya Pradesh Yoga Parishad

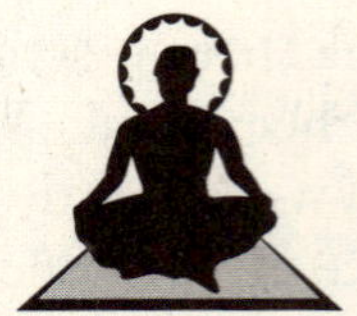

Introduction

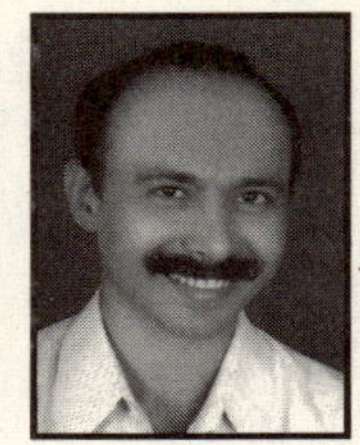

I bow in salutation to Alakh Niranjan Lord Shiva 1008 Shri Adinath, who is the pioneer of imparting knowledge since the beginning of creation. I also bow in reverence to His Divine Omkar Divyaghosh, who manifested in the form of Mother Saraswati till the reign of Veer Prabhu, and was called as Mata Jinvani.

The same profound knowledge was passed on in its totality by the great saints, mahatmas, sages, medicants and acharyas to their disciples. It is because of this tradition that the Indian culture has flourished till this day and has made its unique place in the world.

'This bright light of knowledge is wholly their blessing.'

I first received the light of spiritual knowledge from my father. He had many encounters with many enlightened souls. By the grace of god, I too started moving towards spiritual development day by day. My inquisitiveness towards spirituality started increasing. I studied many subjects. Since the subject of spirituality is quite vast and deep, I met different gurus to learn and study different topics and continued to practise as a learner. Even today, if I come across a camp based on spirituality or yoga being organised, I enroll myself as an innocent child without introducing myself, and humbly imbibe the knowledge and processes that are taught. This is a subject where the more we learn, the more our knowledge develops.

I would like to name all those great saints, acharyas and yogis from whom I got this knowledge directly or indirectly.

First and foremost, I would like to pay my respect to Gautam Gandharacharya. I also pay my respect to Shri Kundkundacharya, Shri Shubhchandracharya, most respected Acharya Vidyasagarji, most respected Dhyan Sagarji Maharaj, Maharishi Patanjali Maharaj, Rishi Gherund, Muni Vashishthji, Swami Shivanand, Swami Satyanand Saraswati, Shri B.K.S. Iyengar, Shri Barfani Baba, Swami Vishuddhanand Paramhans 'Gyanganj', Gopinath Kaviraj, Swami Kartikeyaji, Swami Dheerendra Bramhachari, Paramhans Niranjananand Saraswati, Dr K.M. Ganguliji, Baba Ramdev, Shrimati Shashi Sood, Shriman S.D. Sood and Dr Phoolchand 'Yogiraj'. This book is a manisfestation of the blessings from all of you, because your soul and profound vision is also directed towards the well-being and good health of people.

I pay my respect to esteemed Pt. Rajkamalji, who motivated me to move on the spiritual path.

I am grateful to the entire team of Trilok Prachya Vidya Research Centre. I express my heartfelt gratitude to late Ajay Kumar Verma, Dr H. Malvi, Shri M.P. Yadav, Dr (Shri) Ashok Janvade, Dr Subhash Atre (Ex. D.G.P.), Shri Manoj Kulkarni, SP Shri Hemant Chauhan, Dr Mahesh Bhargav, Shri Chandragopal Jethwani, Shri Devendra Sharma (Cartoonist), Dr Shobhit, late Savita Saini (didi), Neha Tripathi (PG Food and Nutrition), Dr Pramod Shankar Soni, Shri Sanjeev Dubey, Dr Akshay Jain, Rachna Jain and Lakhan Haldkar.

We have established Trilok Prachya Vidya Research Centre with a vision of not only keeping alive the ancient knowledge of Indian culture, but also to promote more research in this field, so that the whole world can benefit from it. This centre has been working efficiently for many years. In order to accumulate maximum knowledge and facts in this research centre, we have collected information and facts from many yogis, hath yogis, astrologers, vastuvids, ayurvedacharyas, tantra-mantra, tratak experts etc. on kundalini jagaran vidya, mysterious supernatural objects/places, siddha lands, parad vigyan, svarna tantram, rare jadi bootis, surya vigyan (where we can transform one object into another), manuscript of jyotish shastra, parapsychology etc. We have collected and preserved the rare experiences of all these people and the ancient knowledge on these subjects, and we aim to bring all these experiences/experiments to our inquisitive readers.

Our endeavour is to bring about materialistic, spiritual, physical and mental happiness and prosperity to the readers and to the whole world. We have worked very hard to prepare this book. This has been possible by the encouragement and support of people who demand more knowledge on the subject. We have tried our best to get them acquainted with the prevalent and popular names of the asanas. Yet, it has been observed, that the same asana has been given different names by different acharyas according to place and time. It has also been noted that by bringing a slight variation, the same asan is given a different name. This is our humble request to the readers that they should not pay much attention to these differences and variations, rather get acquainted with the benefits of those asanas and help others gain its benefit. Keep the feeling of self-improvement and well-being of others in mind. It is our humble request to the students as well that they should take guidance regarding the names, illustrations, methods etc. of the yogasanas from a yoga trainer. Though we have tried to keep many things in mind while preparing this book, we would still request that before adopting any procedure, please consult a yog trainer/guru. In case of any suggestion, or error in this book, please do not hesitate to bring it to our notice. We shall ever be grateful to you.

Rajeev Jain 'Trilok'
Director – Trilok Prachya Vidya Research Centre
Himalay Yoga Niketan Samiti®
Mob.: 09826530366
rajeevjaintrilok@gmail.com

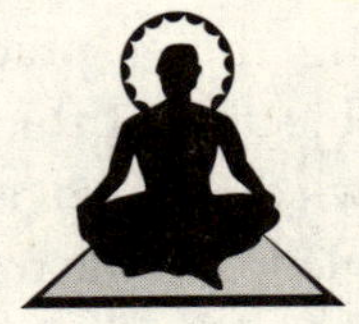

Foreword

The reason for all the maladies of man is ignorance. One can attain happiness only by good conduct. Self-study destroys ignorance. My favourite writer Shri Rajeev Jain 'Trilok' has created a 'heaven on earth' situation by writing his book *Mastering Yoga*. He has very economically expressed much in a few words by enumerating the measures to cure mental, physical and spiritual ailments. This book will work as a physician in every household. Nowadays, yog treatment is becoming very popular. Hence the demand for this book will increase day by day. I have been reading many books on yoga for the last 32 years, but have experienced priceless string of pearls in the form of *Mastering Yoga*. Yoga is a ethereal way of becoming one with the Divine. It is the ultimate bliss which has no form of expression. There is no limit to what one can achieve through yoga; there is no unit to measure it. The book reflects the good intentions of its writer. The laws of the all powerful nature are always active in fulfilling the good intentions of those who have awakened to the call of their conscience.

This book on yoga is absolutely scientific and meant for all. It has no trace of either communalism or a narrow attitude towards any religion. This book has been written by keeping in mind the diversities of place, time, religion and gender, among other things. It is a priceless heritage for mankind. The readers of this book must keep in mind that just as one cannot learn swimming by merely having theoretical knowledge, rather diving into the waters, similarly to gain complete knowledge from this book, they will have to practice what they read. It is possible to acquire true knowledge only by doing things practically, and consecutively finding liberation. The objective of this book is to rediscover and reestablish the lost knowledge of yoga. It is carefully written in order to imbibe the knowledge in the reader's minds. I believe that by studying this book, the practitioner will be able to satisfy all his curiosities because this book has combined the essence of all ancient books. At present, man is continuously troubled by many complicated diseases. The writer has addressed the ways to get rid of these sufferings in a special way. The remedy for physical, mental and spiritual maladies has been mentioned in specific places in this book. This is one of the books which is capable of directing man towards awakening his conscience. This book is written in a comprehensive way to satisfy the inquisitive readers. This book is like a flame of knowledge to expel the darkness of ignorance. The writer has tried to make this book simpler interesting, natural and error free by making some amendments in the previous editions. We believe that this effort will bring forth the facts to the forefront and satisfy the curious readers. The reason for man's sorrows is that he believes that illness and disease are his destiny and he has no option but to suffer. Whereas good health and happiness are actually his birth right. So, in order to come out of this collective insanity/misconception of diseases and ailments, and to experience health, happiness and completeness in our lives, it is important that we introduce systematic yoga in our daily routine. Both, the root cause of diseases as well as the systematic yogic treatment for those causes are enumerated in this book. The practitioners who wish to get quick relief by following the path of yoga, must keep in mind the intensity and duration of their disease. They must not try to do the treatment all by themselves by merely reading the book, but also consult an expert yoga doctor and get it done. This book has been written with the objective of motivating all those who are suffering from ailments caused by physical, natural and materialistic factors; those who are surrounded by ill health and wish to get above this situation by adopting yogabhyas.

This book is filled with such an energy which, when generated through regular practice, proves to be a capable medium of coming out of all our sufferings. This book is a message and a guide to all those doctors who are in search of new methods of treatments. It is my desire that this book should be used with the grace of the self-sufficient, victorious, master of the three worlds and the endless universal power of the Divine.

Dr L. J. Pachauri
Govt. Medical Officer,
Prakritik Aur Yoga Chikitsa Vigyan,
Bhopal (MP)

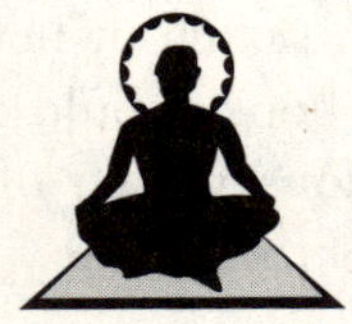

Preface

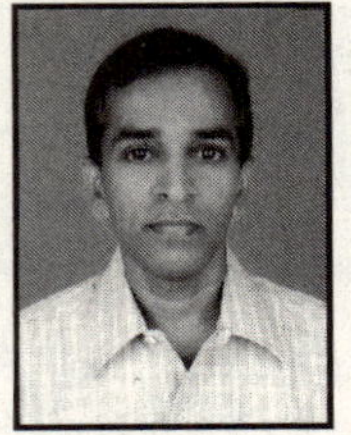

Shri Rajeev Jain 'Trilok' has included all his experience in his book *Mastering Yoga* and created a book which is very useful for the common man. It is also beneficial for the students of yoga. Though many books are available on yoga, *Mastering Yoga* actually lives up to its name.

Yogic approaches and natural treatments not only cures the diseases of people, but is also helpful in their all-round development. These approaches are not only free of any side effects, but they are also very easy, effective, and give quick results.

Today, Yoga and natural treatment are in demand everywhere because they have reached people in the form of medical cure. What we need is a well-researched literature, which has been written with absolute authority. *Mastering Yoga* plays a significant role in this direction.

The book has been presented well, and illustrations have enhanced its utility all the more.

Dr Rajiv Rastogi

Asst. Director (Pra. Chi)

Central Council for Yoga and Naturopathy Treatment Research, New Delhi

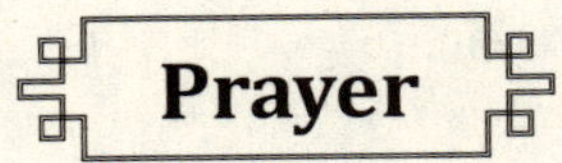

Prayer

योगेन चित्तस्य पदेन वाचां,
मलं शरीरस्य च वैद्यकेन।
योऽपाकरोतं प्रवरं मुनीनां,
पतञ्जलिं प्राञ्जलिरानतोऽस्मि।।

Hari-Har-Brahmā, Buddha, Jineshwar, Supreme Sire, Allah-Tālā, Wāh-e Guru!
I pray to you that may I always remain a being with a compassionate heart.
May I never ever hurt an innocent being or get corrupted mentally,
Even if I am offered a rosary of gems that can convert iron into gold.
May my compassion manifest upon helpless and suffering beings,
May I be helpful for the needy at the right moment and may I own patience with courage.

May I learn to smile in adversities and may I possess a fear of sinful deeds,
May I live in the present and may I embrace my death with the Lord's name on my lips.

Let me treat others in the way I want to be treated myself,
May I shower my love upon the youngsters and treat my elders with due respect.
May I practice yoga daily to keep myself healthy and fit,
And with the help of DHYAN-YOGA, may I end all diseases.

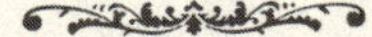

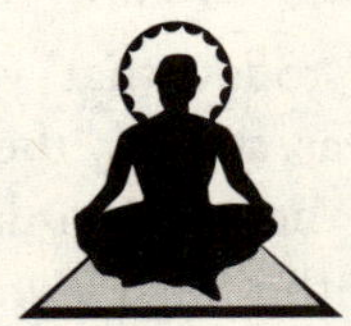

Introduction to Yoga

An Ideological Perspective

From a historical point of view, it is very difficult to express when, how and where the knowledge of yoga initiated. If we take a look at the ancient texts, we will find a mention of yoga vidya in the Vedas and the religious texts of Jainism. Therefore, we can say that the tradition of yoga has been in existence since ancient times. The knowledge of yoga has been prevalent since such knowledge were not written about but passed on by word of mouth from one guru to the other and from the guru to the disciple. But it is not so important to debate on when the knowledge of yoga initiated, rather, the important question is who expounded the knowledge on yoga first, and when? Yog has maintained its superiority in the world for thousands of years. It has touched the lives of people of all types and given the right direction to humankind.

In fact, yoga is a 'universal and global religion'. According to yoga, religion is a science, but even if we study it without connecting it to any religion, we will find that we are actually studying a text akin to our own religion, while reaffirming our faith and religious feelings for the sake of the welfare and upliftment of the humankind. In this way we can try to understand the secrets of yoga with more clarity.

Sages who had connected with their souls, advocated Yoga which was directed and interpreted by the laws of their own spiritual conduct followed in a systematic manner. It makes the practitioner capable of achieving his goals. Thus in practical terms, yoga is a symbol of knowledge and universal well-being.

It's a popular belief today that yoga was introduced by Maharishi Patanjali, whereas, actually the first guru of yog is Lord Shiva. Some people are of the opinion that *Yoga Darshan* written by Patanjali is based on the *Yoga Sutras* written by Hiranya Garbh. Maharishi Patanjali propagated the Ashtang Yoga, which is conceived as Yam, Niyam, Aasan, Pranayam, Pratyahar, Dharana, Dhyan and Samadhi. Indian Literature has greatly contemplated on the subject of Yoga. Lord Krishna said in *The Bhagvad Gita* -

तपस्विभ्योऽधिको योगी ज्ञानिभ्योऽपि मतोऽधिकः।
कर्मिभ्यश्चाधिको योगी तस्माद्योगी भवार्जुन।। (6/46)

O Arjuna! Be a yogi, because amongst the sages, wise men and those indulging continuously in their work towards fulfilling their desires – the yogi is the best.

Lord Krishna says to his friend Uddhav in *Shrimad Bhagvat Mahapuran* -

जितेन्द्रियस्य युक्तस्य जितश्र्वासस्य योगिनः।
मयि धारयतश्चेत उपतिष्ठन्ति सिद्धयः।। (11/15/1)

Dear Uddhav! When the yogi gains control over his senses, breath and mind, and starts concentrating his thoughts on me, he gains mastery over many *siddhis*.

It is clear from this that all the siddhis (Anima, Mahima, Laghima, Prapti, Prakamya, Ishita, Vashita, Kamavasayita) can be automatically mastered by practicing yoga. However, the ultimate achievement of yoga is not limited to the mere mastery of the siddhis, but acquiring the knowledge of the self and self-esteem.

The main objective of the various approaches and prayers of yoga is to cleanse the mind from the negative emotions of attachment and jealousy, and purify its tendencies by infusing the divine qualities in it. Yoga is a journey from knowing of the self to mastering of the self. Yoga is the only means to awake the inherent conscience.

The significance of yoga in character-building is also apparent. When the inherent divine nature of the humankind is awakened by practicing yoga, they become an epitome of humanistic qualities. The main factors of character-building lie in nothing else than in forgiveness, pity, compassion, knowledge and detachment.

Types of Yoga

In the ancient texts, many types of yoga are mentioned. According to preferences, there have been many followers of those types. In Yoga Pradeep, yoga is believed to be of many kinds, such as Raj Yoga, Ashtang Yoga, Hatth Yoga, Laya Yoga, Dhyan Yoga, Bhakti Yoga, Kriya Yoga, Mantra Yoga, Karm Yoga and Gyan Yoga. Lord Krishna had preached three kinds of yoga – Gyan Yoga, Karm Yoga and Bhakti Yoga.

Meaning and Definition of Yoga

The general meaning of yoga is to join, combine, be one with, or to collect. In Sanskrit, the word yoga is said to have originated from the root word 'yuj'. The word 'yoga' is constructed by adding 'karan' after the root word 'yuj' and by adding the prefix 'dhan' in 'bhaav vachya'. In Sanskrit, the root word 'yuj' has been used for 'samyog' in the 'Rudhadigan' as 'yujir yoge[1]'. In 'Divadigan', it has been used for 'samadhi' as 'yuj samadhau[2]'. In 'Churadigan', it has been used for 'samyaman' as 'yuj samyamne[3]'. By adding the prefix 'dhan' to the explanation of the root word 'yuj' in these meanings, the word yoga has been formed.

The practical meaning of the word yoga is very comprehensive. Its scope is also very wide. Thus, we find many different meanings of yoga.

1. 'Yujir yoge' siddhant kaumudi dhatukram no. 1444
2. 'Yuj samadhau' siddhant kaumudi dhatukram no. 1177
3. 'Yuj samyamne' siddhant kaumudi dhatukram no. 1807

Yoga is the practical form of Sankhya. It is a universal religion devoid of all religious, communal and ideological sentiments, which teaches us to realise the soul through the experience of the 'self', guiding the practitioner to his ultimate goal (salvation).

In the present times, there are many misconceptions about yoga. If we try to understand it in simpler words, then, yoga is the journey from 'imperceptible to subtle' and from 'without to within'. We move towards the perceptible due to the tendencies or thought waves of the mind; in other words, the mind focuses on the outer world instead of becoming stable. The more unstable we become, the more the *Raj* and *Tam* increase in our lives. But as we train our mind to focus on our inner self, the level of *Sat* or profound knowledge and philosophy accordingly manifest to attain self-realisation and reach a stage of absolute clarity.

In the second sutra of the Samadhi part of Yog Darshan, Patanjali has defined Yoga as:

योगश्चित्तवृत्तिनिरोधः ।।2।।

that is, yoga means to control the tendencies of the mind.

Shri Patanjali further writes:

तदा द्रष्टुः स्वरूपेऽवस्थानम् ।।3।।

Which means that (having gained control over the senses), one is established in one's own nature/form.

वृत्तिसारूप्यमितरत्र ।।4।।

In another situation (not being established in one's own nature), one sees one's image as per one's tendencies.

In the above sutra, only the term 'chittavritti nirodh' term has been used, instead of 'sarv chittavritti nirodh'.

In this way the sutra's composer has enumerated both, sampragyat and asampragyat samadhis, as yoga. Undoubtedly, the Asampragyat Samadhi, where all the tendencies or thought waves are brought under control, is yoga. However, the Sampragyat Samadhi, in which pure concentration is maintained, also falls under the characteristics of yoga. This means that when the deluded shroud of *Raj* and *Tam* is removed from the mind and the concentration thus received is illuminated by the light of *Sat*, such a condition should also be considered as yoga.

Different Definitions of Yoga and Their Comparision in Different Text

★ **According to Vedant:** Yoga is the complete union of Jeevatma with Paramatma.

★ To give up all thoughts related to the physical body, or in other words, to give up all desires of the physical body and to generate a longing for soul is yoga.

★ **According to Sankhya philosophy:**

'पुंप्रकृत्योर्वियोगेऽपि योग इत्यभिधीयते'

The condition of establishing separate entities of Purush and Prakriti, and by keeping them apart when the Purush establishes himself in his own nature is yoga.

★ **योग कर्मसु कौशलम्:** The skill of duty is yoga. ।। Gita ।।

★ The combination of Pran and Apan, meeting of the Sun and the Moon, and the union of Shiv and Shakti is also called yoga.

★ **According to Yoga Bhashya:**

'योगः समाधिः स च सर्व भौमश्चित्तस्य धर्मः ।'

★ **In the words of Mahatma Yagyavalk:**

'संयोग योग इत्युक्तो जीवात्म परमात्नो ।'

★ **According to Yoga Shastra:**

'सर्व चिंता परित्यक्तो निश्चिन्तो योग उच्यते ।'

★ **According to Pratyabhigyan Darshan:**

'The absolute knowledge of the oneness of Shiv and Atma is yoga.'

★ **According to Yoga Vashishth:**

'The means by which one can sail across the ocean of the world is yoga.'

★ **According to Shri Bharti Krishnateerth:**

'The means by which the Nar and the Narayan become one is yoga.'

★ **According to Shri Arvind:**

'Yoga does not mean the mere attainment of the Divine, but it is the act through which the awareness of Divine presence is expressed and, through which one becomes a part of God.'

★ **Sampoornanand (Chid Vilas) has written:**

'Yoga is the only way to self-realisation.'

★ **Lord Shri Krishna has said:**

नात्यश्नतस्तु योगोऽस्ति न चैकान्तमनश्नतः ।
न चाति स्वप्नशीलस्य जाग्रतो नैवचार्जुन ।।
युक्ताहार विहारस्य युक्त चेष्टस्य कर्मसु ।
युक्त स्वप्नावबोधस्य योगो भवति दुःखहा ।। Geeta 6-16/17

'He, who eats a lot, cannot master yoga. He, who remains without food, cannot master yoga either. He, who over sleeps, cannot master yoga, and he, who never sleeps/sleeps less, cannot master yoga either.

He, who remains perfectly balanced in his diet, other conduct, in sleep and while being awake, his yoga becomes a source of joy and happiness for him (that is, a source to eradicate sorrow).'

★ **According to the author of this book (Rajeev Jain 'Trilok'):**

'Yoga is the profound way of self-realisation in its true nature.'

★ **According to Shrimad Yoga Gita:**

'प्राणापानसमायोगो योगश्चित्तात्मनोस्तथा
यत्र जीवेशयोर्योगस्तं योगं विद्धि भूपते।।'

Bramhanand says, 'O King! The method by which Pran and Apan become one, mind and soul become one, and the living and the Divine become one, is known as yoga.'

★ **According to Shri Yashovijayakrita 'Dvatrinshika':**

'मोक्षेण योजनादेव योगो ह्यत्र निरुच्यते।'

It means that all methods which lead to the purification of the soul and towards salvation (moksh) are yoga.

It is further written in Yashovijayakrita 'Dvatrinshika':

'समितिगुप्ति धारणं धर्मव्यापारत्वमेव योग त्वम्।'

It means that the religious business (job) of gaining control over the mind, words and body (the three kinds of samiti) is none other than yoga.

★ **A certain yogi has said:**

'योगं वदान्यै बल बुद्धि श्रेष्ठं
पौरुष भवेत सदचित्त सौख्यं।
आत्मं परमात्मं भवतां नरेणं
क्षेमं च श्रेय योगं सुधीनः।।'

It means that in our lives, yoga is the only way by which a man can achieve the five great qualities of strength, intelligence, excellence, vitality and good character.

It is only through yoga that humankind can become capable of rising above the ordinary and reach the soul and the Divine. And by this medium alone they can achieve their goals of welfare, goodness and awareness.

The Need of Yoga in the Present Context

Yoga is needed today more than ever. In the past, our environment, atmosphere, food habits, lifestyle, etc. were natural to a great extent. But today our polluted environment and atmosphere, fast food and tinned food, food devoid of proteins and vitamins, changing lifestyle and perverted mentality have affected our health. Today, while the scientists have provided us with many facilities, their adverse effects have also had a negative impact on our health. Owing to these reasons, it's very important to get acquainted with yoga today. Through yoga we can generate right thinking and provide guidance to the present generation and the generations to come.

What Does Yoga Do

It is very difficult to say what Yoga does. It can be understood only after putting it to practice. However, we have tried to explain it in a few words.

When you adopt the path of yoga sadhana, you resolve problems of the abdominal region, such as indigestion, loss of appetite, constipation, gas and acidity. By following the diet mentioned in yoga, one can keep away fatal diseases, such as blood pressure, diabetes and heart diseases. The feeling of peace and contentment automatically starts permeating into our lives. The practitioner stays away from treachery, falsehood, theft and bad character. This results in the development of his moral character at both, individual and social levels.

Yoga grants us physical well-being as well as mental peace which results in freedom from stress. We can enhance our memory by doing yoga nidra and meditation. Yoga brings about a remarkable increase in our working skills and working capacity.

Yoga makes our circulatory system, digestive system, respiratory system and reproductory system active and functional. It has been proved by scientific experiments that the physical degeneration and instability of mind caused due to advancing age can be cured by the practice of yoga. We can drive away negativity and develop immunity through it.

In this way, it is an indisputable fact that yoga is a scientific approach, and not merely a type of physical exercise. While on one hand, its *asanas* and *shatkarmas* make our body disease free, well-built and enhances our immunity; on the other hand, pranayama and meditation among other things, enhances our concentration, vigor and glow of the body.

Almost all Indian philosophies have accepted this fact: Until the mind and conscience is not clear, one's aspirations does not abate, and one cannot realise their true self and attain true knowledge. Yoga is the best means of self-development. It purifies both, the body and the mind.

The science of yoga is the true guide to lead an ideal life. Since knowledge is directly related to life itself, practical and experimental science is needed in every field. Yoga is an absolutely practical psychology. In this way, yoga leads to one's all round development. Apart from being a science, yoga is also a lifestyle.

What is Yoga?

If we consider the word YOGA on the basis of the four letters of the English alphabet, we can clearly see what each individual letter conveys:

Y ield	:	What results does yoga yield for us?
O btain	:	What new achievements can we obtain from yoga?
G ive up	:	What are the things that we can give up by adopting yoga?
A ttain	:	What can we finally attain through yoga?

Yield (What results does yoga yield for us?)

- It strengthens the control over our breath.
- Meditation provides stability of mind. It helps to achieve emotional balance – one remains unaffected by sorrow, happiness, appreciation and insult.

- We feel psychologically sound, remain happy in life, connect to the society in a positive way, and draw a sense of satisfaction from serving to others.
- We are able to imbibe all the moral values, which make our life happy and joyful. Following this path leads to experiencing spirituality in life.

Obtain (What new achievements can we obtain from yoga?)

- By adopting yoga, a meaningful life can be built by giving it a meaningful direction.
- By adopting yoga, one is able to maintain awareness, consciousness and alertness. It makes one knowledgeable about their deeds and thoughts, allowing them to live as a conscious, principled and good human being.
- Yoga enhances concentration. One gives up their false pride and surrenders to the presence of the Almighty.
- Yoga helps develop the ability to work in an organised and planned way.
- Yoga helps develop creativity, positive attitude, and a feeling of detachment.

Give up (What are the things that we can give up by adopting yoga?)

- By adopting yoga, we can give up all those things which create numerous problems and cause harm, such as bad habits, wrong tendencies, intake of intoxicants, and shattered personality.
- Our negative and destructive mentality gradually disappears and we start gaining the true knowledge about ourselves.
- Our attachment towards worldly objects, greed for money, craving for respect and fame, worry for the fulfillment of our needs start vanishing gradually.
- We can give up all unnecessary and illogical activities which not only harm us, but also disrupt the social order. Hence, by doing Yog, the purity of mind is enhanced.

Attain (What can we finally attain through yoga?)

- One attains overall good health – the body becomes nourished, the mind becomes calm, one experience happiness from many sources and moves towards spirituality.
- One develops various skills, enhances the quality of life, acquires the qualities of a good human being, sees goodness everywhere, finds every appearance attractive, finds life very interesting, has a feeling of fulfillment, and his life is filled with love.
- One's mind is always joyful. One respects the life of every creature, enjoys life and is able to emotionally participate.
- One gets rid of the worries caused due to negativities and feels relaxed and peaceful. The mind and the heart move into a state of absoluteness, all confusions and violent thoughts cease, the disorders of the body vanish and one gains a lot of strength.
- Along with all these things, one starts considering oneself as a successful person and starts feeling victorious. One understands the true value of one's soul.

The Art of Living Through Yoga

People often misunderstand the meaning of Yoga as only a form of exercise, yogasan, pranayama or physical activity. But if we understand yoga with greater depth and observe its true benefits, we would be able to accept it as the greatest achievement of our life. We do not achieve mere physical, mental and material excellence through yoga, but become capable of making our life happy and prosperous, giving the right objective to our family as well. By adopting yoga, we can reach the ultimate level of spirituality.

Whenever I organise a yoga camp, I always inspire the participants to enhance their living conditions along with teaching them about yoga. In my lectures, I also teach about the art of living, so that the practitioner can imbibe positive qualities.

- It has been observed that whatever we think, manifests in our body accordingly. For example, we have seen that when we get angry, our appearance and expressions starts changing. Eyebrows shoot up, blood circulation becomes rapid, and muscles tighten. The energy stored in the body is wasted unnecessarily, which increases the mental stress. The environment around us also turns unfavourable. Our impression of the world deteriorates and there is a lot negativity in our life. A kind of poison is created in the body which is very harmful. When we are constantly in a state of anger, the immune system weaken and we start feeling frail; the body is susceptible to diseases. Many other things happen in our life. We become physically and mentally ill, which affects our economic condition. As a result we build the same kind of friendships. Many a times, we form bad habits, such as taking intoxicants. Intoxicants take away the glow from our face. We may eat healthy food but their positive effects are not visible on the exterior. We deteriorate day by day. Families disintegrate; children do not develop good character. The society starts looking down upon us. As a result, we start feeling neglected. We are fed up of the world and life seems to be meaningless to us. We keep worrying from morning to evening, and are unable to sleep in the night. Life becomes totally dependent on medicines. There is dejection all around us. Were we born to go through all this? Would we able to do anything for the rest of our life?

Who says that you will not be able to do anything? Who says that you are a nobody?

You are special.

You are still as God had created you. You are a source of tremendous power. Your soul is pure. All that is impure has entered your being from the outside. You have immense knowledge within yourself. You are a true human being. You have immense potential. You should develop them. You are a store house of happiness. So get up without delay. Get up with enthusiasm. Don't worry about the world. The world will be with you when you win its confidence.

Struggle alone. There are invisible powers within you. The light of your ancestors illuminates your life. Pledge to yourself that a new energy will generate within you right now.

Promise to yourself that you will begin a new life from today; you will not be driven by anger; you will not eat non-vegetarian food; you will not indulge in intoxicating substances; you will not use foul language. Promise to yourself that you will give up pride; that you want deliverance from illusion and that you shall give up greed.

Take a vow that you shall live a pure life.

Determine that you will treat everyone with love and affection. You will not neglect anyone and will be affectionate towards all. Once you make this decision, you will notice that there is peace all around you; the environment is pure and you are getting more respect. When you smile, the whole world smiles along with you.

After some days you will observe that your body has become healthier and that you are also enjoying better mental health. You have better self-esteem and are able to get respect from others. You have become a better person in every way.

The reason behind giving this little example was to prove that just as you think, so are the chemical elements that your body produces and releases. If your thoughts are good, then the chemicals which are life-giving and nourshing will be produced in your body till your last breath. So, why not change your lifestyle today and make *yam*, *niyam*, and others a part of your daily life?

- Upnishad says, 'यथा पिण्डे तथा ब्रह्मांडे'. This small phrase has numerous meanings. Our physical body is the expression of the universe. The powers and elements which have also created the universe have created our physical body, brain and the microscopic body. We have seen that the nature is becoming imbalanced. As a result, the whole universe has become disease-stricken and we can see natural calamities striking everywhere. Similarly, if our food habits and lifestyle is imbalanced, we will also become disease-stricken. We will become slaves to the external elements. That is why, we should live balanced lives, and become free of worries. In this way, we can change the way we live, adopt yoga and make this life a successful and beautiful one.

Scientific Reasons of the Benefits of Yoga

Benefits from Yogic Sookshm Vyayam, Yogic Sthool Vyayam, Pavan muktasan Samooh, kriyas to control the air and exercises of Shakti Bandh: In the morning, the body is generally rigid. It is not ready for the advanced order of exercises. Hence, by doing light exercises, all the parts of the body become flexible and supple. Light exercises open up all the joints of the body. The blood starts flowing in sufficient quantity, and we do not face any problem doing the yogasanas.

The body becomes swift. It becomes light. A lot of freshness can be felt. As the joints of the bones open up, the air trapped in them moves out of the body due to the increase in the speed of blood circulation. A wonderful feeling of new energy and awareness is generated in the body. As the brain receives abundant supply of blood, it becomes active. In this way, all the parts of the body, right from the big toe of the feet, ankles, calves, knees, thighs, buttocks, pelvic region, waist, abdomen, back, spine, lungs, fingers of the hands, elbows, shoulders, neck, eyes, head, to parts of the digestive system become active and all the disorders are cured, thereby making us disease free.

Benefits of the Asanas Related to Padmasana and Meditation: By doing Padmasana and the asanas related to Padmasana, the energy generated in our kundalini starts flowing in the upward direction and we are able to absorb the energies from all the chakras – from *Mooladhar* to *Sahasrar* – and gain all their benefits. A new zeal and awareness is generated in our life. We attain self realiaation by doing meditation in this posture. Padmasana gives stability to our spine. Therefore, we do not have to face the problem of a bent back in old age. We can sharpen our memory through the state of *Dhyana* and *Dharana,* using the Padmasana posture.

Benefits from Asanas Related to Vajrasana (Thunderbolt pose): When we sit in Vajrasana, it regulates the blood circulation in our pelvic region, reproductive organs and the parts of the digestive system, making them strong. It is beneficial in containing diseases of the reproductive organs. It is helpful in curing diseases like hernia, early discharge, problem of less sperm count, piles, enlarged testicles, hydrosol, and irregular periods in women.

Benefits of Asanas Done in Standing Posture: The muscles of the calves and the thighs get strengthened by doing these asanas, as a result we get rid of diseases, such as arthritis, trembling of limbs, pain in the calves, and problems in the knees. When we do the asanas in the standing posture, the muscles of the back are thoroughly stretched through which they are also rectified and repaired.

Benefits of Asanas Done by Bending Backward: When we do asanas by bending backwards, our lungs expand and are able to take in more oxygen and thus, grant us youth. When we bend backwards, our abdominal muscles are stretched, which makes our digestive system healthy and strong. It gets abundant blood supply along with appropriate massage.

When we bend backwards, the nerves of our spine also become strong. Our entire body is connected to the spine. Therefore, the whole body is set in balance and diseases, such as slip disc, sciatica, spondylitis and many other diseases of the spine are cured.

Benefits of Asanas Done by Bending Forward: Such asanas cause contraction in the abdominal region due to which pressure is exerted on the abdomen. The nerves and cells of the back expand. The spine receives abundant blood supply and therefore, is able to carry out its functions efficiently. Due to the contraction in the abdominal region, the related parts get a thorough massage and the diseases of the digestive system are cured. The kidneys, liver, pancreas, among others, become strong and free of diseases.

Benefits of Asanas Done by Twisting the Spine Sideways: If the spine – the supporting pillar of our body – is healthy, our body will look well-built like the trunk of a tree. When we do asanas by twisting the spine, the internal organs and the muscles of our body get massaged. The spine becomes more flexible and supple. When we do such asanas, parts of our digestive system also gets a good exercise, thereby becoming active and efficiently functional.

Benefits of Asanas Done by Balancing the Body on the Head: When we do asanas by balancing the body on the head, the brain receives abundant blood supply, resulting in complete nourishment of the head. The pituitary gland starts functioning better. So, our power of thinking and understanding is enhanced. The blood circulation is increased in the entire body. The heart functions better and purifies the blood more efficiently. The internal parts of the abdominal region and the back are strengthened, making them function better. We can say that whether it is the issue of mental health, problem of hair fall, facial beauty, or any issue related to the body, the asanas done by balancing the body on the head and shoulders can bring about a total transformation in the body.

The Effect of Yogasanas on the Various Systems/ Organs of Our Body (A Scientific Approach)

It is a known fact that our ancient sages had immense knowledge of all sciences. But the problem with us is that we start comparing their knowledge with ours, and try to prove them wrong by unnecessary debates and logic. Or, we believe in what the western scientists have to say. If they say that our ancient sages were wrong, then we believe that the sages were wrong; and if they say that our sages were right, then we believe they were right. We simply do not want to use our brains in a positive way. Let us consider the issue of yoga. Yoga had been a part of our Indian tradition for thousands of years. We stopped considering yoga as a part of our daily life many decades back due to our ignorance and laziness. So much so, that if someone did yoga, we made fun of them, and they too would feel ashamed and eventually, give it up. Now that the people of the western countries have started doing yoga, we too have awakened to this art.

This was as far as yogasanas are concerned, but there are many other useful and practical things which we do not follow. For example, the wise people of our country had claimed that we should not eat late in the night, should not indulge in alcohol and non-vegetarian food. We can take the example of our dinner. The scientific reason behind the statement that dinner should be taken before sunset or at least by 7.30 p.m., is that meals should be taken at least four hours before we go to bed. If we sleep immediately after dinner, the food will not be digested. It will remain undigested in the stomach throughout the night and will rot. Our digestive system will not be able to absorb the proteins and vitamins and undertake other routine jobs. The stomach will have to work round the clock without any rest. When the food is not digested, harmful gases are formed, which is the reason for many diseases and disorders.

That is why gurus suggest taking meals at least four hours before going to bed. If we see it scientifically, we will understand that in those four hours, we would be active, which would help us digest our food easily.

Regarding vegetarian diet, the acharyas have explained that it is absolutely easy to digest and it gives us a lot of physical, mental and spiritual energy. It also prevents us from doing many bad things. We can avoid the emergence of *tamasik* elements in our body. As the saying goes, 'as you eat, so shall you be'. Pure food leads us to pure thoughts. The family atmosphere becomes happy, peaceful and prosperous and positive.

When we indulge in too much of worldly desires, we become prone to many diseases. The glow and aura of our body are destroyed. The face loses its charm, develops wrinkles and the body becomes weak. Our mental strength and memory also affected. Our weakness starts being reflected in our eyes. Our hands and feet also become weak.

Thousands of such useful hints and suggestions have been given by our respected sages, saints and gurus. If we imbibe them, we can bring about a tremendous positive transformation in our lives.

Now we shall explain the effects of yogasanas on our body, in a scientific manner.

Digestive System

It is a rule on Earth, that all those things which lie unused for a long time, deteriorate and their potency eventually decreases. With the advent of many modern gadgets, the potential and capability of the human body to do work has decreased. Subsequently, the potential of the various parts of the body to carry out their functions has also deteriorated.

The digestive system has also been tremendously affected by all these factors. This has resulted in the emergence of various diseases, such as constipation, indigestion, acidity, gas disorders, malfunctioning of the liver, pancreas, the malfunctioning of the intestine, ulcers, diarrhea, and piles.

We must do asanas which exerts pressure on the abdominal region, such as asanas done by bending forward. For example: Pashchimottanasana, Yogmudrasana, Naukasana, etc.; asanas Dhanurasana, Bhujangasana, Matsyasana, Chakrasana, etc., which are done by bending backwards and asanas which exert pressure on both the sides of the abdomen like Katichakrasana, Ardh Matsyendrasana, Tiryak Tadasana, Tiryak Bhujangasana, Uttan Mandukasana, etc. By doing the above mentioned asanas, all the parts of the digestive system get a good massage. Blood circulation increases and all the blockages in the circulatory system are removed. The digestive system starts functioning properly. The problems caused due to our indiscipline and irregular lifestyles start vanishing. The working capacity of the abdominal region increases by doing these asanas. The front abdominal muscles get good exercise. Therefore, the digestive system is able to absorb the nutrients, such as vitamins and proteins in abundance from the food that we eat, and gives us good health by keeping us protected from diseases.

Similarly, the lungs and the stomach begin to function well when we do Pranayama (by doing Antara kumbhaka, and Bahir kumbhaka).

By practising these mudras with the three locks (bandhs) and nauli along with other kriyas of purification, all the parts of the digestive system start functioning efficiently. By sitting in meditation postures, many minor disorders of the abdomen can be cured. In these postures, the front abdominal muscles are slightly stretched, which benefits the entire abdominal region. Hence, we can say that yoga kriyas assist the digestive system function effectively.

Respiratory System

We all agree that now, the entire atmosphere is polluted. The environment has become impure, and if we ask a very busy person to do yogasana, they will comment that they don't even have the time to breathe, how can they do yoga? To this, all we have to say is: At least try to breathe in the correct manner, otherwise, how will you live? This may be a statement on the lighter side, but this joke proves that the life of the common man has deteriorated.

It is important to know the art of breathing, otherwise not only will the heart, lungs, among others become weak, but the entire functioning of the respiratory system will be affected. Not only this, there are about 600 trillion small and big cells in our body which need fresh air (oxygen) to remain healthy. Therefore, by doing yogasana and the specific kriyas of Pranayam, we can grant good health not only to our lungs and cells, but to the whole body.

The asanas which are beneficial for the respiratory system are Chakrasana, Mayurasana, Sarvangasana, Halasana, Shalabhasana, Pashchimottanasana, Mandookasana, among others. All these asanas exert pressure on and stretch the abdomenal region along with the chest, and activate the muscles related to the process of respiration.

Our yogacharyas have suggested that Pranayama also strengthens the respiratory system. The objective of all the different Pranayamas is almost the same. Antara kumbhaka, Bahir kumbhaka, Deergha, Poorna and Samgati are kriyas which massage the parts of the respiratory system. The blood is purified and the blood circulation is regularised and increased, enhancing the vital force of life. The lungs become strong, more functional and flexible. These asanas and Pranayamas establish a balance between all the nerve centres and provide benefit to the patients of high blood pressure and low blood pressure.

Kriyas, such as Uddiyana Bandha, Bahya and Antara kumbhaka, Kapal-bhati, Nadi-shodhana Pranayama, Nauli, Neti, and Dhauti keep the entire restpiratory sytem disease free. As a result, the body does not suffer from diseases related to respiration, such as Asthma, cold, flu, high blood pressure, low blood pressure and impurity in the blood.

Blood Circulatory System and the State of the Heart

Heart is the pump to the blood-transport mechanism. The asanas exert pressure which regularise the blood supply in the related areas, improving the immunity of that body part against any infection. One must do the following asanas to enhance and regularise the blood circulation – for the upper part of the body, we should do Vajrasana, Gomukhasana, Mandookasana, Bhadrasana, Shashankasana, etc. For the waist, we should do Padmasana, Yogmudrasana, Baddha Padmasana, Matsyasana, etc. For the abdominal region, we should do Shalabhasana, Dhanurasana, Pashchimottanasana, Halasana, Sarvangasana, Mayurasana, Chakrasana, Moola Bandha, Nauli, Kunjal, and Sheershasana and related exercises, Vipreetkarni, Trikonasana, Pashchimottanasana, Shashankasana, Uttana Mandookasana, Tolangulasana, Dvipada Kandharasana, etc. help in the regularisation of blood circulation.

Asanas like Sheershasana and Sarvangasana, in which the position of the legs is upward, rectify the slow pace of blood circulation and regularise it in all the nerves and arteries, regulating the blood pressure of the body. Often when we are mentally and physically fatigued, an unnecessary tension is created in our heart rate and blood pressure. This can cause harm to our heart. In such cases, Shavasana, relaxation processes, asanas of meditation, Pranayama, etc. prove beneficial. Problems like heart attack or other diseases related to the heart do not arise and our body stays healthy.

Nervous System

It needs a lot of deliberation to keep this body, made of 72,000 nerves, healthy. However, mere thinking is not enough. One must take the right action too. Just as a defect in even a small part of the television can disrupt the clarity of the picture on screen, similarly, a small disruption in a body part can cause harm to the body. We have to take care of the body as long as the soul resides in it.

All the asanas which affect the nervous system have proven to be very effective, but a few which are more beneficial deserve a special mention: Surya Namaskara, Uttaanpadasana, Pashchimottanasana, Lolasana, Kukkutasana, and Dhanurasana. We can also benefit from Dharana and Dhyanasanas and from Shavasana and Sithilikarana.

By doing the above mentioned asanas, we can get rid of maladies like tension, insomnia, worry, restlessness, irritation, fury, anger, and other mental disorders. One becomes calm, spiritual, good-humoured and of a serious disposition.

Lymphatic System

Since only those asanas are effective on the lymphatic sytem which work well on the circulatory system, refer to the asanas related to the circulatory system.

Asanas Which Affect the Endocrine Glands

(1) Penial gland: It is affected by doing Surya Namaskara, Yoga Mudrasana, Padhastasana, Bhramari, Kapal-bhati, Trataka, Neti and Sheershasana.

(2) Pituitary glands: It is affected by doing Sheershasana.

(3) Thyroid gland: This gland is activated by doing Sarvangasana, Halasana, and Vipareetkarani.

(4) Liver: It is affected by doing Matsyendrasana (by turning the spine to the right-hand side).

(5) Spleen: It is affected by doing Uddiyan Bandha and Nauli kriya.

(6) Chlome: It is affected by doing Matsyendrasana (by turning the spine to the left-hand side).

(7) Adrenal: It is affected by doing Mayurasana, Simhasana, Neti and Ujjayi Pranayama.

(8) Kidney: It is affected by doing Bhujangasana, Surya Namaskara, Maarjaari asana, Shashankasana.

(9) Ovaries: They are affected by doing Siddhasana, Padmasana, Vajrasana, Moola Bandha, Vajroli Mudra and Yoni Mudra.

Asanas That Affect the Various Body Parts

The parts of the entire abdominal region, such as liver, spleen, intestines and stomach: Vajrasana, Sarvangasana, Halasana, Pashchimottanasana, Bhujangasana, Shalabhasana, Matsyendrasana, Sheershasana, Uttanpadasana, Pavanamuktasana, Shakti Bandha asanas.

Heart: Sheershasana, Sarvangasana, Shavasana, Yoga-nidra, Nadi-shodhana Pranayam, Surya Namaskara.

Lungs: Chakrasana, Mayurasana, Sarvangasana, Halasana, Shalabhasana, Pashchimottanasana, Uddiyana Bandha, Nadi-shodhana Pranayam, Kapal-bhati.

Head/Brain: Asanas of the Sheershasana group, Sarvangasana, Matsyasana, Padmasana, Siddhasana, Yogmudrasana.

Eyes: Sheershasana, Surya Namaskara, Sutra Neti, Jal Neti, simple Trataka.

Nose, teeth, ears: Surya Namaskara, Sarvangasana, Matsyasana, Simhasana, Nadi-shodhana, Bhramari Pranayam.

Asanas That Affect the Air, Bile and Phlegm

Ayurveda is one of the most ancient systems of treatment in India. According to Ayurveda, the root cause of all diseases is tridosha. If these doshas are in balance, then the body remains healthy, and if even one of them becomes imbalanced, then diseases related to that dosha start emerging. There may be one or two congenital or hereditary diseases in a person which are governed by one's body constitution. Therefore, asanas according to specific body constitutions are mentioned below:

Bodies with air as the predominant factor

Kriyas of the Pavana Muktasana group, asanas of Shakti Bandha, Vajrasana, Veerasana, Matsyendrasana (Ardha and Poorna), Dhanurasana, Chakrasana, Sarvangasana, Shankh-prakshalana, Nauli, Uddiyana Bandha, Surya Namaskara, Marjari asana

Bodies with bile as the predominant factor

Naukasana, Bhujangasana, Shalabhasana, Uddiyana Bandha

Bodies with phlegm as the predominant factor

Sheershasana, Sarvangasana, Pashchimottanasana, Uttanpadasana, Kapal-bhati, Uddiyana Bandha

Ayurveda mentions all three factors. They can be considered as ek-doshaj – when only one factor is predominant in the body. Furthermore, there are three types of dvi-doshaj, where two factors are predominant – vaat-pitt prakriti (air-bile), vaat-cough prakriti (air-phlegm) and pitt-cough prakriti (bile-cough). In such cases, asanas pertaining to both the factors should be done. The fourth nature is called Sannipatic. In this case, asanas related to all the three doshas should be done under the guidance of a yoga guru. In this way, we can keep our body healthy and disease free through yogabhyasa.

Asanas to Calm the Gas, Bile and Phlegm

To calm the vaata (gas) dosha

1. Tadasana
2. Utkatasana
3. Trikonasana
4. Hast Padasana
5. Surya Namaskara
6. Janusheershasana
7. Pashchimottanasana
8. Meru Vakrasana
9. Ugrasana
10. Yogmudrasana
11. Naukasana (done by lying down on the stomach as well as on the back)
12. Vipareetkarni
13. Halasana
14. Shalabhasana
15. Shavasana

Asanas to calm the pitta (bile) dosha

1. Marjari asana
2. Naukasana, Vipareeta Naukasana
3. Parvatasana
4. Sarvangasana
5. Vipareetkarni
6. Ashvasanchalana asana
7. Janusheershasana
8. Ugrasana
9. Pashchimottanasana
10. Hast Uttanasana
11. Setubandhasana
12. Bhujangasana
13. Supta Vajrasana
14. Akarna Dhanurasana
15. Shavasana

Asanas to calm the kapha (phlegm) dosha

1. Hasta Uttanasana
2. Parvatasana
3. Tadasana
4. Vrikshasana
5. Trikonasana
6. Veerasana

7. Bhujangasans
8. Shalabhasans
9. Ugrasans
10. Ashvasanchalanasans
11. Setu Bandhasans
12. Naukasans
13. Dhanurasans
14. Chakrasans
15. Akarn Dhanurasana
16. Shavasana

Great yogis do not do different kriyas,
rather they do every kriya with a positive attitude.

–RJT

Yoga helps in building purposeful life and
giving it a new direction.

–RJT

Ashtanga Yoga
(Eight-limbed approach)

योगाङ्गानुष्ठानादशुद्धिक्षये ज्ञानदीप्तिराविवेकख्यातेः । (Patanjali Yog Darshan 2/28)

Meaning: By practising the various features (parts) of Ashtanga Yoga, the impurities are destroyed and life is filled with the light of knowledge and wisdom.

Explanation: By putting into practice the eight features of Ashtanga Yoga as mentioned below, the impurities of the mind are destroyed and it becomes absolutely pure and clean. In such a situation, the power of the yogi's mind reaches up to the greatest height (vivek khyati, or pragya buddhi – the highest of the seven kinds of awareness). In other words, he is able to clearly see his soul surpassing the perception of intellect, pride and senses.

The Functions and Significance of Ashtanga Yoga

If we consider them closely, the functions of the eight parts of yoga are not so simple and ordinary. These eight parts are the result of deep thinking of our sages. It is their blessing that they first disintegrated these eight parts and then wove them in the form of a string of pearls for our easier comprehension. Each of these eight parts has a different function which show us the path of managing our bodies from head to toe, reaching right up to the goal of salvation. This is a great achievement for us and a valuable gift from the great sages to the humankind. So, let us express our gratitude by imbibing them in our lives.

There are eight parts of Ashtanga Yoga (*yama, niyama, asana, pranayama, pratyahara, dharana, dhyana* and *samadhi*).

1. **Yama (Social Ethics):** It teaches us to how live our social and religious life, which in turn enhances our moral and ethical values.
2. **Niyama (Personal Ethics):** It transforms the working pattern of our entire life. It polishes our character and teaches us to live with discipline.

3. **Asanas (Postures):** It keeps us healthy till our last breath and helps in the development of our body.
4. **Pranayamas (Breathing techniques):** It renews our life. It teaches us the skill of breathing and helps us develop and elevate our life force.
5. **Pratyahara (Inward senses):** It teaches us how to gain control over our senses and how to win over ourselves. It helps us in our mental progress.
6. **Dharana (One-pointed focus):** It teaches us to concentrate and helps us in our intellectual progress.
7. **Dhyana (Meditation):** It grants us many achievements. We need to master the state of dhyana in almost all areas of our life. We can even achieve self-realisation through dhyana.
8. **Samadhi (Highest state of consciousness):** In this state, we can transform our dormant mind into an awakened one and experience bliss, which is the ultimate goal of life.

In this way, we learn to live our life in a disciplined and righteous manner by following the Ashtanga Yoga.

Parts of Ashtanga Yoga

यमनियमासनप्राणायामप्रत्याहारधारणाध्यानसमाधयोऽष्टावङ्गानि ।

(Patanjali Yog Darshan 2/29)

Meaning: Yama, niyama, asana, pranayama, pratyahara, dharana, dhyana and samadhi are the eight parts of yoga. They play their part in two ways:

1. External (bahiranga)   2. Internal (antaranga)

Yama, niyama, asana, pranayama and *pratyahara* are considered as external because their functions are associated with external activities. *Dharana, dhyana* and *samadhi* are considered internal because they are related to the mind.

Given below are the interpretations of these parts:

Yama

अहिंसासत्यास्तेयब्रह्मचर्यापरिग्रहा यमाः । (Patanjali Yog Darshan 2/30)

Meaning: Ahimsa (non-violence), satya (truth), asteya (not stealing), bramhacharya (celibacy) and aparigraha (not hoarding) are the five yamas.

1. Ahimsa (Non-violence)

अहिंसा प्रतिष्ठायां तत्सन्निधौ वैरत्यागः । (Patanjali Yog Darshan 2/35)

Meaning: When the emotion of non-violence becomes absolute in the yogi, even the most violent creatures around him give up their feeling of hatred and enemity. To not cause any pain to anyone with our thoughts, words or actions is called ahimsa. In Jainism, the five yamas are called as Panch Mahavrat. They are considered as the foundation of the religion. It is written in the religious texts that to interact with everyone with tolerance and self-restraint is called ahimsa. We should not hurt or make anyone hurt other living creatures knowingly or unknowingly. Those who kill others or encourage those who kill, in turn create enemity for themselves in this world. It has been said that 'ahimsa parmo dharma' and 'live and let live'.

Therefore, not to cause pain to anyone in ideas, words or actions is ahimsa, and to forgive and forget the wrong doings and shortcomings of others also come under the perview of ahimsa.

2. Satya (Truth)

सत्य प्रतिष्ठायां क्रिया फलाश्रयत्वम। (Patanjali Yog Darshan 2/36)

Meaning: We should always be alert and give up all falsehood while speaking. We must only say what is beneficial for others. When the truth is firmly established in our speech, it starts manifesting in our actions. The yogi acquires the power to bless, give boon or to curse someone.

3. Asteya (Not stealing)

अस्तेय प्रतिष्ठायां सर्वरत्नोपस्थानम् । (Patanjali Yog Darshan 2/37)

Meaning: When the quality of non-stealing is firmly established in the character of the yogi, various priceless gems appear in front of him. Irrespective of the object being living or non-living, less or more, without the owner's permission, the 'sadhak' with self-restraint will neither take it himself nor instigate anyone else to take it. He will not agree with the act either. We should not accept anything from others, which is not given to us directly.

4. Bramhacharya (Celibacy)

ब्रह्मचर्य प्रतिष्ठायां वीर्यलाभः । (Patanjali Yog Darshan 2/38)

Meaning: Bramhacharya is the root of a religious life. That is why, the sages always strive to follow bramhacharya. When the sadhaka observes bramhacharya in its totality, immense power is generated in his body, mind and soul.

5. Aparigraha (Not hoarding)

अपरिग्रह स्थैर्ये जन्मकथन्तासंबोधः । (Patanjali Yog Darshan 2/39)

Meaning: Aparigraha means not to indulge in hoarding. To avoid hoarding of things in more than the required quantity is aparigraha. The sages do not practice any kind of collection. The person who practices aparigraha gets excellent results in yoga sadhana and religious activities.

Niyama

Every sadhaka should follow certain rules in their life. Whether the person wants to enjoy the materialistic pleasures or spiritual bliss, he/she should follow high-quality rules in their life. According to Patanjali, the five basic rules of life are:

1. Saucha (Cleanliness)
2. Santosha (Contentment)
3. Tapas (Austerity)
4. Swadhyaya (Study of self)
5. Ishwarapranidhana (Surrendering to the Divine)

1. Saucha (Cleanliness)

शौचात्स्वाङ्गजुगुप्सा परैरसंसर्गः । (Patanjali Yog Darshan 2/40)

Meaning: Those who follow the rules of saucha become free of the attachment towards their body and of the desire to indulge in physical activities with others. This means that one does not have any attachment towards one's own or somebody else's body. By cultivating the feeling of friendship, or by doing 'japa-tapa', or by any other sadhana, one can cleanse one's inner self and get rid of attachment, hatred, jealousy. Restlessness of the mind can be put to an end, and one can always remain happy. Distraction ends and concentration sets in. One is able to command control over one's senses. Hence, one becomes capable of self-realisation.

2. Santosha (Contentment)

संतोषादनुत्तमसुखलाभः । (Patanjali Yog Darshan 2/42)

Meaning: There is no happiness greater than contentment. A great personality has said that one should drink the nectar of contentment, which means that contentment is like nectar, and we must imbibe it in our life. When the sadhaka develops contentment, his thirst for desire gets quenched, and he gets rid of attachments. A renowned poet has said:

गोधन, गजधन, बाजधन और रत्न धन खान।
जब आवै संतोष धन, सब धन धूरि समान।।

3. Tapa (Austerity)

कायेन्द्रियसिद्धिरशुद्धिक्षयात्तपसः । (Patanjali Yog Darshan 2/43)

Meaning: The impurities are destroyed by practising tapa. One gains mastery over the body and senses. There are many types of tapas, but that which gives you an insight into the self and thus purifies and elevates the within and without is called tapa.

4. Swadhyaya (Study of the self)

स्वाध्यायादिष्टदेवतासम्प्रयोगः । (Patanjali Yog Darshan 2/44)

Meaning: Swadhyaya leads to the vision of the Lord. In Jainism, it is said that 'swadhyaya parama tapah', which means that self-study is the greatest of penances. 'Sva' means self; to study, think and reflect on the self is swadhyaya.

5. Ishwarapranidhana (Surrendering to the Divine)

समाधिसिद्धिरीश्वर प्रणिधानात् । (Patanjali Yog Darshan 2/45)

Meaning: One can attain mastery over Samadhi by taking refuge in God. When the sadhak surrenders his will – actions and every such thing which strengthens his arrogance – to God, such a state is called ishwarapranidhana. When he surrenders himself selflessly to God, he attains the ultimate state of Samadhi. When he sees the sentient and the insentient in the light of his understanding, he attains the power of profound vision and is thus able to see the Supreme with his power of divine sight. This is ishwarapranidhana.

Asanas (Postures)

The third aspect of Ashtanga yoga is Asana. According to Maharishi Patanjali:

स्थिरसुखमासनम् । (Patanjali Yog Darshan 2/46)

To sit joyfully and firmly in any given posture is called asana.

Explanation: The position in which one is able to sit firmly (without moving) and comfortably for a long time is called asana. A firm and comfortable physical posture leads to mental balance. The distractions of the mind can be checked. The yogi wins over his body and mind by practising yogasanas and thus his life is blessed. The sadhaka knows that a healthy mind resides in a healthy body. He rids himself of physical limitations and mental obstacles by regular practice of asanas. He does not look up to the sky, or wander in the mountains to meet God. He feels the Supreme within himself by these practices.

प्रयत्नशैथिल्यानन्तसमापत्तिभ्याम् । (Patanjali Yog Darshan 2/47)

Meaning: By efforts, relaxation and meditation on the Supreme, one can gain mastery over asanas. Then, the sadhaka does not neglect or ignore the body and the mind, neither does he try to destroy them. He considers them as an instrument to gain knowledge.

ततो द्वंद्वानभिघातः। (Patanjali Yog Darshan 2/48)

Meaning: It is further said that once the asanas are mastered, the difference between cold and hot, hunger and thirst, victory and defeat, gain and loss, respect and insult, mind-body, body-mind, come to an end. The sadhaka reaches the fourth step of the path of yoga, which is Pranayama.

Pranayamas (Breathing techniques)

(For more information, see the detailed explanation further in the book.)

तस्मिन् सति श्वासप्रश्वासयोर्गतिविच्छेदः प्राणायामः। (Patanjali Yog Darshan 2/49)

Meaning: After mastering the asanas, the holding of inhalation (shvasa) and exhalation (prashvasa) is called Pranayama.

Shvasa: The drawing in of breath from the nose is called shvasa (inhaling).

Prashvasa: The expelling of air from the nose is called prashvasa (exhaling).

The process of controlling the breath by doing Rechak, Purak and holding the breath inside and outside is called pranayam. Pranayama should be done after mastering the asana. It is clear from this that those who do pranayama without practising the firmness or stability of the asana, do it the wrong way. It is important to have a firm posture while doing pranayam.

बाह्याभ्यन्तरस्तम्भवृत्तिर्देशकालसंख्याभिःपरिदृष्टोदीर्घसूक्ष्मः। (Patanjali Yog Darshan 2/50)

Meaning: Pranayama is of three types: Bahya vritti, Abhyantara vritti and Stambha vritti. It is prolonged or short when considered from the point of view of desh (place), kaal (time) and sankhya (number).

Bahya Vritti Pranayama

To expel the air inside the body and to check its natural flow is called rechak or bahya vritti.

Abhyantara Vritti Pranayama

To draw the breath in from the nostrils and check its natural flow is called puraka pranayama or abhyantara vritti pranayama.

Stambh Vritti Pranayama

To hold the breath in its place by checking both the inhalation and exhalation is called stambh vritti pranayama or kumbhaka pranayama.

The explanation of pranayama as per the desh, kaal and sankhya is as follows:

1. **Desh Paridrishta (Region or part of the body)**

   Measuring the breath by the region of the body is called desh paridrishta. To bring the breath up to the nose in rechak, to draw in the breath up to the Mooladhar in purak and to hold the breath in the navel area in kumbhak are examples of desh paridrishta.

2. **Kaal Paridrishta (Time)**

   To consider the breath from the point of view of time, like inhaling for a given duration, holding the breath and exhaling for certain time duration, is called kaal paridrishta. For example, rechak for 2 seconds, purak for 1 second and kumbhak for 4 seconds.

3. **Sankhya Paridrishta (Counting)**

   To breathe according to a count is called sankhya paridrishta (You should keep track of the counting in your mind.). To do the first pranayama for a given number of counts, then the second pranayama for another number of counts, then the third pranayam, and so on is sankhya paridrishta. This kind of pranayama is prolonged and light.

   As the sadhaka increases his practice, the rechak, purak and kumbhak, all the three types of pranayama become successively prolonged and light in the context of desh, kaal and sankhya.

Now the fourth type of pranayama is explained as:

बाह्याभ्यन्तरविषयाक्षेपी चतुर्थः। (Patanjali Yog Darshan 2/51)

Meaning: That which gives up or criticises the subjects of the inside and the outside is the fourth type of pranayama.

In this state, the sadhaka gives up thinking about the subjects of the inside and the outside, or in other words, he does not worry whether his breath is being drawn in or expelled out or is being held. He only focuses his mind on the Supreme. This state, without the realisation of desh, kaal and sankhya, when the prana involuntarily pauses in a particular region, then this is called the fourth pranayama. This pranayama is totally different from the other three pranayamas. In this type, the flow of the prana automatically halts due to the calm state of the mind.

The Benefits of Pranayama

ततः क्षीयते प्रकाशावरणम्। (Patanjali Yog Darshan 2/52)

Meaning: By the practice of that pranayama, the shroud of ignorance that covers the light of knowledge vanishes.

According to the Panchashikhacharya:

तपो न परं प्राणायामात् ततो विशुद्धिर्मलानां दीप्तिश्च ज्ञानस्य।

Meaning: There is no penance greater than pranayam. As a result, karmas are purified and the light of knowledge illuminates the practitioner.

According to Bhagavan Manu:

Just as metals of gold are purified by fire, and their impurities are cleansed, similarly the impurities of the senses are cleansed by doing pranayam.

He also mentions another benefit of pranayama:

धारणासु च योग्यता मनसः। (Patanjali Yog Darshan 2/53)

Meaning: Our mind becomes capable of dharana.

Explanation: By doing pranayam, mind becomes stable and thus becomes capable of dharana.

Pratyahara (Inward senses)

The characteristics of pratyahara are explained as:

स्वविषयासम्प्रयोगे चित्तस्वरुपानुकार इवेन्द्रियाणां प्रत्याहारः। (Patanjali Yog Darshan 2/54)

Meaning: When all relations with the materialistic subjects are given up, and one follows the true form of the inner self, such a state is called pratyahara of the senses.

Explanation: The writer says that by doing pranayam, all the external subjects of the five sense organs and the mind gradually become pure. The sadhaka starts becoming introvert and materialistic desires vanish. This is called pratyahara. This is the fifth state of a yogi. He burns all the external materialistic desires of the senses with the flame of his inner knowledge, and gains divine and profound vision.

The benefits of pratyahara are further explained as:

ततः परमा वश्यतेन्द्रियाणाम्। (Patanjali Yog Darshan 2/55)

Meaning: With this pratyahara, the senses are controlled to the optimum.

Yagyavalka writes about the characteristics of pratyahara as: 'To forcefully withdraw the senses, which are indulged naturally in their respective matters is called pratyahara.'

When the same state of concentration that the mind acquires when it is free from materialistic subjects is acquired by the senses too, then this is called pratyahara.

The creators of the Goraksha system explain that to give up the subjects of the five senses – smell, vision, taste, hearing and touch – gradually through practice in the correct sequence, or in other words, to turn the senses away from the astringency of their subjects, is pratyahara. After mastering asanas and pranayam, to remove the materialistic disorders of the mind and to remain constant in one's original state is called pratyahara. It is further stated that just as a turtle withdraws and hides its limbs within its shell, similarly yogis should withdraw their senses from materialistic matters and devote or divert their inherent characteristics towards the 'atma' or the soul. The soul causes itself great harm by indulging in materialistic pleasures. Therefore, people must give this up and move towards his own well-being, therein lies the true meaning of pratyahara.

In the previous section, the five external practices yama, niyama, asana, pranayama and pratyahara have been explained along with their benefits/results. Now, the rest of three internal practices dharana, dhyana and samadhi are being explained. When the body is mastered and put in order by the practice of the asanas, when the mind is purified in the fire of pranayam, and when the senses are controlled through pratyahara, then the sadhaka attains dharana, the sixth state of Ashtanga Yoga.

Dharana (One-pointed focus)

देशबन्धश्चित्तस्य धारणा। (Patanjali Yog Darshan 3/1)

Meaning: To restrict the mind to various regions by mere instinct or will is called dharana.

Explanation: Here, region is referred to any of the part of the body such as the waist, abdomen or forehead. These are regions inside our physical body and to visualise them in your mind as any of the external objects such as the Sun, Moon or in the form of any deity is called dharana. (also see Dharana chapter).

Dhyana (Meditation)

तत्र प्रत्ययैकतानता ध्यानम्। (Patanjali Yog Darshan 3/2)

Meaning: To maintain the same focus on Him is dhyana.

Explanation: The disposition with which the mind focuses on its goal, when it is so unbreakable that no other thought emerges in between, then that state is called dhyana. Many preceptors or scholars have explained dhyana in many ways: (also see Dhyana chapter).

Vachaspati Mishra says:

The concentrated and unidirectional state of mind is dhyana.

According to Shri Vishwanath of Nyaya Sutra-Vritti

प्रणिधानम चित्त एकाग्रमिदम।

Meaning: The mind becomes focused in the state of pranidhana.

Dhyana is the state of stability of the mind in which the fluctuating dispositions of the mind are restrained or controlled. Where the feelings of attachment and hatred do not exist, Rajoguna and Tamoguna virtually come to a naught, and the state of sanity, insanity and foolishness vanish. The fourth state of the mind is concentration where the Satoguna being dominant, the mental powers are focused on one and only one object or region. Where there is no distinction between the mind, intellect, pride, love and hatred, and all the internal powers are dedicated to the Supreme Cosmic Power either in surrender or in service. Then, the awareness of 'I' and 'mine' vanishes and one attains the state of dhyana.

Samadhi (Highest state of consciousness)

तदेवार्थमात्रनिर्भासं स्वरूपशून्यमिव समाधिः। (Patanjali Yog Darshan 3/3)

Meaning: When in the state of dhyana, one glimpses only at the goal, and the self comes to naught, then this state is called samadhi. When this state of dhyana is focused upon, the self becomes null by its own enlightened form due to the nature of dhyana, and such a state is called samadhi.

The last state of dhyana is samadhi, which is the ultimate state of the stable mind. Only dhyana similar to self-oblivion is samadhi. When the sadhak becomes oblivious to the self while doing dhyana when the only achievement that one receives is the authority of the supreme goal and the authority of the self is forgotten; when the separation of the self from the goal is not perceived, that stable state of mind is called samadhi. There can be no state of self-realisation without samadhi. Samadhi is end of the search of sadhana.

त्रयमेकत्र संयमः । (Patanjali Yog Darshan 3/4)

Meaning: Dharana, Dhyana and Samadhi, these three are collectively called Samyama or abstinence. The classical language for all the three is Samyama. Therefore, in this book, wherever samyama is mentioned, it should be interpreted as Dharana, Dhyana and Samadhi.

तज्जयात्प्रज्ञालोकः । (Patanjali Yog Darshan 3/5)

Meaning: In Samadhi, with the mastering of samyama, the light of the intellect shines forth. This means that the more one masters the minutest subjects, the more the intellect is purified. In other words, the sadhaka's intellect is blessed with the power of supernatural knowledge. The meaning of pragyaloka is the light of the true form of knowledge, not the knowledge regarding the worldly matters. The essential knowledge related to the receiver, received, and worth receiving is the stairway to kaivalya or salvation. This is mainly called pragyaloka.

तस्य भूमिषु विनियोगः । (Patanjali Yog Darshan 3/6)

Meaning: Samyama should be applied in various areas.

Explanation: The writers expound that those who have not won over the following subjects, they cannot cross over or over-step the later subjects to gain benefit. In other words, first gain control and mastery over the simpler subjects and then subsequently gain control over other issues and continue to move forward.

त्रयमन्तरङ्गं पूर्वेभ्यः । (Patanjali Yog Darshan 3/7)

Meaning: Dharana, Dhyana and Samadhi these three internal aspects of Sampragyata Yoga are mentioned in compared to Yama, Niyama, Asana, Pranayama and Pratyahara.

Explanation: Dharana, Dhyana and Samadhi are the internal aspects of Sampragyata Yoga, because having acquired the clarity of knowledge regarding all the elements or all the facts through Samadhi, the knowledge is sustained in the concentrated mind and called Sampragyata.

तदपि बहिरङ्गं निर्बीजस्य। (Patanjali Yog Darshan 3/8)

Meaning: Yet the three internal aspects of Dharana, Dhyana and Samadhi are the external means of Nirbeeja Samadhi (Asampragyata Samadhi). Its internal aspect is only ascetism, as in this state, even the Sampragyata ceases to exist or is brought under control. When viewed from the point of view of control of instincts, Sampragyata and Asampragyata, both are considered as Yoga or Samadhi, but when viewed from the point of view of Sabeeja Samadhi, Asampragyata mean external Samadhi.

Yoga develops the art of living.

–RJT

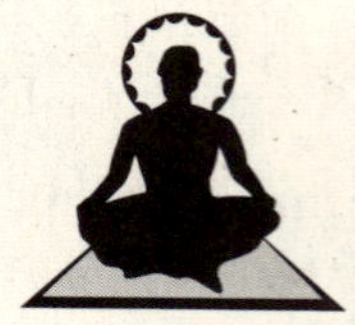

Names of the Yogasanas

A Mysterious Argumentative Viewpoint

Under the Hatha Yoga, various yogasanas have been expounded. Our preceptors have given different names to various asanas. These asanas have been given very meaningful names. The names of some asanas are related to birds, Bakasana (Heron), Mayurasana (Peacock), Kukkutasana (Cock) and Hansasana (Swan). Some asanas have been named after insects: Vrishchikasana (Scorpion), Shalabhasana (Locust), etc.

Some names are based on the names of animals: Shvanasana (Dog), Ushtrasana (Camel), Singhasana (Lion), Gomukhasana (Cow), Vatayana (Horse), etc. Some names are based on trees and flowers: Vrikshasana (Tree), Tadasana (Palm), Padmasana (Lotus), etc. Some have been named on aquatic animals and amphibians: Matsayasana (Fish), Kurmasana (Tortoise), Bhekasana (Frog) and Makarasana (Crocodile).

Asanas which resemble reptiles, such as the snake were named as Sarpasana or Bhujangasana. Asanas, such as Hanumanasana, Veerasana, Mahaveerasana and Buddhasana, were named after the gods and great sages like Kapil (Kapilasana), Vashishtha (Vashishthasana), Vishwamitra, Bhagirath, etc. They were named so to help us imbibe their memories in our culture. What was the reason that our great sages thus named the asanas?

A simple logic can be that while performing these asanas,

when we reach the final stage, the form or shape of the asana resembles the name given to it. Like when we execute Mayurasana, our body looks like a peacock. To make the sadhaka feel attached to the peacock could also have been one of the reasons.

There can be several logic behind this. I personally feel that while the sadhaka takes the form of these creatures, he feels that he should not have any hatred in his heart towards these creatures, because he knows that it is the same supreme power that takes innumerable forms and breathes through all the creatures of the universe, right from the smallest creature to the greatest of sages. The 'formless' is the greatest form of the supreme power.

There is another logic, that God has given at least one special feature to every living being. So much so, that each plant and tree has its own specialty. Since man wants to acquire maximum skills and qualities, he aims to achieve them from those asanas, along with the benefits gained by doing that particular asana. Another apparent reason for naming the asanas after plants and animals is: The acharyas wanted to bring us closer to nature so that we can imbibe the qualities of nature in our lives.

Yoga helps one attain new achievements in life.

–RJT

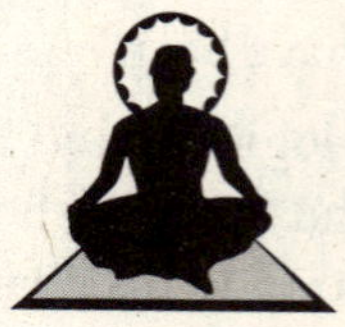

Yoga: Precautions/Rules

A practitioner is required to observe many precautions and rules, therefore every practitioner must make note of the following points. As while building a house we pay special attention to the foundation and make it strong so that the building constructed on it can remain safe and stable for a long period of time, similarly, if we adopt the rules and precautions pertaining to yoga in our life, many problems will be solved automatically.

Sequence of Practice

- Yogasana and the yoga process should be done under the guidance of an able yoga trainer.
- Do any yogasana, but the sequence of the process while returning to the original position should be opposite to what it was while attaining the last position.
- Yoga practice will be more beneficial if done in sequence and as prescribed.
- While doing yogasanas and the entire process, the focus should be on the practice alone.
- Do not do yoga either to imitate or to impress others.
- Yoga practice is meant for the self, as you do, so will be the benefit.
- Follow the time limit and speed specified for yoga practice, otherwise it could do more harm than good.

- Pay special attention to the practice of yama and niyama.
- Decide which yogasana to do and which not to do only after reading the entire book thoroughly.
- No asana should be performed without prior preparation. The correct sequence to be followed is: First do light exercises, lighter asanas, followed by a little advanced asanas or asanas related to pavanmuktasana so that the rigidity of the body is removed and the body becomes supple and the muscles become flexible. Only then it is advisable to do pranayama (beginners, medium, advanced) and meditation.
- Do not do any asana forcefully. By regular practice, it automatically becomes easy to perform.
- Always remember to do shavasana after every yoga practice. Shavasana helps remove any stress that might have been caused due to the practice and one starts feeling happy and relaxed.
- If you do a forward-bending asana, then, after a moment's rest, do a backward-bending asana (Please use your wisdom by keeping in mind your age and diseases, so that no complications arise.).

Inhalation – Exhalation

- While doing any yoga kriya, be cautious about the inhalation and exhalation.
- Always inhale through the nose, not through the mouth.
- Every asana has its own sequence of inhalation and exhalation. Be sure to keep it in mind.

Diet

- The urinary bladder and the intestines should be empty before doing the asanas.
- In case of constipation, one should do the Shankhprakshalana process given in this book under the guidance of a guru or after consultation. Yogabhyasa should be done only after that.

- In order to keep our body agile, fit, beautiful and ever youthful, one should give as much importance to diet as one gives to yogasana.
- One should not eat too sour, pungent, heavy, stale food or food that takes too long to digest. Contemporary scientists agree that our food should be sattvik, vegetarian, fresh, pure and simple.
- One glass of fresh and cool water can be taken sometime before doing the asana as it is very helpful in removing the toxins from the joints.
- The sadhaka/practitioner should not take intoxicants such as alcohol, opium, bhang, tobacco, bidi, and cigarettes.
- If you are suffering from any disease, consult an expert regarding the asanas and diet.
- One must do yogabhyasa half an hour before and at least four hours after meals.
- If constipation is very severe kind, this disorder (ordinary digestion disorder) can be cured with yogabhyasa. However, shankhprakshalana must be done at least once or twice in a year.
- Tamsik food like eggs, fish, meat, etc. should be given up because it is said, 'As you eat, so shall be your mind.'

  "जैसा खाओ अन्न, वैसा बने मन।"

Bathing

Take bath with fresh clean water before and sometime after doing asanas (according to season and physical condition).

Clothing

- Do not wear tight clothes while doing asanas. Wear loose, comfortable, and convenient cotton clothes.
- Use a blanket or rug to do asanas.
- The electric current generated in the body during yogabhyasa is not destroyed when you use a blanket.
- Male sadhakas must wear a loin cloth or a kuchchaa.

Time

- The practice of yogasanas is considered to be more beneficial if done during sunrise.
- The energy emitted from the Sun in the early morning gives us new strength as this energy is revitalising in nature.
- Probably yet another reason for doing yoga in the morning is that a person is stress-free.
- Set the time limit for every asana according to your physical condition.
- People do not have paucity of time in the morning.
- If a person does yoga in the morning, he feels fresh and energetic the whole day. Hence, the person does work joyfully. If due to any reason you do yogabhyasa after being out in the scorching Sun, rest a while and then proceed.
- Yogabhyasa becomes more effective when done in a set place and at a same set time.

Place

- The place for yogabhyasa should be clean, airy, peaceful, joyful to the mind, good and pollution free.
- The place for yogabhyasa should be leveled.
- If you are doing yogabhyasa in a closed room, keep the doors and windows open.

Direction

- For asanas performed in lying position, it is best to keep the legs pointing towards North or East direction.
- For asanas performed in standing position, facing towards the East gives special benefits.
- If one chooses to face the North-east direction while praying, we gains quicker health benefits.
- Direction is also significant because it awakens our awareness and provides many other benefits along with spiritual benefits.

Eyes

- In the beginning, do not close your eyes. Only after you get accustomed should you close your eyes. Nonetheless, do not let your mind remain idle or restless.
- Even while your eyes are closed (as per the instructions of your yoga trainer), keep your mind alert towards the yoga kriyas.

Physical Condition/Age

- Though there is no set age limit for yogasanas, people must apply their wisdom to consider their age, physical condition, practice, etc. for doing yogabhyasa.

For People Suffering From Illness

- The kriyas related to yogasanas are no doubt meant to get rid of ailments and become healthy, but the patient should not do asanas which aggravate their pain or intensity of the disease. For example, people with high blood pressure should not do sheershasana or sarvangasana.
- In a given illness, to know which asana should be done and which asana should not be done, you must see the relevant chapter. Also, in case of illness, consult an able trainer and only then proceed with doing the asanas.

Focus

- While doing yogabhyasa, focus with a positive mind on the illness for which you are doing the yoga kriyas, while imagining that your illness is being cured.
- During yogabhyasa, keep your mind free of disturbing feelings, such as worry, anger, hatred, nervousness, jealousy, fear, pride and vengeance.

Special Tips to be Kept in Mind During Yogabhyasa

- Use the yoga kriyas with absolute wisdom.
- Maintain absolute faith, patience and positive thoughts.
- Do not harbour jealousy, anger, hatred and sorrow in your heart.
- Do not indulge in intoxicating things and dirty mentality.
- If you encounter any problem during the practice of any asana, seek the guidance of an able guru and apply your own wisdom.
- Give up heavy food, non-vegetarian food, excessive lust and staying awake till late in the night.

A sadhaka who practises yoga must follow all the precautions and rules, otherwise it could lead to the development of many disorders in the body, like dislocation of the bones, increase in joint pain, increase or decrease in heart rate, constipation or loose motion, muscular pain, irregularity in breathing, fatigue etc. Along with these, there are chances of many kinds of physical, mental and financial losses too.

Do the kriyas related to yogabhyasa with
self confidence and believe that you shall certainly
obtain spiritual and physical benefits.

–RJT

Every person must do yoga sadhana in his life,
but it is advisable that the sadhaka must first learn
and understand about all the facts related to
yogabhyasa and then implement them.
This way, he will be able to reap more benefits.

–RJT

SUBTLE YOGIC EXERCISES

(Subtle Exercises/Easy Kriyas)

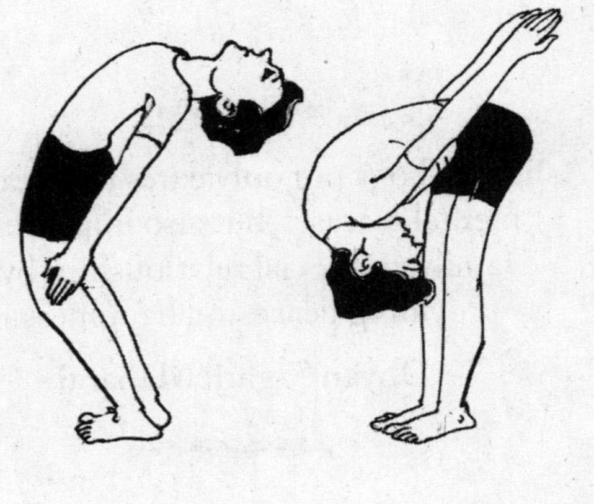

Ashtanga Yoga not only cures physical and mental diseases, but also improves family and social relationships by providing peace and happiness.

– Dhyan Sagarji Maharaj

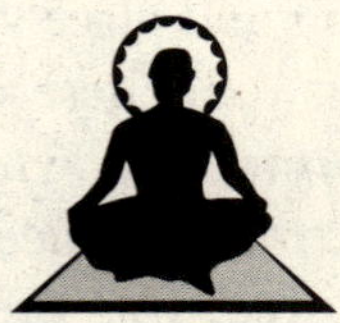

Subtle Yogic Exercises

(Easy/Light Exercises)

We have to understand this one fact that nothing is done or achieved immediately. A lot of practice is needed, whether it is yogasana or any other form of exercise. The body is very rigid and stiff in the morning, so we find it difficult to do yogasanas. Therefore, in order to make the body flexible and ready for the yogasanas, we must do some 'sookshma vyayama' or light exercises so that it becomes easier to do the yogasanas and the body does not experience any ill effects. However, according to yogacharyas, 'sookshma vyayama' develops the 'sookshma prana' regularly and as the name suggests, it keeps the body well-balanced.

Since almost all these asanas fall under the group of Gatimaya Vayunirodhaka (Pavanmuktasana) and Shaktibabdha exercises, we have included them in sookshma vyayama and hence not given them any separate definition. Sadhakas can make use of them and gain benefit thereof (the writer has visited many yoga centres and observed that in some places they are called as pavanmuktasana and in some places as sookshma vyayama).

Yogacharya Gurudev Phoolchand Yogiraj learnt these yogic exercises from his Guru Swami Dheerendra Bramhachari and he imparted this knowledge to me. Gurudev says that Swami Dheerendra Bramhachari always said that these sookshma vyayamas must reach the common man and they should benefit from them. I express my gratitude towards my Gurudev, Swami Kartikeyji and Swami Dheerendra Bramhachari.

1. Yogic Prayer

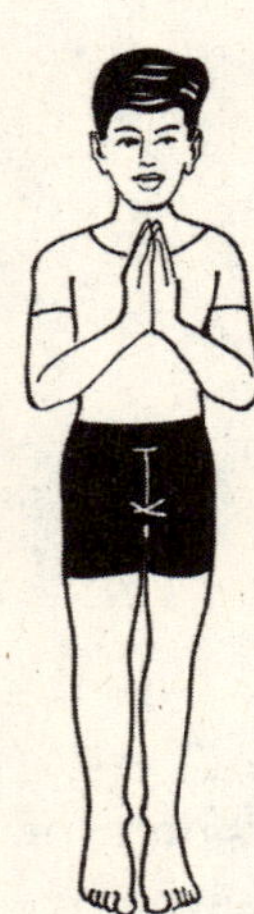

Method: Stand with the feet together (Samavastha*), join your palms and place your thumbs at the base of the neck. Press your chest with your arms. Keep your breathing normal and when the mind is focused, loosen your arms, and meditate on God for at least half a minute. Keep your breathing and mind focused.

Benefits:

- Increases the concentration of the mind.
- Beneficial for mental peace and self-awareness.
- Since pressure is put on the nerves carrying sensation to the mind, it helps in controlling the mind.
- Mental diseases are cured.

2. Uchcharana Sthala and Vishuddhi Chakra Shuddhi (Treatment of the vocal chord)

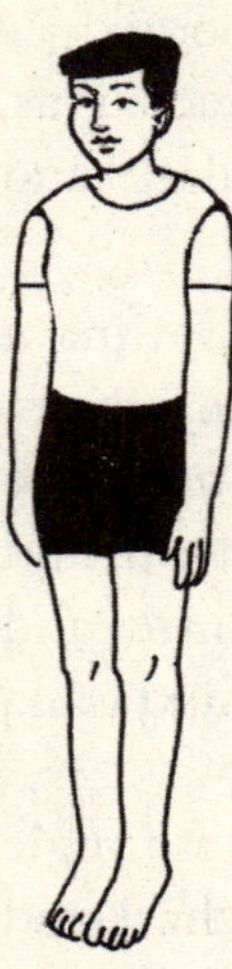

Method: Stand in samavastha. Place the little finger, ring finger, middle finger and the index finger on the throat, palms facing inwards. Invert and place the right index finger on the left; arms should be at the level of shoulders and keep the neck straight. Bring the hands down to the original position. Inhale and exhale from your chest 25 times, and after finishing the process, focus on the Vishuddhi chakra or the throat.

Benefits:

- All the impurities of the air, bile and phlegm which get accumulated in large quantity in the blood vessels of the throat are directed towards

---

*Samavastha means to stand with the feet together, looking ahead. The toes and the heels should be together and the arms should be close to the thighs. Palms should face inwards. Keep your body, from your feet to shoulder, straight with ease. This position is called samavastha.

the stomach and are eliminated from the body by doing this kriya.

- Speech starts becoming clearer. Disorders like stammering and stuttering are cured. Harsh voice turns into a melodious one.
- It is specially beneficial for musicians.
- Disorders of the head/brain can be cured.
- The power of thinking is enhanced.

3. Buddhi Tatha Dhriti Shakti Vikasaka Kriya (Developing the mind and willpower)

Method: Stand in samavastha. Gradually raise your neck. Fix your gaze in between your eye brows and while doing this kriya, visualise that ill thoughts are being eliminated. Your mind and willpower are developing and sharpening. Inhale and exhale 25 times from your chest. Focus on the crown of your head.

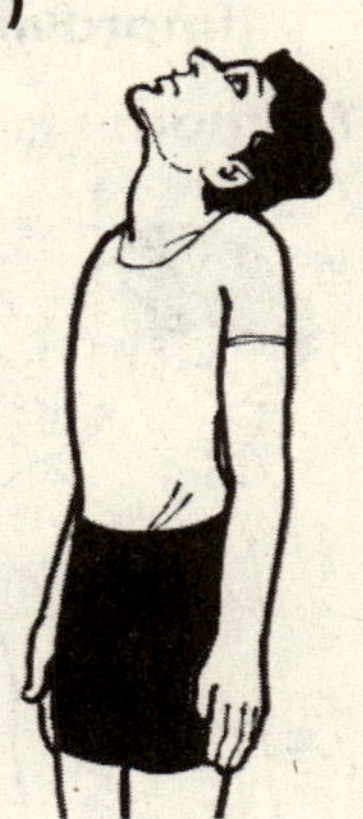

Benefits:

- Diseases of the crown are cured.
- The intellect/brain develops.
- The physical and mental capability is enhanced.
- Determination or willpower develops.
- A poor intellect is transformed into a sharp brain and analytical power of the brain is enhanced.

4. Smarana Shakti Vikasaka Kriya (Increasing memory power)

Method: Stand in samavastha. Fix your gaze approximately 4-1/2 ft ahead of the toes of your feet. While doing this kriya, imagine that amnesia is being cured and your memory power is being enhanced, sharpened and is being continuously developed. Inhale and exhale from your chest 25 times. Keep your focus on the glottis.

Benefits:

- All the parts of the body from the glottis to the crown are cured of the phlegm disorders.
- Mental fatigue and forgetfulness are cured.
- It is helpful in treatment of insanity.
- Power of the mind is enhanced.
- Increases memory power and reduces tensions.

5. Medha Shakti Vikasaka Kriya (Improving memory and concentration)

Method: Stand in samavastha. Place your chin at the sternum notch. Keep your eyes closed. Inhale and exhale 25 times from your chest. Keep your focus on the back of the neck (Medha Chakra). After completing the process, come back to the original position.

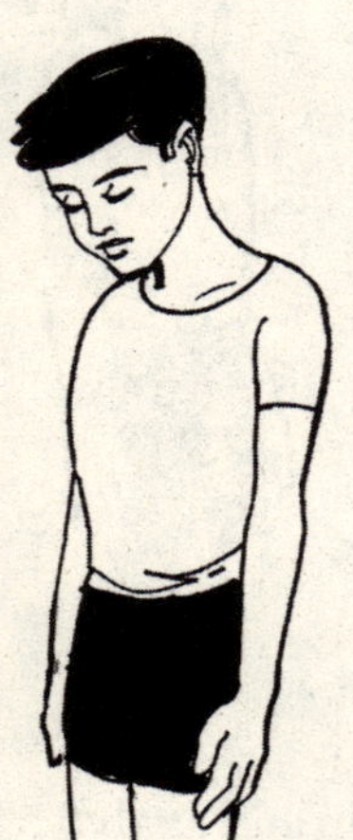

Benefits:

- All the glands of the throat are purified.
- The nectar secreted from the Sahasrar Chakra helps in the development of the body and mind.
- Illnesses like laziness and sleepiness are cured from the body and energy level is raised.
- Phlegm disorders are cured and amnesia and weak intellect are also cured.
- The body of the sadhaka becomes swift and attractive.

6. Netra Shakti Vikasaka Kriya (Improvement of eye-sight)

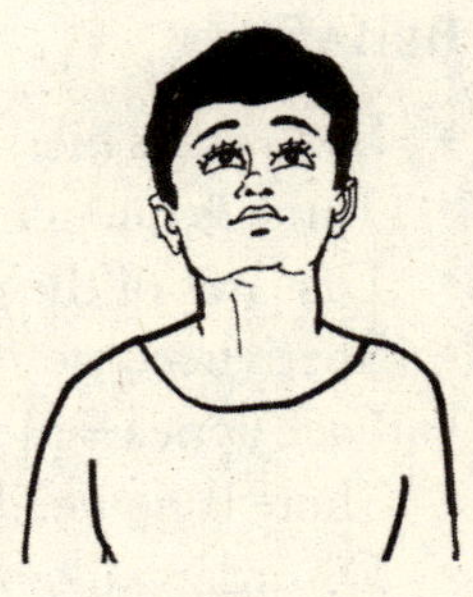

Method: Stand in samavastha. Bend your neck backwards while looking at the tip of your nose. Now fix your gaze without blinking on the area between your brows till tears flow out. Let the tears dry on their own. Breath normally and gradually come back to the original position. Keep your focus on your eyes.

Benefits:

- Eye sight is enhanced. Disorders like too much tears and poor eye sight are cured.
- A person develops the power of attraction and gets the capacity to impress others.
- It is helpful in Trataka kriya. The mind becomes focused and purified.
- By increasing the duration of practice of this kriya, one can get rid of spectacles.

7. Kapola Shakti Vikasaka Kriya (Development of the cheek muscles)

Method: Stand in samavastha. Join the tips of your fingers together, close the nostrils with your thumbs and raise your neck. Now, form your lips in the shape of a crow's beak while whistling. Inhale from your mouth for eight counts and immediately close your mouth. Blow your cheeks. Keep your eyes closed; place your chin at the sternal notch. Hold your breath for 32 counts and then release your thumbs from your nostrils. Straighten up your neck and exhale from your nose for 16 counts. Keep your little fingers on the chest while holding the breath. Arms should be in line with the shoulders. Repeat the procedure three times.

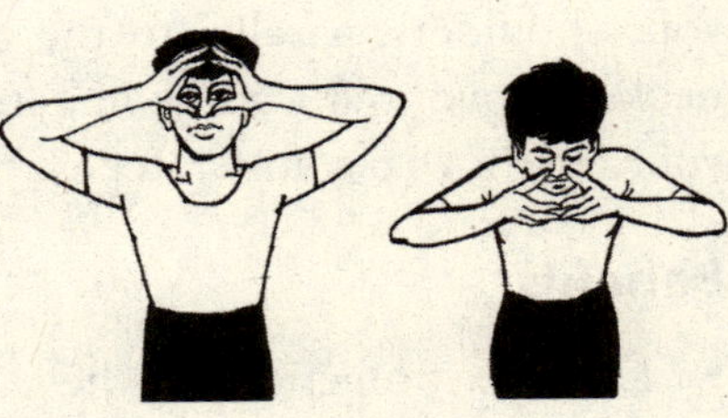

Benefits:

- Sadhaka is blessed with a long life.
- Thirst is quenched.
- Diseases of the mouth are cured.
- Teeth become stronger and foul smell is eliminated.
- Face appears pleasant and wrinkles boils, etc. are cured.
- There is no need for cosmetics.
- Disorders like headache, problems of the eye, heat in the stomach, premature graying of hair, hair fall, etc. are cured.

8. Karna Shakti Vikasaka Kriya (Strengthening the ears)

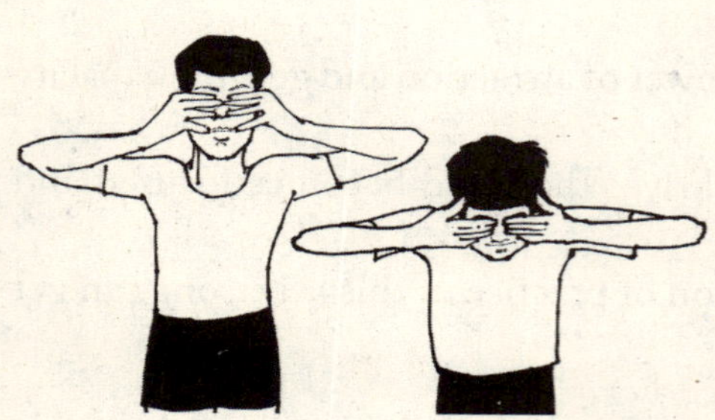

Method: Stand in samavastha. Close your ears with your thumbs, eyes with your index fingers and nose with your middle fingers. As in kriya no. 7, raise your neck and inhale from your mouth till eight counts and blow your cheeks. Place your chin at the sternal notch and hold the breath for 32 counts. Keep your arms in line with your shoulders, parallel to the ground. Now straighten up your neck, remove your middle fingers from your nose and exhale from your nose for 16 counts. Repeat the procedure three times.

Benefits:

- Ear wax, infection of the ear, hearing problems, and other disorders of the ear are cured.
- The power of the ear drums is awakened and they are strengthened.
- By closing the ears, nose, eyes and mouth, the path of the Sushumna nadi is purified. As a result, one is able to hear various sounds (naad or dhvani).
- It is specially beneficial for pranayam.

9. Greeva Shakti Vikasaka Kriya-I (Strengthening of cervical)

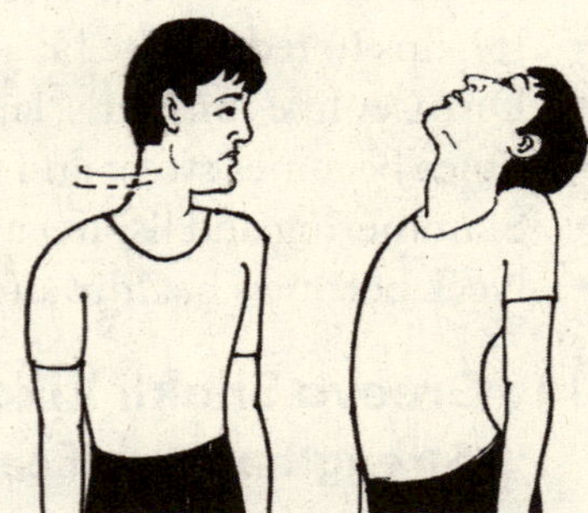

Method: Part I: Stand in samavastha. Inhale and turn your neck towards your left shoulder and then towards the right shoulder. Exhale and turn your neck towards the right shoulder. Repeat the procedure ten times.

Part II: Inhale and bend your neck backwards. Look up, exhale and bend your neck towards the base of your neck.

Benefits:

- All the disorders of the neck are cured.
- It helps to reduce the fat around the neck.
- Diseases like tonsillitis, laryngitis etc. are cured.
- Voice becomes sweet and melodious; stammering and lisping are cured.
- Neck becomes healthy and strong.

10. Greeva Shakti Vikasaka Kriya-II (Strengthening of cervical-II)

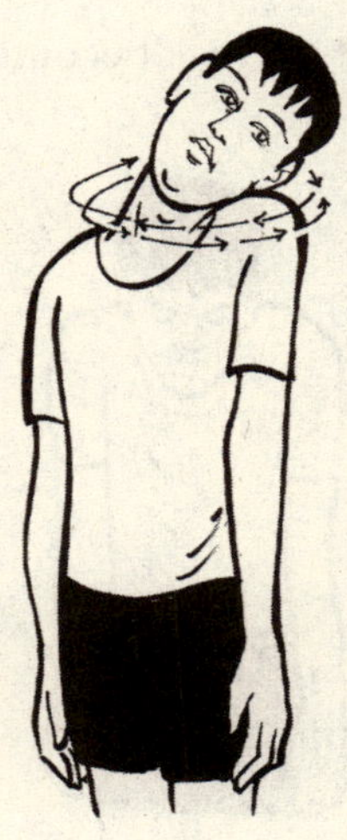

Method: Stand in samavastha. Place your chin at the sternal notch. Keep your eyes open. Inhale and hold your breath. Rotate your neck from the left shoulder to the right shoulder and bring it forward. Exhale, then inhale and rotate your neck from the right shoulder to the left shoulder and come back to the original position. Exhale after the rotation is completed. Try to touch your shoulders with your ears while doing the neck rotation. Repeat the procedure thrice.

Benefits:

- All the disorders of the neck are cured.
- It helps to reduce the fat around the neck.
- Diseases like tonsillitis, laryngitis etc. are cured.
- Voice becomes sweet and melodious.
- Stammering and lisping are cured.
- Neck becomes healthy and strong.

11. Greeva Shakti Vikasaka Kriya-III (Strengthening of cervical-III)

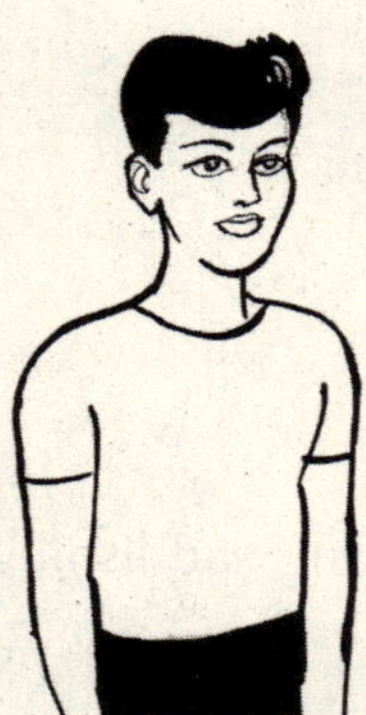

Method: Stand in samavastha. Exhale and contract your stomach. Then inhale, blow out your stomach and stretch the veins of your neck. Repeat the procedure ten times.

Benefits:

- All the disorders of the neck are cured.
- It helps reduce the fat around neck.
- Diseases like tonsillitis, laryngitis etc. are cured.
- Voice becomes sweet and melodious.
- Stammering and lisping are cured.
- Neck becomes healthy and strong.

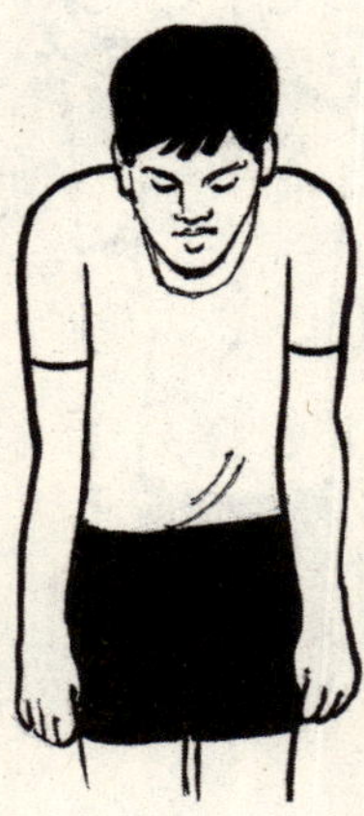

12. Skandha Tatha Bahu Mula Shakti Vikasaka Kriya (Strengthening the shoulder blades and joints)

Method: Stand in samavastha. Form a fist with your thumbs tucked in and the back of your fist facing outwards. Like exercise 7 and 8, bend your neck backwards. Pout your mouth forming the shape of a crow's beak. Close your mouth, blow it out and place your chin at the sternal notch. Close your eyes. Without bending your elbows, rotate your shoulders up and down for 32 counts. Keep your hands straight. Do not use your elbow to bend the hands. Now straighten up your neck and exhale from your nose for 16 counts. Stop moving your shoulders. Repeat three times.

Benefits:

- The bones and muscles of the shoulders become strong.
- The shoulders become well-toned and well-shaped.
- Shoulder pain is cured.
- Disorders of the neck are cured.

13. Bhuja Bandha Shakti Vikasaka (Strengthening the upper arms)

Method: Stand in samavastha. Form a fist with your thumbs tucked in. Bend your arms and keep them parallel to the ground from the elbow to the fist. Inhale and bring the arms up straight in line with the shoulders, fists facing inwards. Exhale and bring the arms back to the original position. Repeat the procedure five to ten times.

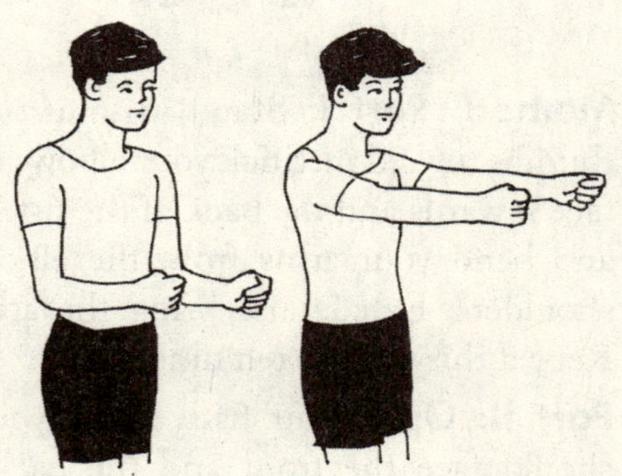

Benefits:

- Pain of the arms and shoulders is cured.
- Upper arms are toned; arms become strong.
- It is beneficial for guards and soldiers.

14. Kohni Shakti Vikasaka Kriya (Strengthening the elbows)

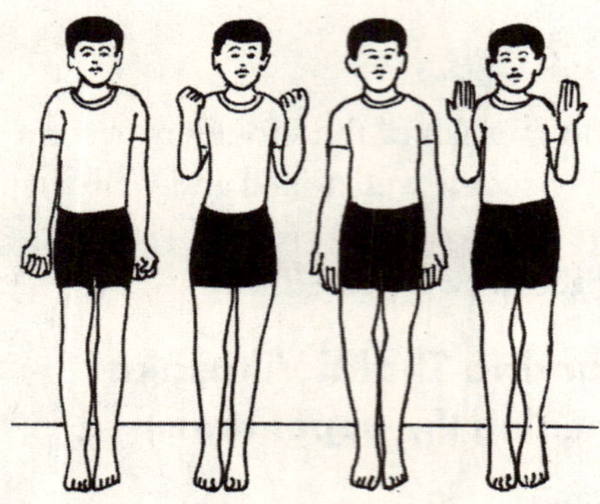

Method: Part I: Stand in samavastha. Form a fist with your thumbs tucked in. Stick your elbows to your waist. The fist should face inwards and the back of the fist should face outwards. Inhale and bend your arms from the elbow and bring them to your shoulders. Exhale and bring the arms to the starting position. Repeat this process ten times.

Part II: Open your fists. Bring your fingers closer. The palms should face the front and the back of the hands should face backwards. Stick your elbows to your waist. Perform the steps given in part I ten times.

Benefits:

- Elbow pain is cured.
- The bone joints are strengthened.
- Elbows become beautiful and attractive.

15. Bhuja-balli Shakti Vikasaka Kriya (Strengthening the forearms)

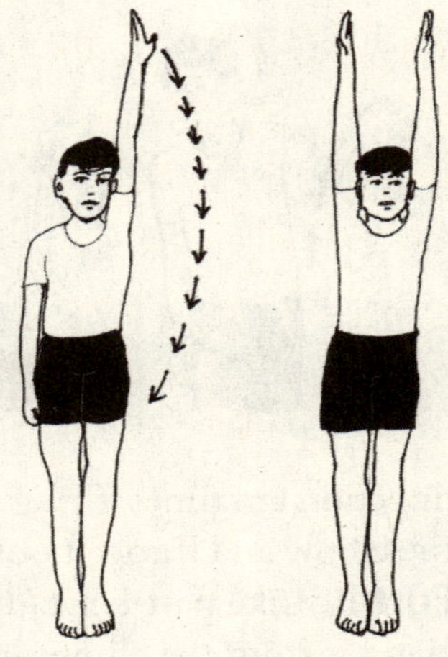

Method: Part I: Stand in samavastha. Inhale and raise your left arm above the shoulder from your side, upper arms should touch your ear. Left arm should be facing outside. Exhale and bring the arm back to the original position. Repeat this process ten times.

Part II: Inhale and raise your right arm above the shoulder from your side, upper arm should touch your ear. Right palm must be facing outside. Exhale and bring the arm back to the original position. Repeat this process ten times.

Part III: Inhale and raise both the arms above the shoulders, upper arms touching the ears. Exhale and bring the arms back to the original position. Repeat this process ten times.

Benefits:

- Arms become toned and strong.
- The part from the elbow to the wrist becomes balanced and painless.
- Arms become strong and the working capacity of the arms is enhanced.

16. Purna-bhuja Shakti Vikasaka Kriya (Developing the arms)

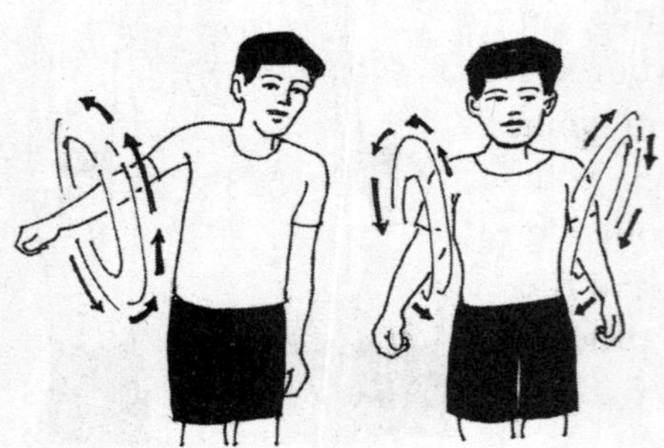

Method: Part I: Stand in samavastha. Form a fist with your thumbs tucked in. Raise your left arm to shoulder level, parallel to the ground. Inhale and hold your breath. Now, swing your arm in circular motion in clockwise direction ten times. Bring your arm close to the waist, bend it from the elbow and throw it out forward forcefully while exhaling.

Part II: Like part I, rotate your left arm anti-clockwise ten times. Bend it from the elbow and throw it out forward forcefully while exhaling.

Part III: Form a fist with your right hand, thumbs tucked in. Raise your arm to shoulder level, parallel to the ground. Inhale and hold your breath. Now, swing your arm in anti-clockwise direction ten times. Bring your arm close to the waist, bend it from the elbow and throw it out forcefully while exhaling. Repeat by rotating the right arm clockwise.

Part IV: Form a fist with both the hands with thumbs tucked in, and as in part III, rotate both the arms downwards to upwards ten times. Then, rotate from upwards to downwards ten times.

Part V: Form a fist with your hands, thumbs tucked in. Raise your arms to shoulder level, parallel to the ground. As in part I and part III, rotate both the arms from downwards to upwards ten times. Then, rotate from upwards to downwards ten times.

Benefits:

- All the wind-related problems of the body are cured.
- The pain in the veins and nerves and in the joints of the arms are cured.
- Hands become beautiful; arms become toned and strong.
- Shoulders become strong.

17. Mani-bandha Shakti Vikasaka Kriya (Developing the wrists)

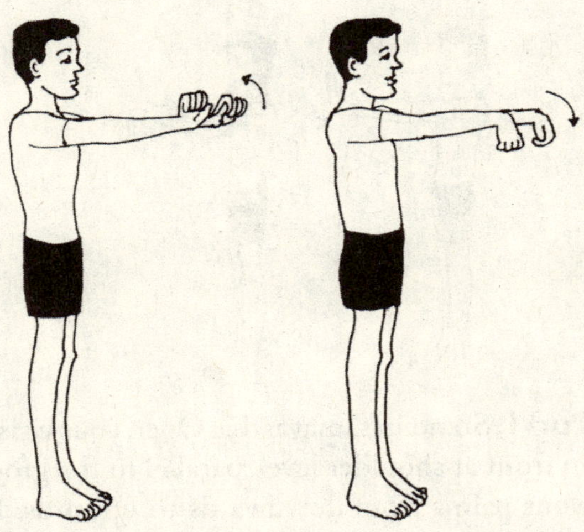

Method: Part I: Stand in samavastha. Form a fist with your thumbs tucked in. Bring your arms in front till your shoulder is parallel to the ground. Let your palms face down. Inhale and bend your wrist upwards with force. Exhale and bring them downwards with force. Repeat five times.

Part II: Raise your arms in front, parallel to the ground. Tuck your thumb in and form a fist. Bend your arm from the elbow and do the rest of the procedure as given in part I.

Benefits:

- By doing all these exercises, the wrist, back and front of the palm, and the fingers are toned and developed. The palms become strong.
- By doing these exercises, the psychosomatic nerves are affected. As a result, the body and the mind become more focused and spiritual.
- The trembling of the hands is cured; joint pain is removed.
- People working on the computer gain special benefits.

18. Kara-prishtha Shakti Vikasaka Kriya (Developing the back of the hands)

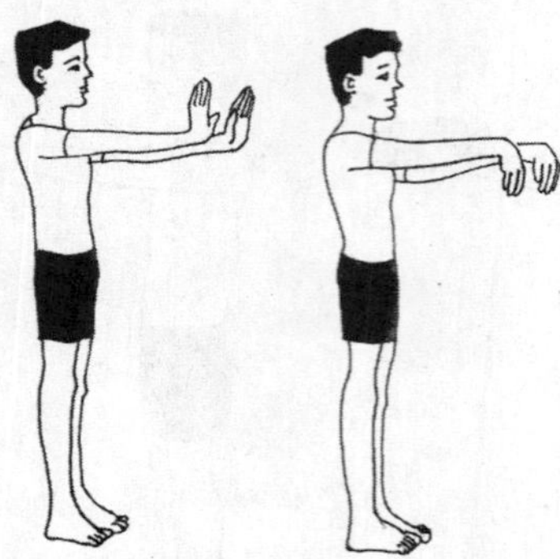

Method: Part I: Stand in samavastha. Open your wrists and raise your arms in front at shoulder level, parallel to the ground. Inhale and move your palms from downwards to upwards. Exhale and bring your palms from upwards to downwards. Repeat five times.

Part II: Raise your arms in front, parallel to the ground. Bend your elbows, palms facing down. Repeat rest of the procedure as given in part I.

19. Kara-tala Shakti Vikasaka Kriya (Developing the palms)

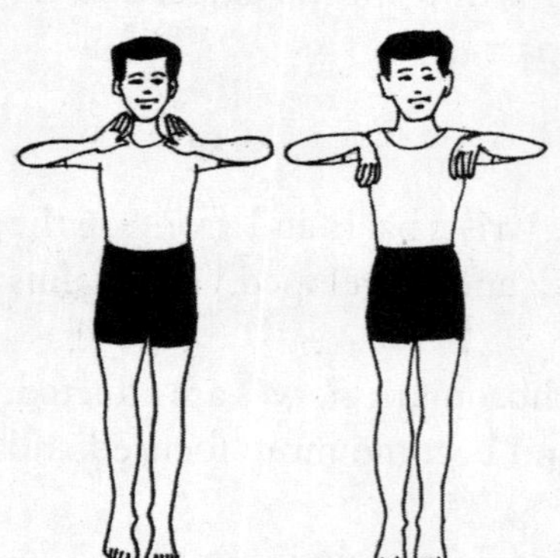

Method: Part I: Stand in samavastha. Raise your arms in front to shoulder level, parallel to the ground. Spread your fingers, palms facing down. Inhale and move your fingers down and up with force. Exhale and move your fingers up and down with force. Repeat five times.

Part II: Bend your elbows, keeping your arms at shoulder level, parallel to the ground. Spread your fingers, palms facing down. Repeat the rest of the procedure five times as given in part I.

20. Anguli-mula Shakti Vikasaka Kriya (Developing the finger joints)

Method: Stand in samavastha. Raise your arm in front to shoulder level, parallel to the ground. Keep your arms stiff, palms loosely facing down. Keeping your breath normal, move your fingers back and forth 10-15 times.

21. Anguli Shakti Vikasaka Kriya (Strengthening the fingers)

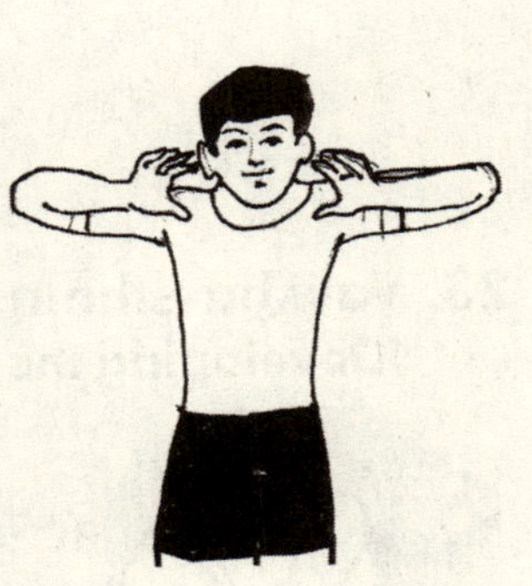

Method: Part I: Raise your arms in front, at shoulder level, parallel to the ground and spread your fingers. Breathe normally and move your fingers forcefully up and down 10 to 15 times.

Part II: Bend your elbows and keep your arms in front at shoulder level parallel to the ground. Spread your fingers and move your fingers forcefully up and down 10 to 15 times.

Benefits of doing exercises 17 to 21:

- By doing all these exercises, the wrist, back of the palm, and fingers become toned and well-developed.
- By doing these exercises, the psychosomatic nerves are activated due to which a person becomes spiritually awakened.
- Trembling of the hands is cured, joint pain is cured and these exercises are specially beneficial for people who work on the computer.

22. Vaksha-sthala Shakti Vikasaka Kriya 1 (Developing the chest I)

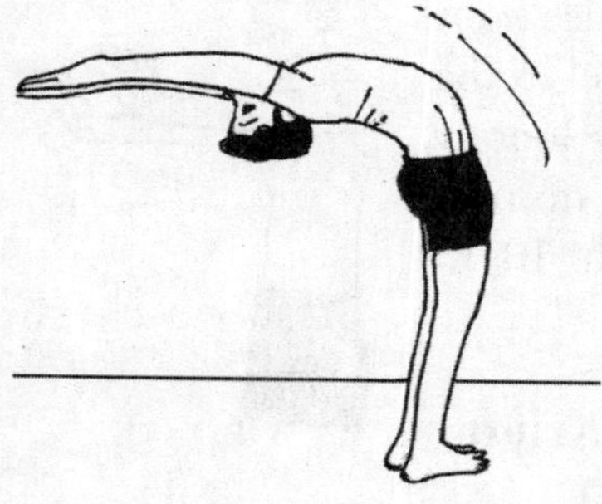

Method: Stand in samavastha. Place your hands in front of your thighs and turn your palms inward. Inhale and take your arms up, keeping your head in between your arms. Look up and lean back from your chest. Remain in this position for some time. Exhale and come back to the original position. Repeat the procedure thrice.

23. Vaksha-sthala Shakti Vikasaka Kriya 2 (Developing the chest II)

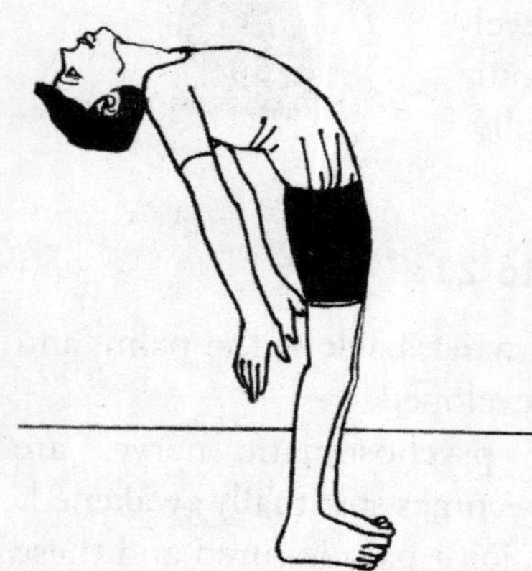

Method: Stand in samavastha. Keep your hands by your sides, close to your thighs. Inhale and stretch your arms at the back, look up and blow your chest out. Exhale and come back to the original position. Repeat the procedure thrice.

Benefits of both the exercises:

- Lungs get strengthened and lungs-related diseases are cured.
- Heart diseases are cured.
- Tuberculosis, asthma, cough phlegm, etc. are cured permanently.
- Deformity of the backbone is cured.
- Chest becomes broad and toned.

24. Udara Shakti Vikasaka (Ajgari) Kriya 1 (Developing the abdominal muscles I)

Method: Stand in samavastha. Exhale and contract your stomach till it touches your back. Hold your breath for as long as you can hold it comfortably and then, gradually inhale and blow your stomach out. Hold your breath (antahkumbhaka). Breathe out and relax. Repeat this procedure thrice.

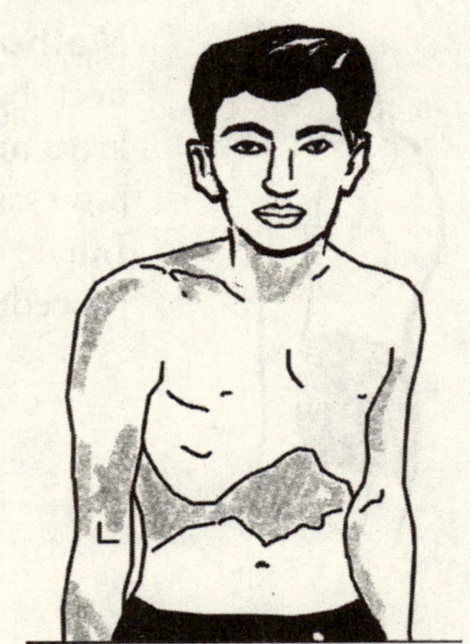

25. Udara Shakti Vikasaka Kriya 2 (Developing the abdominal muscles II)

Method: Stand in samavastha. Place the fingers of your left hand on the neck as in sookshma vyayama kriya number 2. Invert and place the index finger of the right hand on the left index finger and keeping the neck in the same position, bring both the hands down by the sides (keep your neck about one inch above normal) and exhale. Contract your stomach and then inhale and distend or blow your stomach out, keeping the focus on your stomach. Repeat this procedure 25 times without break.

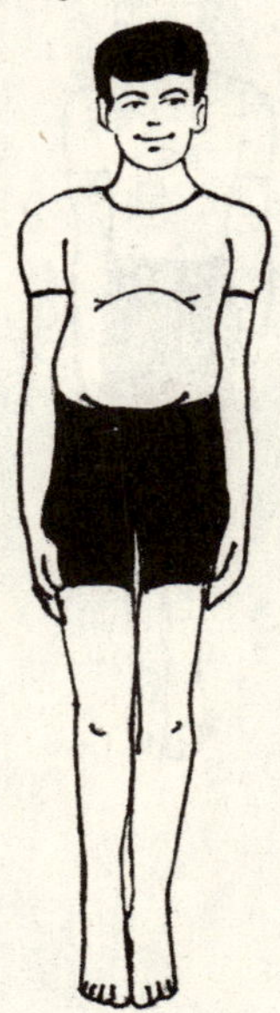

26. Udara Shakti Vikasaka Kriya 3 (Developing the abdominal muscles III)

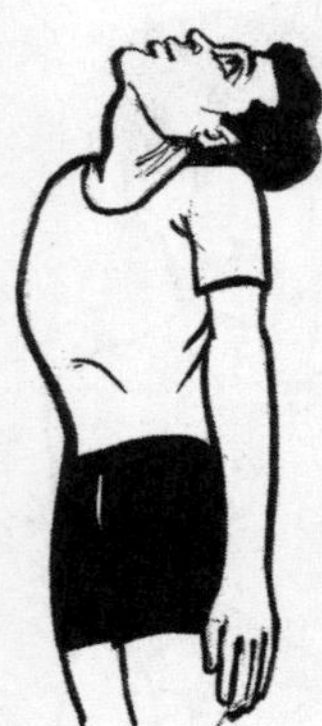

Method: Stand in samavastha. Bend your neck back gradually as in sookshma vyayama kriya number 3. Fix your gaze in between your brows. Exhale and contract your stomach. Inhale and distend your stomach. Do this procedure 25 times without a break.

27. Udara Shakti Vikasaka Kriya 4 (Developing the abdominal muscles IV)

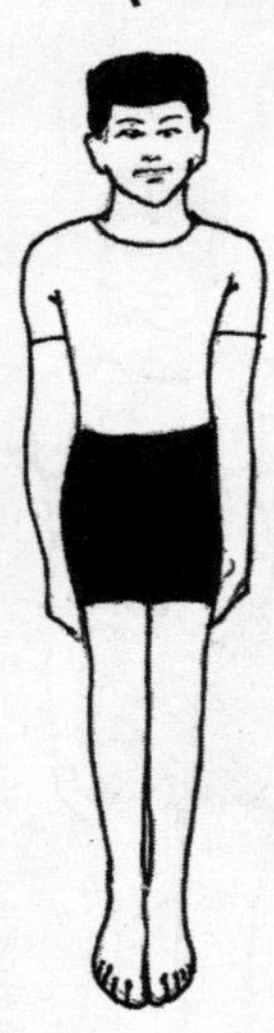

Method: Stand in samavastha. Fix your gaze about four and a half feet away from your toes as in kriya number 4. Exhale and contract your stomach. Inhale and distend your stomach. Repeat 25 times without a break.

28. Udara Shakti Vikasaka Kriya 5 (Kumbhaka) (Developing the abdominal muscles V)

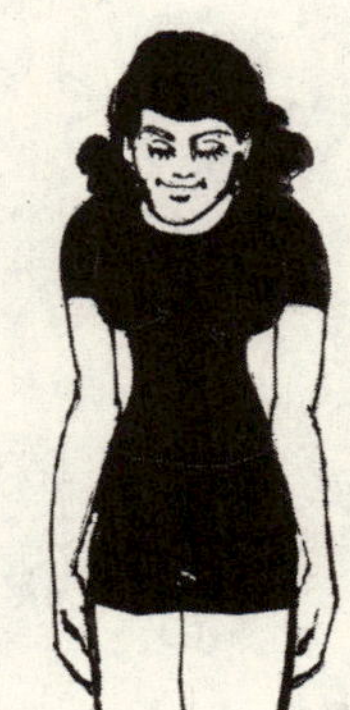

Method: Stand in samavastha. Slowly raise your neck as in kriyas 7 to 12. Form a crow's beak with your mouth and breathe in for 8 counts. Immediately close your mouth, blow your cheeks out and rest your chin on the sternum. Hold your breath for 32 counts and exhale slowly for 16 counts. Do this only once.

29. Udara Shakti Vikasaka Kriya 6 (Developing the abdominal muscles VI)

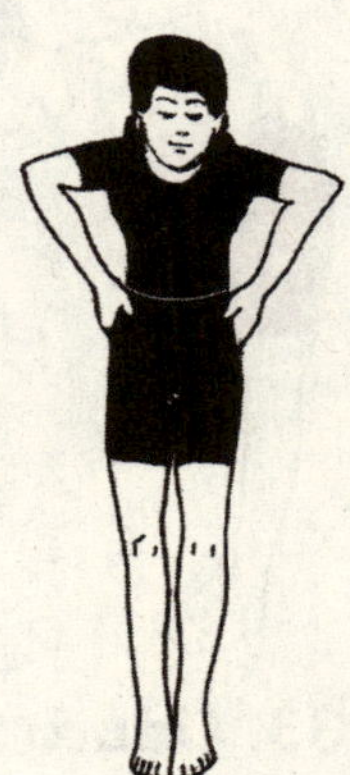

Method: Stand in samavastha. Place your hands on the waist, thumbs in front. Bend from your waist at an angle of 60 degrees; look in front. Exhale and contract your stomach. Inhale and distend your stomach. Do this 25 times.

30. Udara Shakti Vikasaka Kriya 7 (Developing the abdominal muscles VII)

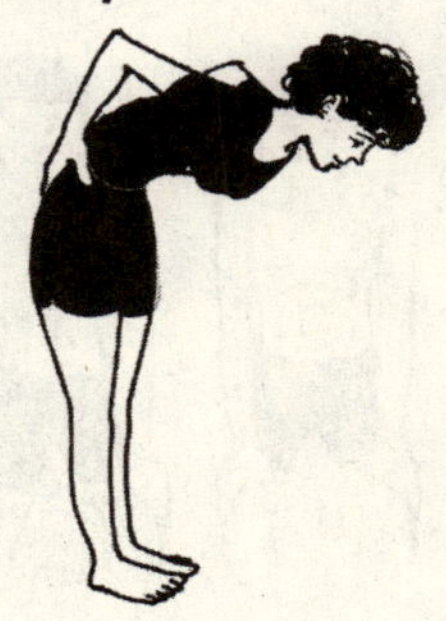

Method: Stand in samavastha. Place your hands on your waist, thumbs in front. Bend from your waist at an angle of 90 degrees. Look in front and exhale; contract your stomach. Inhale and distend your stomach. Do this 25 times.

31. Udara Shakti Vikasaka Kriya 8 (Developing the abdominal muscles VIII)

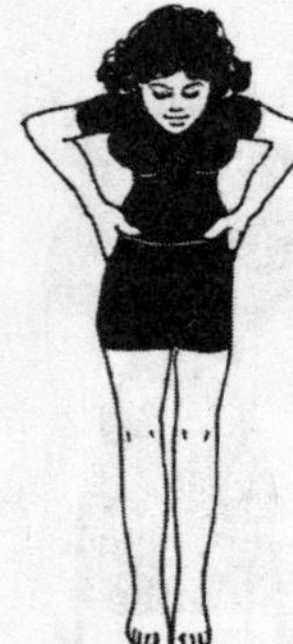

Method: Stand in samavastha. Place your hands on your waist with your thumbs in front. Exhale and bend forward forming an angle of 60 degrees, do bahyakumbhaka and contract and distend your stomach in quick successions. Do this kriya according to your capacity.

32. Udara Shakti Vikasaka Kriya 9 (Developing the abdominal muscles IX)

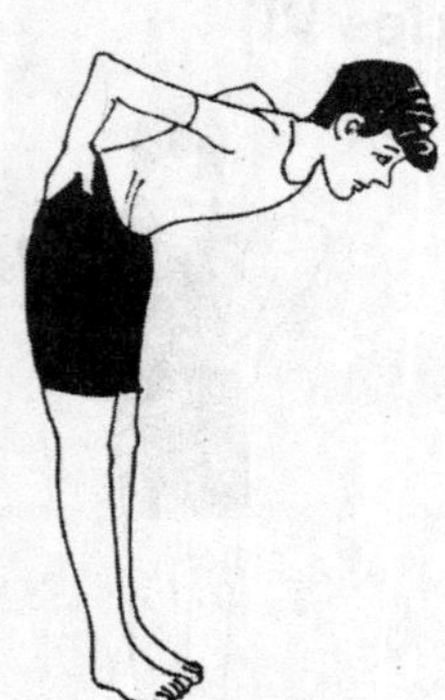

Method: Stand in samavastha. Place your hands on your waist with your thumbs in front. Exhale and bend forward forming an angle of 90 degrees, do bahyakumbhaka and contract and distend your stomach in quick successions. Do this kriya only once.

33. Udara Shakti Vikasaka Kriya 10 (Nauli) (Developing the abdominal muscles X)

Method: Stand with your feet apart. Bend forward and place your hands on your knees.

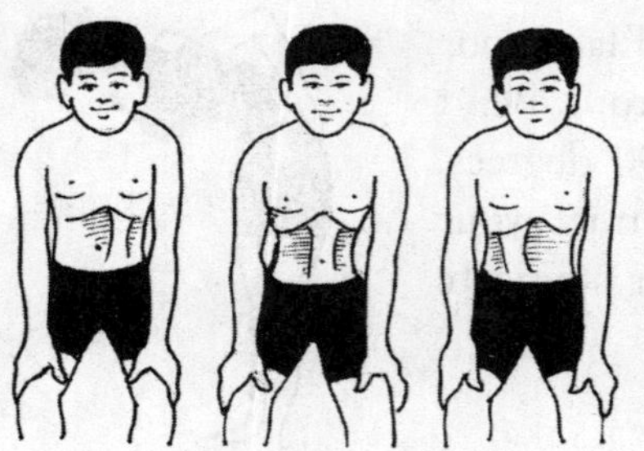

1. Madhya Nauli: Exhale through your nose and empty your stomach. Using your inner strength, move your stomach in and out. Again, using your inner strength, contract your stomach to the maximum and bring out the madhya nauli. Press your left knee with your left hand and bring out the left nauli and similarly press your right knee with your right hand and bring out the right nauli. When you feel liking breathing, stop moving your stomach and breathe in. Do this process three times.

2. Vaama Nauli: Breathe out and empty your stomach. Press your right knee and using your inner strength, rotate your stomach from left to right according to your capacity. When you feel like breathing, stop the process. This is called vaama nauli.

3. Dakshina Nauli: Breathe out and empty your stomach. Press your left knee and using your inner strength, rotate your stomach from right to left. When you feel like breathing, stop the process. This is called dakshina nauli.

Benefits of kriyas 24 to 33:

- All disorders of the stomach are cured.
- All the parts of the stomach become strong.
- Fat around the tummy is reduced.
- Spiritual power is developed.
- The sadhaka gets a long life.
- It is helpful in awakening the kundalini.
- The digestive system starts working effectively.
- Helps in keeping the naval at the centre.
- Blood circulation is improved.
- All the nerves of the body are purified.

34. Kati Shakti Vikasaka Kriya 1 (Strengthening the waist I)

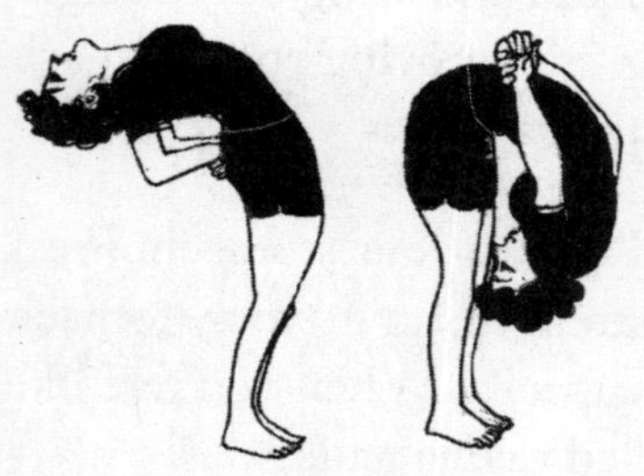

Method: Part I: Stand in samavastha. Bring both your arms to your back, hold the left wrist with your right hand and form a fist with your thumb tucked in. Inhale and bend back from your waist as far as you can. Look up. Exhale and gently straighten up your head, neck and waist. Then, bend forward. Try to bring your head to your knees. Repeat this process three times.

Part II: Hold the right wrist with your left hand and form a fist with your right hand with thumb tucked in. Do the rest of the process as given in part I.

35. Kati Shakti Vikasaka Kriya 2 (Strengthening the waist II)

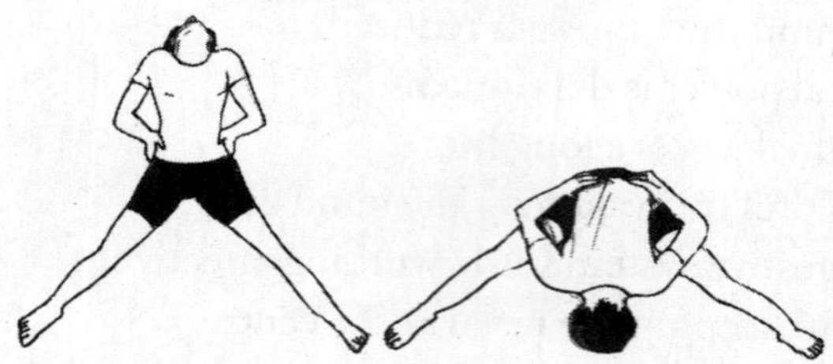

Method: Stand in samavastha. Stand with your legs as far apart as possible. Place your hands on your waist with your thumbs on your stomach. Inhale and bend your neck and waist backward to you maximum capacity. Look up, exhale and bring your neck and waist up. Now, bring your head down as much as you can do comfortably. Repeat the process three times. While doing it for the third time, bring your hands down on the floor and try to rest your head on the floor. Then, keeping your head in the same position, bring your hands back on your waist and hold the position for as long as you can hold it comfortably. Then, jump and come back to the original position.

36. Kati Shakti Vikasaka Kriya 3 (Strengthening the waist III)

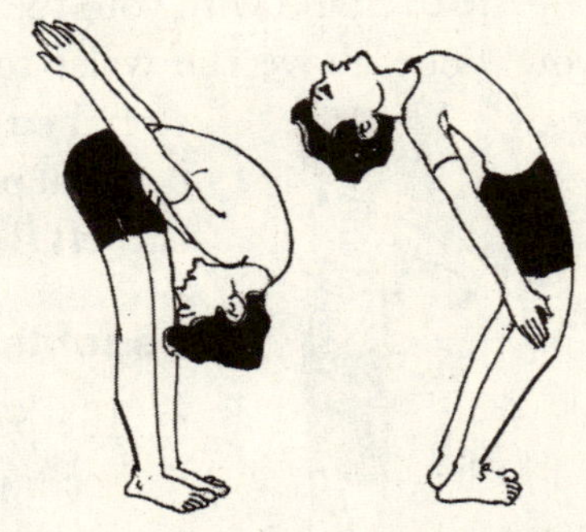

Method: Maintain four-finger-wide distance between your feet. Bring your arms to the sides of your thighs with palms facing inwards. Inhale and bend your neck and waist backward as much as you can and look up. Then, exhale and bend forward to bring your head to the knees while keeping the eyes open and raising your arms towards your back. Do this process in quick succession for about ten times.

37. Kati Shakti Vikasaka Kriya 4 (Strengthening the waist IV)

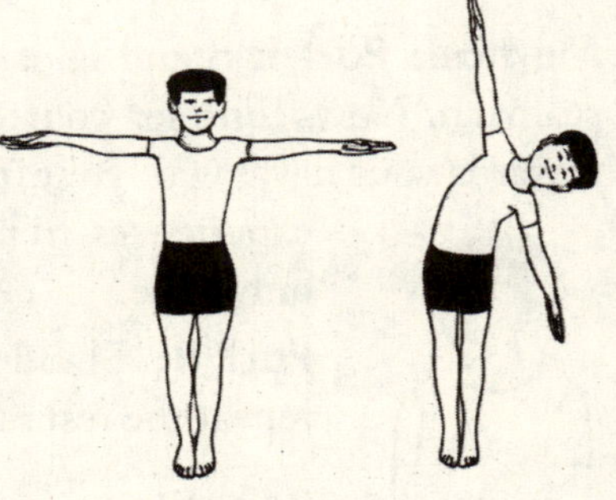

Method: Part I: Stand in samavastha. Raise your arms to the sides, to shoulder level, parallel to the ground, palms facing downwards and fingers together. Inhale and bend down to your left, forming an angle of 30 degrees. Raise your right arm up to an angle of 150 degrees. In this way, both the arms should be kept in one line. Bend your neck and waist. Exhale and come back to the original position. Again inhale and bend to your right to make an angle of 30 degrees with your right arm and raise your left arm to an angle of 150 degrees. Bring both the arms in one line, exhale and come back to the original position. Do this process ten times.

Part II: Maintain one arm's length between your feet. Do the rest of the process as given in part I.

38. Kati Shakti Vikasaka Kriya 5 (Strengthening the waist V)

Method: Stand with your feet about a foot apart. Inhale and turn your body above the waist towards your right, with your arms stretched out. Exhale and come back to the original position. Now, repeat this process on the left side. This can be done 5-6 times.

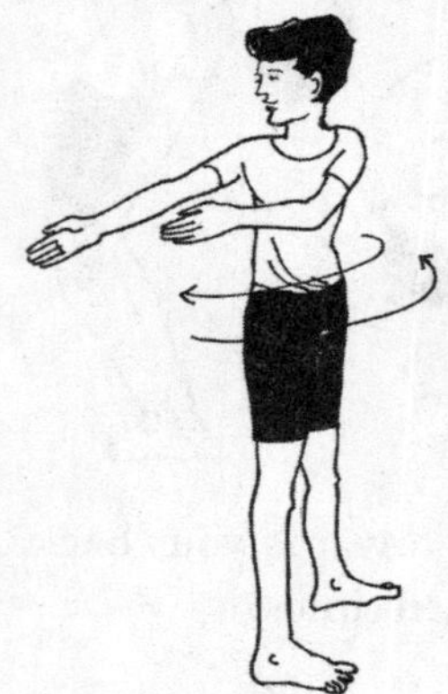

Benefits:

- The pain in the waist is cured; the waist becomes supple and ideal for dancers.
- The body becomes glowing and swift.
- If practised in the first twenty years of one's life, the sadhaka or the practitioner can gain height.

39. Muladhar Chakra Shuddhi Kriya (Toning up and purifying the root chakra)

Method: Part I: Stand in samavastha. Exhale and empty your stomach. Now, contract your anal muscles inward and upward towards your naval with your inner strength and when your body experiences trembling, stop the exercise. Do this only once.

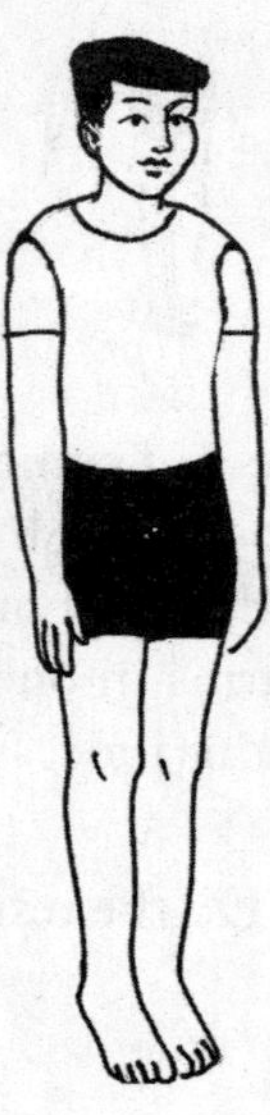

Part II: Stand with your feet apart. Once again repeat the rest of the process given in part I.

Benefits:

- It is helpful in awakening the kundalini because the 'pran' and 'apan' vayu get accumulated together.
- One feels freshness in one's mind.
- Body becomes strong.
- Constipation is cured.
- Piles are cured.
- The body becomes swift and one is gifted with a long life.

40. Upastha Tatha Svadhishthana-chakra-shuddhi (Strengthening and purifying the sacral chakra)

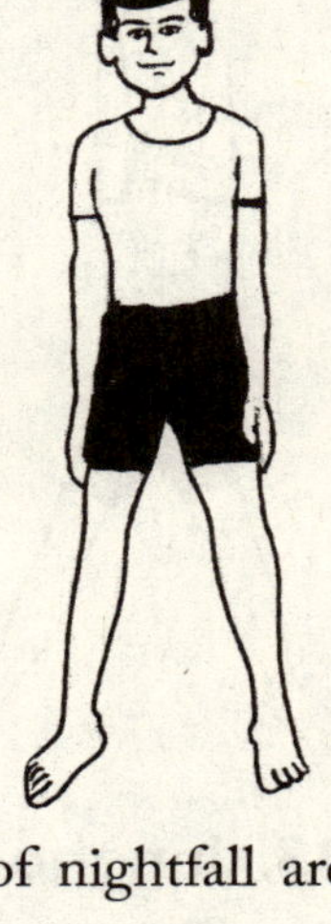

Method: Stand with your feet at an arm's distance. Inhale and pull your genital and anal muscles inwards and upwards towards your naval with your inner strength. Stop when you experience trembling in your legs. Do this only once.

Benefits:

- Diseases of urinary bladder and the anus are cured.
- Diseases like diabetes, fistula, piles, etc. are cured.
- It is specially beneficial for women.
- Diseases related to the uterus and problem of nightfall are cured.
- It is helpful for those practising celibacy.

41. Kundalini Shakti Vikasaka Kriya (Developing the power of the mystic kundalini)

Method: Stand in samavastha. Inhale and strike your buttocks with your left heel. Exhale and come back to the original position. Now, again inhale and strike your buttocks with your right heel. Exhale and come back to the original position. Repeat this ten times.

Benefits:

- It is helpful in awakening the kundalini.
- The body becomes toned and swift.
- Knowledge is enhanced.
- It is helpful for those practising celibacy and who want to attain Moksha.

42. Jangha Shakti Vikasaka Kriya 1 (Developing the thighs I)

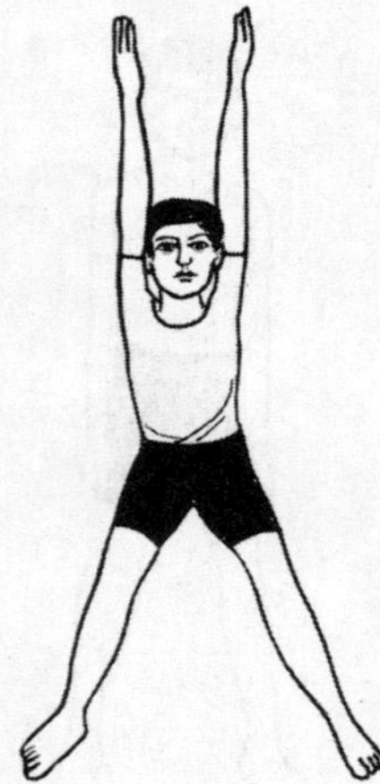

Method: Part I: Stand in samavastha. Inhale and with a jump, throw your feet apart. Raise both your arms above your head. Exhale and with a jump, come back to the original position. Repeat this process ten times.

Part II: Inhale and with a jump, throw your feet towards your thighs. Raise your arms above your head, palms facing outwards. Exhale and with a jump, come back to the original position. Repeat this process ten times.

43. Jangha Shakti Vikasaka Kriya 2 (Developing the thighs II)

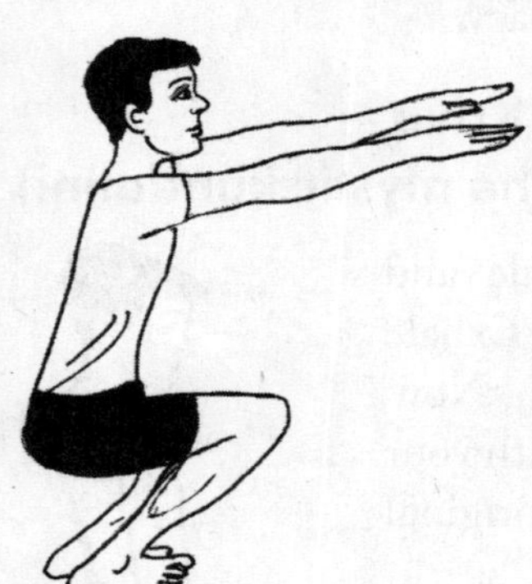

Method: Part I: Stand in samavastha. Spread your arms in the front, parallel to the ground, palms facing downwards. Inhale and bend your knees, as if sitting on a chair. Exhale and come back to the original position. Repeat this process three times.

Part II: Spread your arms on your sides parallel to the ground, palms facing downwards. Inhale, stand on your toes and bend your knees as if sitting on a chair. Exhale and come back to the original position. Repeat this process three times.

Benefits:

- Thighs become strong, beautiful and well-shaped.
- It also helps cure knee pain.

44. Janu Shakti Vikasaka Kriya (Strengthening the knees)

Method: Stand in samavastha. Inhale and bend your left leg back and touch your buttocks with the left heel. Exhale and throw your feet forward as if kicking a football. Repeat with the right leg. Do this process ten times.

Benefits:

- Joint pain and arthritis are cured.
- It is helpful in awakening of kundalini.
- It is ideal for sportsmen.
- Knees become beautiful and well-shaped.

45. Pindali Shakti Vikasaka Kriya (Yogic squats for strengthening the calves)

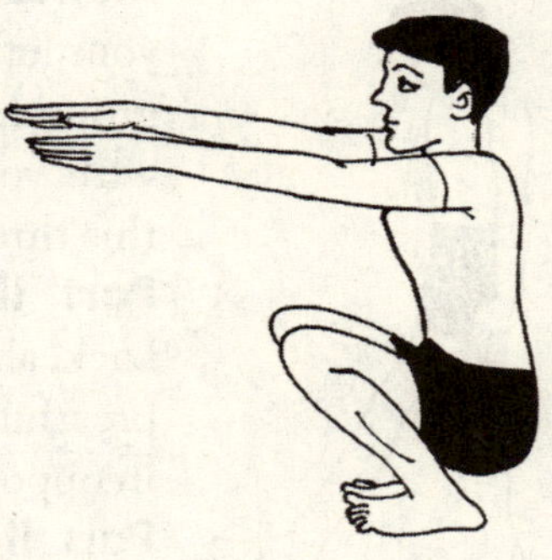

Method: Stand in samavastha. Form a fist with your thumbs tucked in and raise your arms in front of you at shoulder level, parallel to the ground. Palms should be facing each other. Inhale and keeping your knees together, bend your knees to sit completely. Keep your feet firm and flat on the ground. Before you stand up, exhale and by rotating your arms, bring them in front of your chest. Then, bring your arms down and come back to the original position. Repeat this process five times.

Benefits:

- It helps cure leg pain.
- Knees and thighs are toned.
- Celibacy is enhanced.
- It helps cure pain in toes.

46. Padmool Shakti Vikasaka Kriya (Developing the strength of the soles)

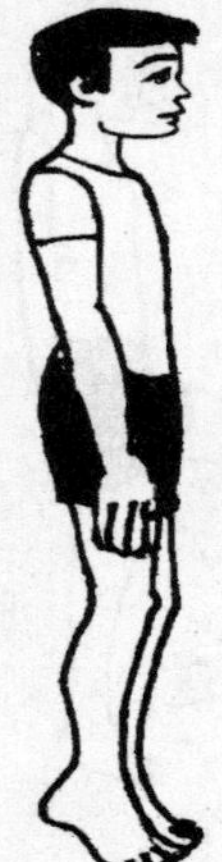

Method: Part I: Stand in samavastha. Raise your heels and stand on your toes. Bounce slowly in your place 10-15 times. Keep your toes fixed on the ground.

Part II: While breathing normally, jump up and down 10-15 times in your place on your toes.

47. Gulpha Padtal, Padprishtha Shakti Vikasaka Kriya (Developing the strength of the ankle and the feet)

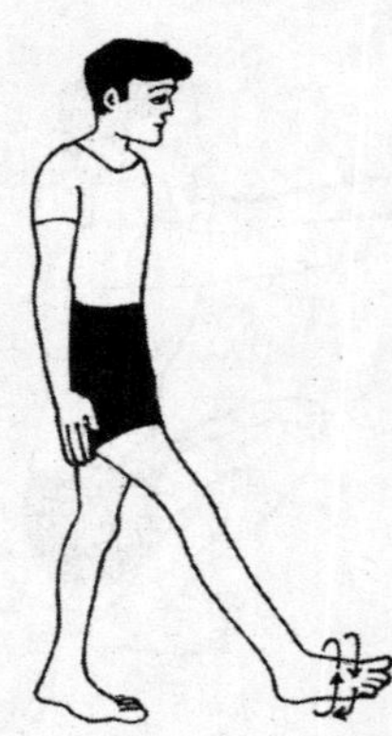

Method: Part I: Stand in samavastha. Raise your left leg in front, about 9 inches above the ground. While breathing normally, make an O with your feet in opposite directions. Repeat this three times.

Part II: Stretch your left leg towards the back, about 9 inches above the ground. While breathing normally, make an O with your feet in opposite directions. Do this three times.

Part III: Repeat the process given in part I with your right leg three times.

Part IV: Raise and stretch your right leg towards the back, about 9 inches above the ground. Rest of the process has to be done three times as given in part II.

Benefits:

- Pain in toes, back of feet and soles are cured.
- Legs become well shaped.
- It is ideal to cure the pain caused by sprain.
- It gives relief from fatigue due to too much walking or running.

48. Padanguli Shakti Vikasaka Kriya (Developing the strength of the toes)

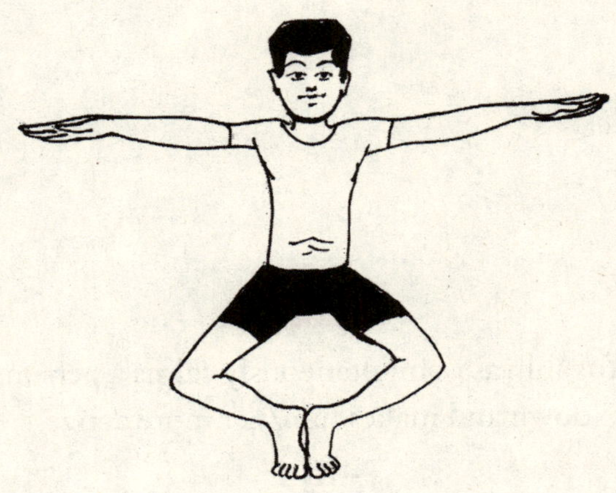

Method: Stand in samavastha. With the help of your hands, bring both the toes together with the soles facing inward. Breathe normally. Jump on your toes and stand up straight. Complete the process in one motion.

Benefits:

- Toes are strengthened.
- Pain in toes and feet are cured.
- It helps resolve the issue of fatigue caused due to walking and runing.
- Feet and toes become flexible.

Yogabhyasa, simultaneously calms a person down and makes him/her more active.

–RJT

By doing yoga sadhana, we can awaken the inherent powers that lie dormant within us.

–RJT

Sthula Yogic Vyayama

(Easy to Execute Yogic Macro Exercises)

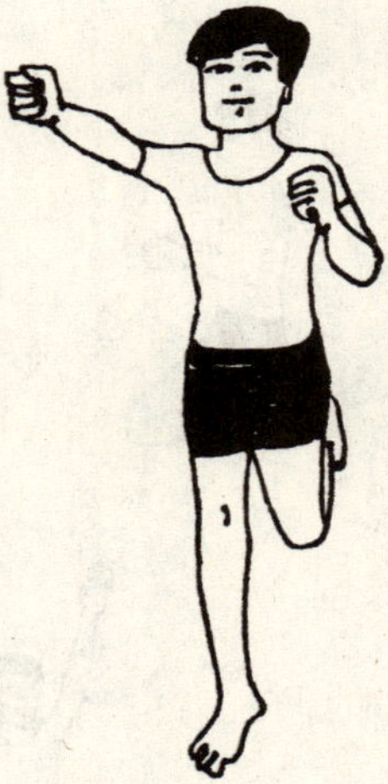

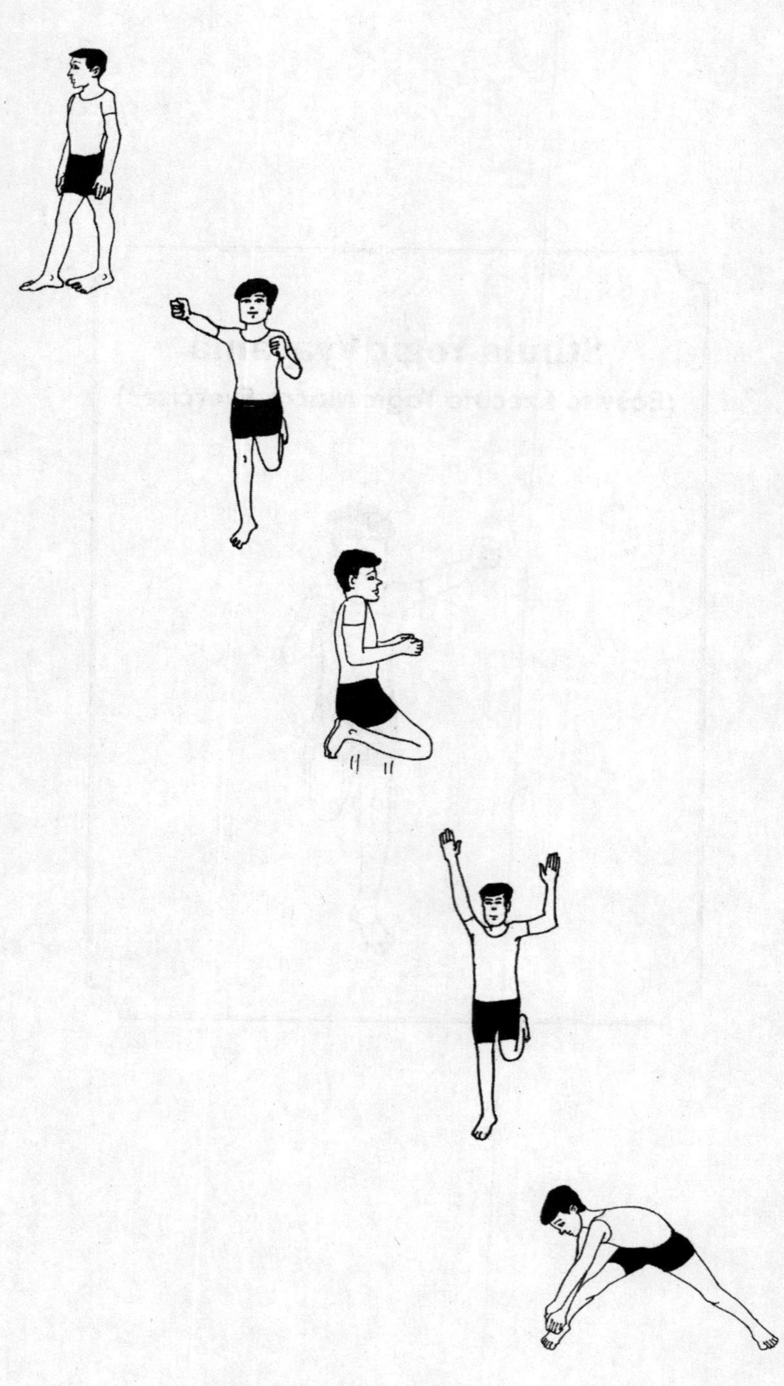

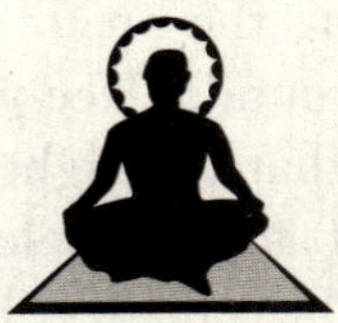

Sthula Yogic Vyayama

(Easy to Execute Yogic Macro Exercises)

Here, we will discuss about Sthula Yogic Exercises. Yoga is a very vast subject and has been prevailed since time immemorial. For example, in Ayurveda, each medicine has its own effect and characterstics depending on weather the medicine taken is cold, warm or taken in powdered form. If we mix up two or three kinds of medicines, its effect will also increase, depending on the combinations. Similarly, any one action associated with yoga if done properly will give us double benefit. If some more actions are mixed (as instrcuted by your yoga Guru), we would not only make our body disease-free but also transform our body. Give your body one hour, and keep diseases at bay for rest of your life. Any kind of yogic exercise, if done chronologically and under the guidance of a Guru will give results better than expected. Yoga makes body strong, beautiful, healthy and well-shaped. If there was even a hint of doubt in this fact, yoga would have disappeared long ago. Yoga is unspoken, but experimented with. Millions today all over the world are benefitting from yoga and transforming their lives.

When lighter exercises are collaborated with yoga, the results are visible in a very short duration. If one practises Engine Run or does execises with vertical movements for two or three minutes everyday, obesity or heart ailments would never bother the practitioner. While subtle exercises help smaller organs, the five kriyas of the macro exercises are advantageous for the whole body.

1. Rekha Gati (Walking in a straight line)

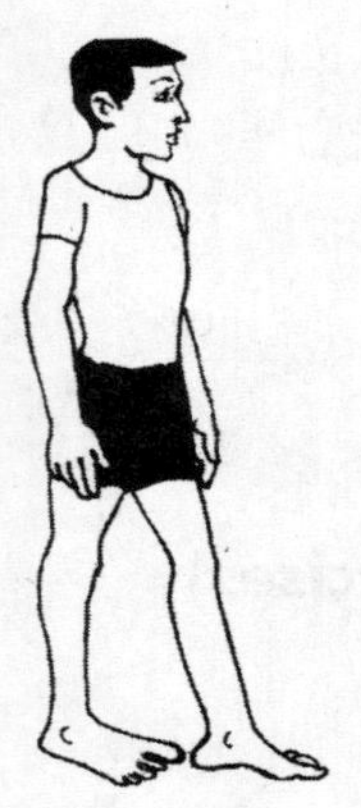

Method: Part I: Stand in samavastha, holding the breath in. With the left foot on the ground, place your right foot in front of it so that the right heel touches the toes of the left foot. Exhale. Repeat the same process with the other leg. The eyes must look in front and not at the feet.

Part II: Inhale, and hold your breath, and with your left foot on the ground, place your right foot at the back, in a way that the toes of your right foot touches the heel of your left foot. Exhale. Walk back ten steps in similar way keeping your gaze in front.

Benefits:

- This exercise increases the power of concentration.
- It also develops memory power, or aids fast recollection.
- It maintains the balance of the body.

2. Hridaya Gati (Engine run)

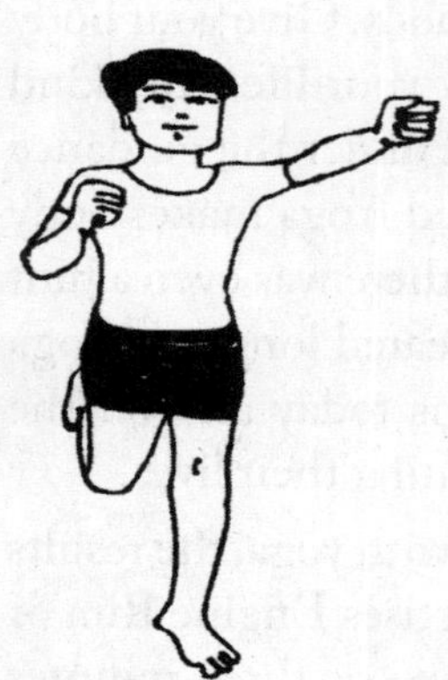

Method: Stand in samavastha. Close your fist with thumb inside. Keep your hands close to your body, bend the left arm from the elbow, parallel to the ground and keep the right arm straight, parallel to the ground. The fists should face each other. Inhale and bend your left foot from the knee at 90 degrees. Bring the right arm forward. Exhale, Inhale and bend the right leg from the knee at 90 degrees. Bring the left arm forward. Exhale and bring the right foot and left arm in the original position. After repeating this with inhalation and exhalation for 10-15 times, run on the spot. Stop when you feel tired.

Benefits:

- This exercise relieves fatigue from hands and legs, and is also a good exercise to shed weight.
- It strengthens the chest, thighs and shingles and relives them of weariness.
- Athletes can specially benefit by doing this exercise.
- The body becomes active and strong.

3. Utkurdana (The jumping exercise)

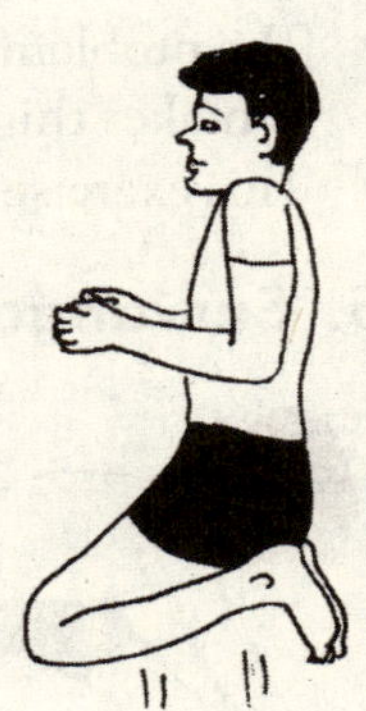

Method: Stand in samavastha, with clenched fists, thumb tucked in and arms stretched in front, parallel to each other. Inhale deeply and keep your palms facing each other. Make a full circle and return to the original position. Jump as high as you can and bend your knees so that the heels strike hard against the buttocks. Exhale, throwing out your arms in front of you, while your feet touch the ground. Repeat this process five times.

Benefits:

- For the first 20 years of one's life, this exercise adds inches to the height.
- It helps awaken the mystic kundalini coil, and also broadens the chest and strengthens the thighs and makes shapely.
- It cures lung diseases.

4. Urdhva Gati (Upward movement)

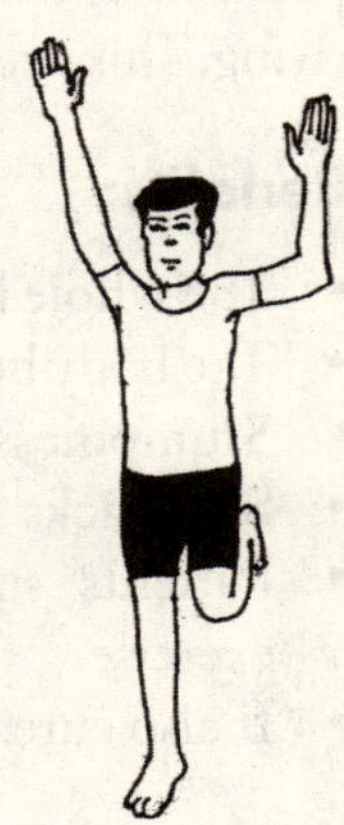

Method: Stand in samavastha. Spread the arms sideways from the shoulders. Keep your gaze up. Breathe in and bend your left leg at 90 degrees. Bend the left arm from the elbow and raise it towards your head. Lift the right arm straight above the head. Let the palms face in front. Breathe out and bring the left foot down. Now, stretch the left arm above the head. Breathe in and bend your right leg at 90 degrees. Bring the right arm down to the shoulder and bend at the elbow. Exhale and rest the right leg on the ground and raise the left arm above the head. Bend the left arm from the elbow and bring it towards the head. Repeat this process for 8 to 10 times slowly. Stop when you feel tired.

Benefits:

- It makes your limbs stronger.
- Kills diseases related to lungs.
- It cures obesity.
- The problem of hands and feet becoming cold is cured.
- It makes thighs well-shaped.
- This exercise is specially beneficial for athletes.

5. Sarvanga Pushti (Developing the entire body)

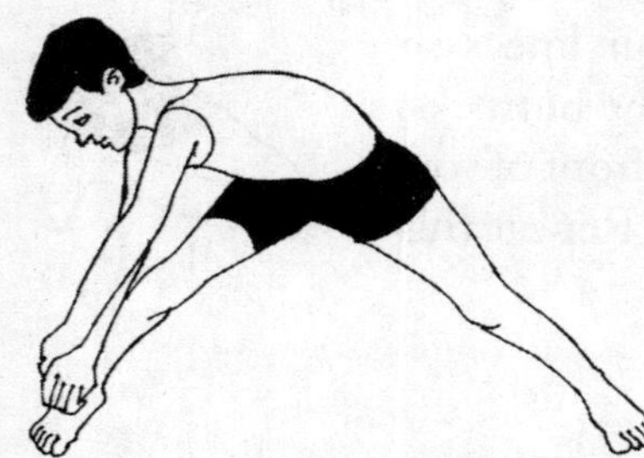

Method: Stand with your feet as wide apart as possible. Form fists with thumbs tucked in. Then, with right wrist upon the left, bend towards the ankle of the left leg. Inhale and slowly raise the arms towards the head, while exhaling on your right. Now, bring left wrist on the right. Inhale again and bring the arms up. Turn to your left and bring your arms down to the left ankle. Exhale and repeat the process three times by changing the position of the wrist. Inhale while coming down and exhale while rising. This execise is to be done very slowly.

Benefits:

- The whole body becomes supple and strong.
- The body becomes flexible.
- Stumpiness is cured.
- Stiff backs are cured.
- Patients suffering from tuberculosis can benefit from this exercise.
- It also cures constipation.

Exercises of the Pavanmuktasana Group

(Air-relieving Poses)

Simple exercises to control the Air for the abdominal area, and for developing strength

All these simple exercises which come under the category of Pavanmuktasan* are taught in almost all the yoga centres. The reason for doing these exercises in the beginning of the program is that they bring flexibility and help in removing rigidity from almost all the muscles and joints of our body. In the previous chapters, a series of Sookshma vyayam (Subtle exercises) and Sthool vyayam (Macro exercises) were explained. All those exercises also bring about stability in the body.

By doing all of the following exercises, the joints of our body open up and we get rid of laziness. The practitioner experiences swiftness and freshness which makes it easier for him/her to do yoga after these exercises.

Even though all these asanas are very simple, they are very effective. They provide a new life force and energy to the body.

Vayu Nirodhak Kriyas

(Air restraining exercise)

Padanguli (Bending of the toes), Padtal (Touching the toes to the ground), Padprishth (Rotation of the toes) and Gulf Shaktivardhak/Vikasaka Kriya (Strengthening the ankle)

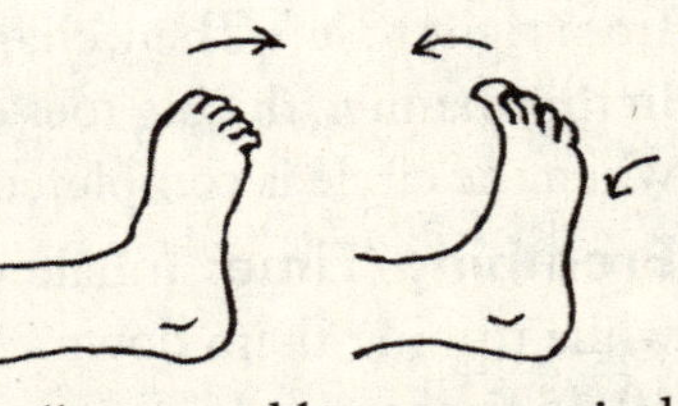

Exercise 1. Padanguli (Bending of the toes): Sit with your legs stretched in front of you. Lean back a little and rest your hands beside your buttocks. Do not bend your spine, neck or head. Do not bend your elbows and keep your mind

*I learnt the intricacies of Pavan muktasana kriyas for the first time from Dr K. M. Ganguli. Then, I learnt them from Dr Phoolchand Yogacharyji and later in a camp from Paramhans Niranjananand Saraswati. I express my gratitude to all the teachers.

stress-free. Shift your entire focus on your toes and bend them forward and backward.

Breathing/Time: Exhale when you bend your toes forward. Inhale when you bend them towards yourself. Do this 10-15 times.

Exercise 2. Padtal (Toes touching the ground)

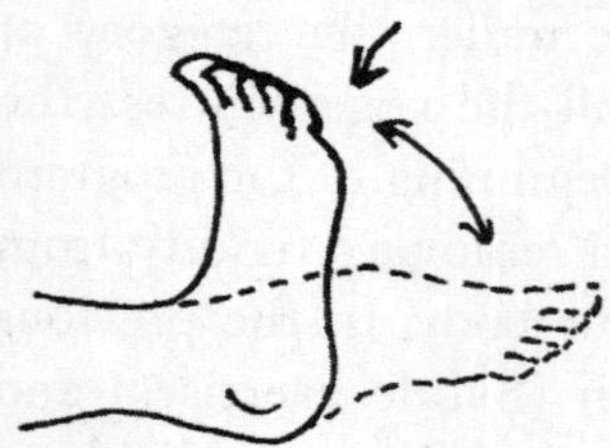

Method: Now bend the toes forward from the ankle, in such a way that they touch the ground. Bend them as far as you can do it comfortably. Then, try to bend them back towards yourself, as much as you can.

Breathing/Time: Inhale when you bend your toes and ankles towards yourself, and exhale when you bend them forward. Do this exercise 10-15 times.

Exercise 3. Padprishth (Toe rotation)

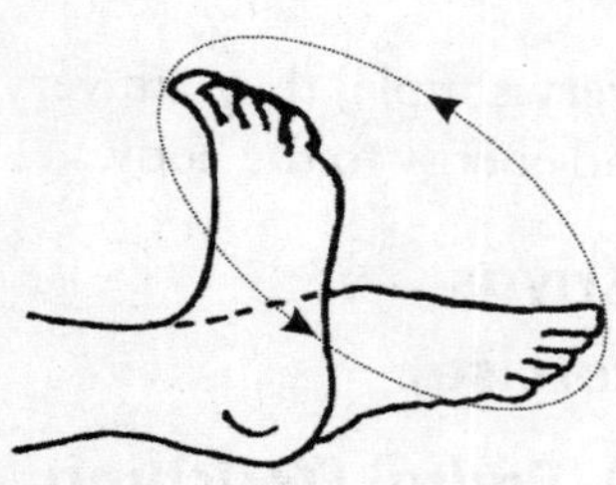

Method: Keep the legs a little apart. First do the exercise with the right leg. Move the right foot from the ankle in circular motion. Move 10-15 times from right to left and then, 10-15 times from left to right. Do the same exercise with the left leg. Now, bring your feet together and do this exercise. Again, keeping some distance between the two legs, move both the feet from the ankle in circular motion but in the opposite directions. Move one foot from left to right and the other from right to left. Then, change the direction. When the legs move in this manner, the big toes of both the feet must touch each other when the circle is completed.

Breathing/Time: Inhale while bringing the feet up and exhale while turning them down. All the above exercises should be done 10-15 times.

Note: We have done this kriya in Sookshma vyayam in standing position. It can also be done in sitting position. It is taught in almost all the yoga centres.

Exercise 4. Gulf Shaktivardhak (Ankle crank)

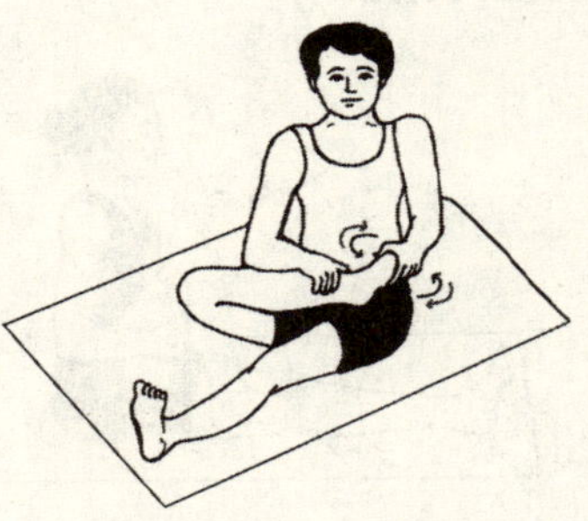

Moving the feet in circular motion can be done in yet another way. Keep one leg straight and bend the other from the knee, placing it on one of the thighs in such a way that the ankle must be facing out. Now, hold the ankle with one hand and with the other, hold the toes. Now, move the ankle in circular motion about 10 times, first from right to left and then from left to right. Do this with the other leg.

Breathing/Time: Same as in exercise 3.

Exercise 5. Supt Janu Sanchalan Kriya (Stretched knees exercise): (Moving the knees forward and backward)

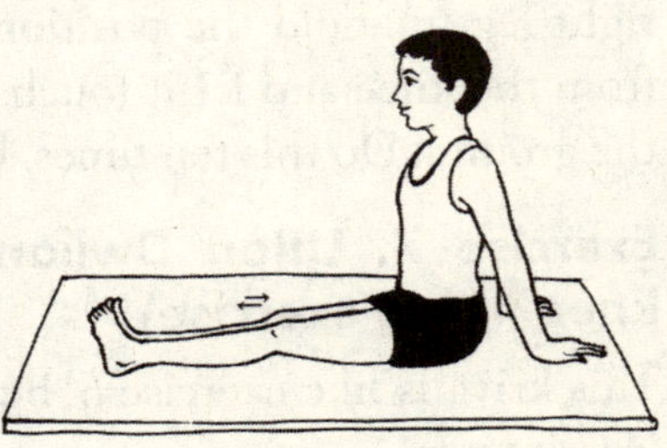

Sit with your legs straight in front of you. Since we have to direct the knees forward and backward, contract the muscles and pull the knees towards yourself. Hold the position for some time and then release the muscles. Repeat this exercise 10-15 times.

Breathing/Time: Inhale while pulling the knees towards yourself and exhale while releasing them.

Benefits:

- The joints of the calves, toes, ankles, knees and fingers become strong and flexible.
- The possibility of developing arthritis in that particular limb is eradicated.
- It relieves pain in the calves and cures muscle pull.

Exercise 6. Uttan Janu Sanchalan Kriya (Raised knees movement)

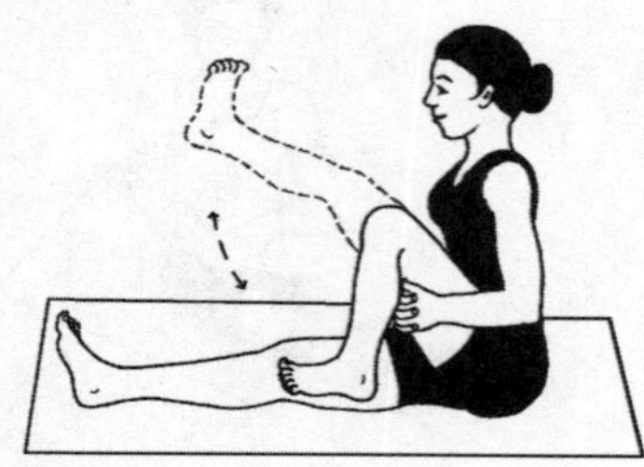

Method: (a) Sit with your legs stretched in front. Hold your right thigh with both your hands, and bending your right knee, let the thigh touch your abdomen and chest. Now, slowly stretch your leg upwards. Hold this position for some time and bring your leg down on the ground. In this exercise, take the leg up as high as you can, to the extent that the leg touches your nose. Meanwhile, the other leg must remain flat on the ground. The spine and the waist should remain straight. Repeat this process 10 times. Then, do the same with other leg.

(b) Now do this process by reversing the order. First take your right leg up, hold the position for some time, and then bend it from the knee and let it touch your chest. Bring the leg down on the ground. Do this ten times. Repeat with the other leg.

Exercise 7. Uttan Dwijanu Sanchalan Kriya (Double knee lifting exercise)

This kriya is like exercise 6, but it has to be done using both the legs at once.

Method: (a) Sit with your legs stretched in front of you. Keep your legs together. Keep both your hands on the sides of your buttocks, slightly at the back. Now bend your knees and bring them close to your chest. Then, straighten your legs while lifting them up, and then slowly bring them down on the ground. Do this kriya 10 times.

(b) Now reverse the order. First, lift your legs straight up. Then, bend your knees to touch your chest and bring them down on the ground. Do this kriya 10 times.

Breathing: Exhale while bending the knees and inhale while straightening the legs.

Precautions: People with severe back ache, heart problems and high BP should do this exercise carefully.

Benefits:

- All disorders of the knees are cured.
- Back ache and pain in the buttocks are cured permanently.
- Restless legs syndrome or related disease do not occur.
- Constipation and poor digestion are cured and appetite is enhanced.
- Fat around the abdomen is reduced.

Exercise 8. Jaanu Chakra Kriya (Moving Knees in circular motion)

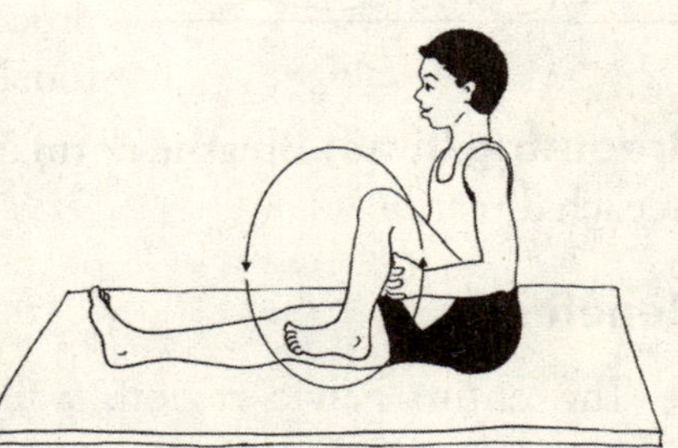

Method: Sit with your legs stretched in front. Since we have to hold each thigh with our hands and move the lower leg, hold the right thigh with both the hands under the knee, the palms of one hand holding the opposite elbow. Now, bring the thighs close to the abdomen and lifting your right leg from the knees, move the lower leg in circular motion from right to left and from left to right, 10 times each. Repeat this process with the left leg.

Breathing: Inhale while taking the legs up and exhale while bringing them down.

Aim: To keep the knees disease free.

Benefits:

- It helps get rid of diseases like arthritis.
- It gives strength to the knee joints and gives relief from pain.
- It regularises the flow of blood by clearing the blockages.

Exercise 9. Shroni Vikasak Evam Shaktivardhak Kriya (Developing and strengthening the pelvic region)

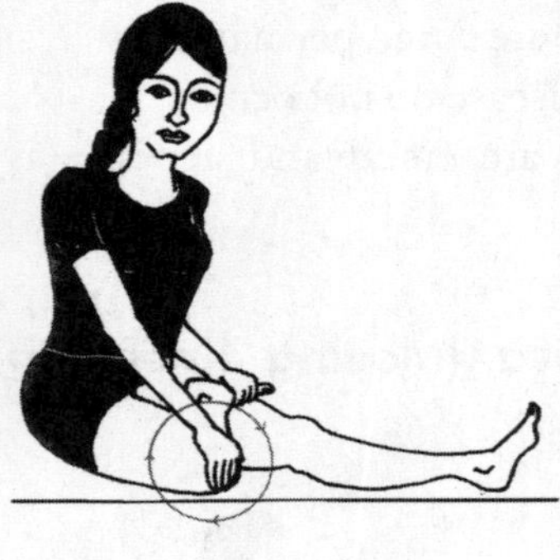

Method: Sit with both the legs stretched in front. Bend the right leg from the knee and place it on the left thigh. Hold the right foot with your left hand and the right knee with the right hand. Now, try to make a big circle with the right knee in one direction. Do this process in the opposite direction too. Repeat it with the other leg.

Breathing/time: Breathe normally and do the process 10 times in each direction.

Benefits:

- The entire pelvic region, waist, buttocks and reproductive organs benefit from it.
- By doing this asana, problems related to these body parts do not occur.

Exercise 10. Gatimaya Ardha Titali Asana (Half butterfly pose)

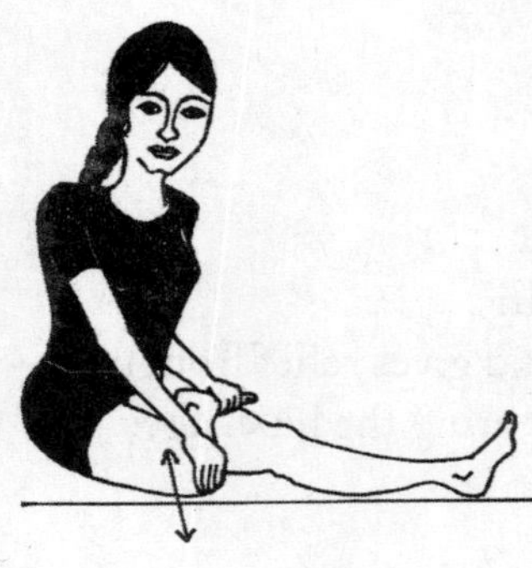

Method: Sit with your lags stretched in front. Keep your waist, spine and neck straight. Bend your left leg and place it on the right thigh. Hold the big toe of the left leg with your right hand so that it stays in place, and hold the knee with your left hand. Now, press the knee down with your hand and then lift it up towards your chest. Do it in such a manner that the knee should touch the ground. Repeat with the other leg.

Breathing: Inhale while lifting your knee up and exhale while pressing it down.

Exercise 11. Gatimaya Poorna Titali Asana (Dynamic full butterfly pose)

Variation 1: Sit with your legs stretched in front. Keep your waist, spine, neck and head straight. Bend your legs and join the soles together and place them close to your genitals. Hold the heels with both the hands and move your thighs up and down. Begin slowly and then gradually increase the speed. Try to touch the ground with your thighs and knees.

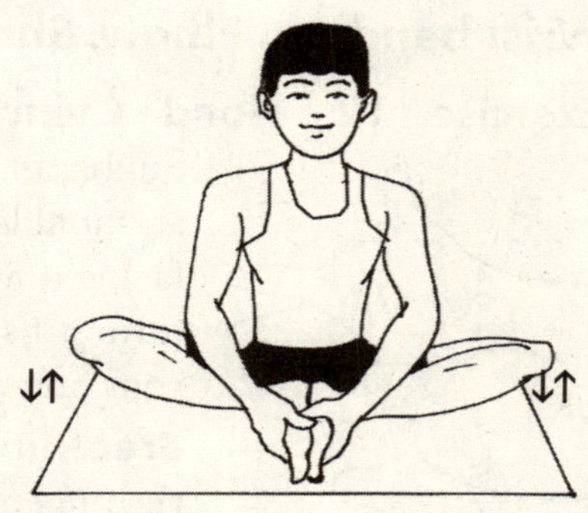

Variation 2: Sit with your legs stretched in front. Keep your waist, spine, neck and head straight. Bend both the legs and join the soles together. Bring them close to your genitals. Place your hands on your knees and slowly start pressing your knees down and then lift them up. Do this kriya 20-25 times. Try to touch the ground with your knees.

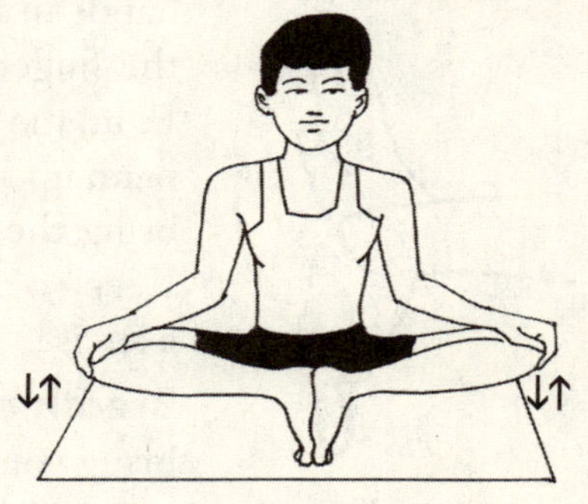

Breathing: Normal

Benefits:

- Knee joints and buttocks become strong by doing this asana, and it reduces the fat in the buttocks and keep them balanced.
- It controls the disorders caused by wind.
- Brings about a new energy in the lower parts of the body.
- Brings about stability in the digestive system.

Precautions: Sciatica patients and those with back ache must do this according to their condition. In case of severe pain, do not do this exercise.

Mushtika, Manibandha, Kohni, Skandh Shaktivardhak/Vikasak Kriya (Hand clenching, Wrist bending, Elbow, Shoulder strengthening)

Exercise 12. Hand Clenching: Sit in any posture of Sukhasana. Stretch your arms in front, at shoulder level. Keep your palms open, facing down. Now, tuck your thumb in and form a fist and then open the fist, spread your fingers and make them rigid.

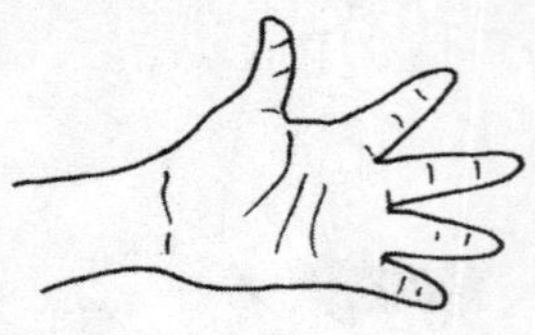

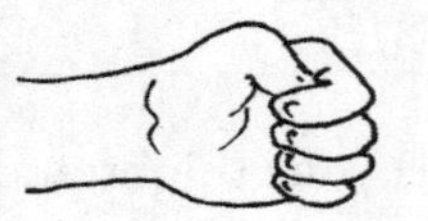

Breathing/time: Inhale while opening the fingers and exhale while clenching your fist. Repeat this exercise 10-15 times.

Exercise 13. Wrist Bending: In the same way, spread your hands in front, keep your palms open, but the fingers should be close to each other. From the joint of the wrist, move the entire palm up and pull it towards yourself. Then, bring the palm down and again pull it up. Keep your hands straight while doing this exercise.

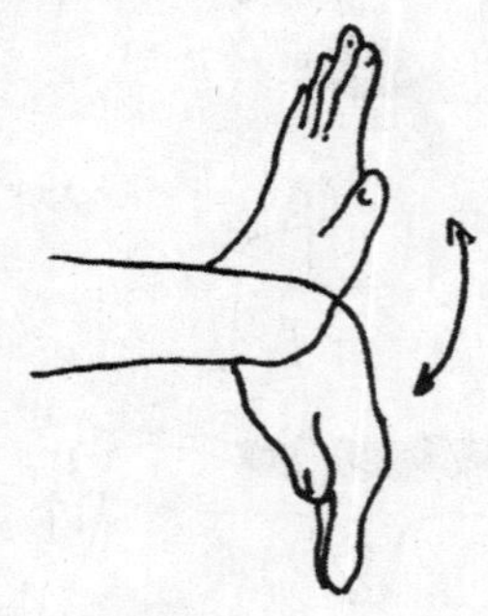

Breathing/time: Exhale when you bring your palm upwards and inhale while bringing it down. Repeat this kriya 10-15 times.

Exercise 14 a. Wrist Joint Rotation: Sitting in the same position, form a fist with your thumb tucked in and rotate your wrist from right to left and then from left to right 10-15 times. Do this with one hand at a time. Keep your arms straight.

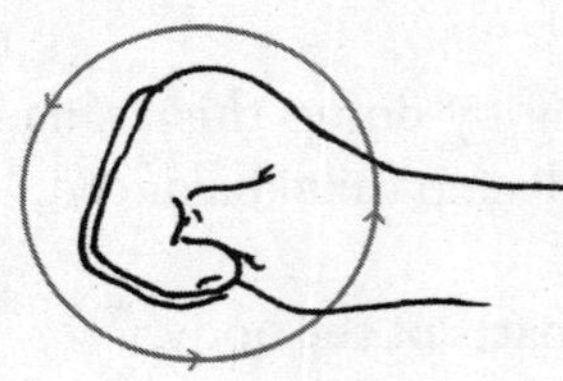

Exercise 14 b. Now, do this kriya with both the hands. Move both the wrists in the same direction. Move them from left to right and then from right to left, 10-15 times each.

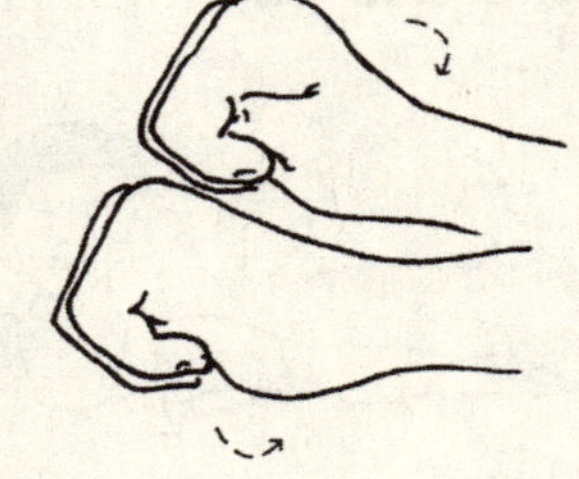

Exercise 14 c. Now, move both the wrist in opposite directions. Move the left wrist from left to right and the right wrist from right to left 10-15 times. Then, reverse the direction of the movement.

Benefits: The joints of the wrist become strong and no diseases occur in fingers. The blood circulation of the hands is regularised.

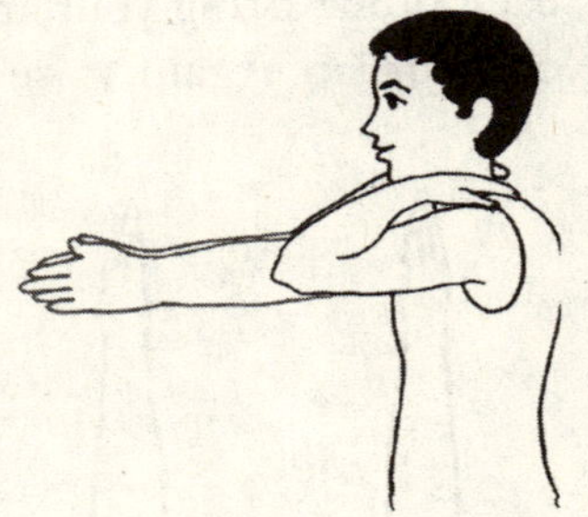

Exercise 15 a. Elbow bending: Sit in any posture of Sukhasana. Raise your arms up to the shoulder level, palms facing either up or towards each other. Now, bend your arms from the elbow and try to touch your shoulder with your fingers. Then, straighten up your arms. Do this exercise 10-15 times.

Exercise 15 b. Sit in the same position. Spread your arms sideways like the wings of bird; palms facing up, arms at shoulder level. Now, bend your arms from the elbow and try to touch the shoulder. Then, straighten up your arms. Do this 10-15 times.

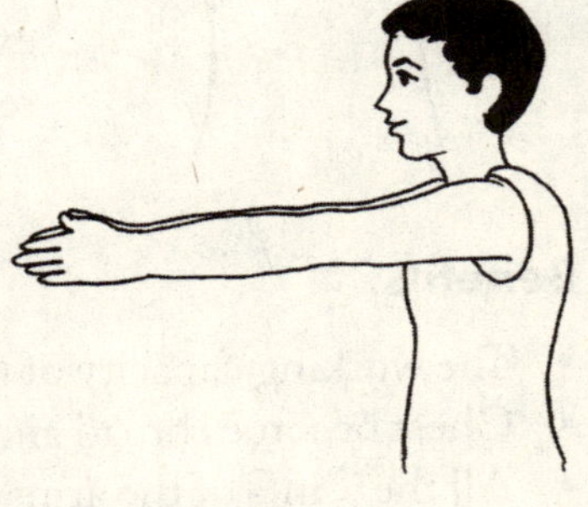

Exercise 15 c. Continue to sit in the same position. This exercise involves swift movement. Spread your arms in front to the level of your shoulders. Palms should face each other. Now, move your arms to the sides and bring them back in front. Again, move your arms to the sides and bring them back in front. Relax your arms and keep them on your lap. Do this 10-15 times. (While moving the arms sideways, the palms should face down and while moving in front, they should face each other.)

Exercise 15 d. Sit in Sukhasana. Spread your arms sideways, in line with your shoulders. Your palms should face down. Now, raise your arms up. Your arms should touch your ears and palms should face each other. Bring your arms back to the shoulder level and down on your lap. Again, raise your arms up to the shoulder level, take them up touching your ears and bring them back to the shoulder level and then keep them on your lap. You can do this exercise while counting. On count one, spread your arms sideways, on count two, raise your arms up, on count three, bring them back to the shoulder level and on count four, keep them on your lap. Repeat this 5-10 times.

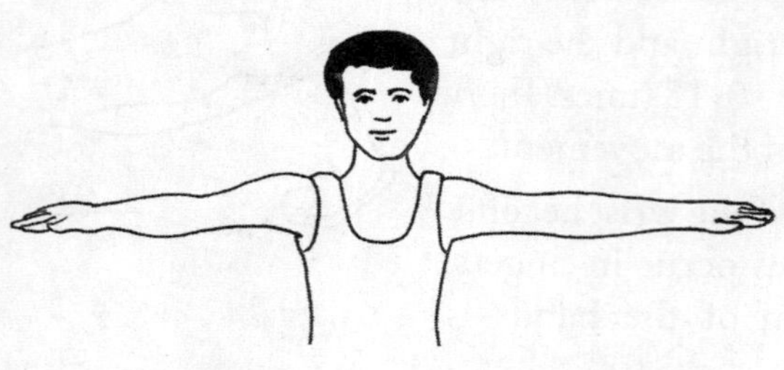

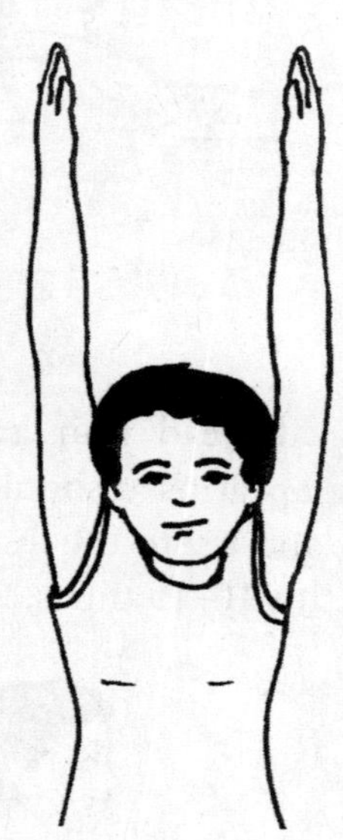

Breathing/time: While spreading your arms and taking them up, inhale and while bending or bringing them down, exhale. All the above mentioned exercises can be done as per individual requirements.

Benefits:

- The working capacity of the lungs is enhanced.
- Chest becomes broad and strong.
- All the joints of the arms start functioning efficiently.
- Shoulders become strong.

Skandh Sanchalan Kriya (Rotating the shoulders)

Exercise 16. Variation 1.

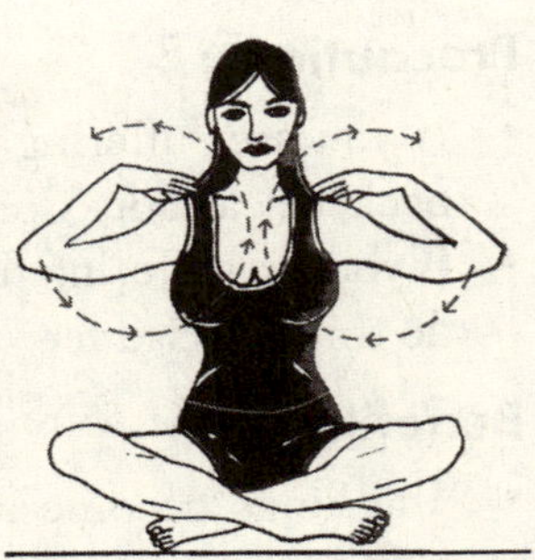

Method: Sit in any posture of Sukhasana. Spread your arms sideways and bend them from the elbow to bring the fingers of the right hand on the right shoulder and those of the left hand on the left shoulder. Now, bring both the elbows in front of the chest and try to make them touch each other. Then lift your elbows and try to touch your ears and then take the elbows back as much as possible, so that the chest may expand. Making the elbows touch the sides, bring them back to the original position. Repeat this rotation of the elbows 10-20 times. Then, do this in the opposite direction too.

Breathing: Inhale while raising your elbows and exhale while bringing them down.

Benefits:

- The chest becomes broad and toned.
- Women can make their breasts shapely by doing this exercise.
- Due to the expansion and contraction of the lungs, their working capacity is enhanced.
- All the shoulder joints become strong.

Variation 2.

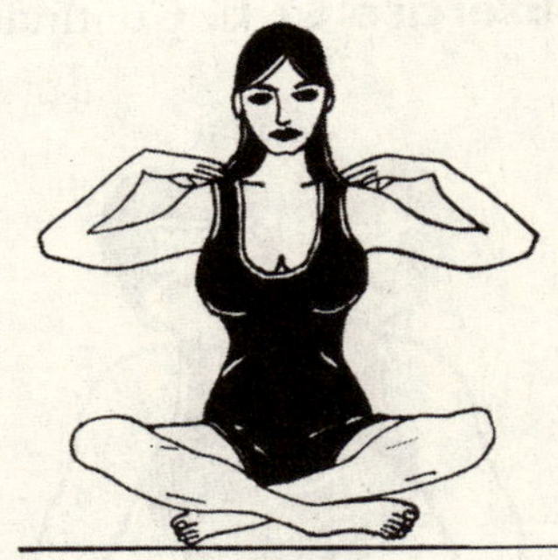

Method: Sit in any posture of Sukhasana. Bend your arms from the elbow and place the hands on your shoulders. Now, slowly turn your torso from right to left and then from left to right. You can do this exercise slowly or quickly. Make sure that while doing this exercise, the head and the gaze remains fixed. Only the shoulders and the chest will move.

Breathing: Exhale while turning towards the right and left and exhale while coming to the original position.

Precautions:

- If you are suffering from any disease or complication of the neck, be cautious doing this exercise.
- If you are suffering from a heart disease or high blood pressure, do this exercise very slowly.

Benefits:

- The lungs become more active and their capacity to receive oxygen increases.
- The neck becomes more flexible and supple.
- It is also helpful in purifying the blood.

Gatimaya Greeva Shaktivardhaka/Vikasaka Kriya (Dynamic neck exercises)

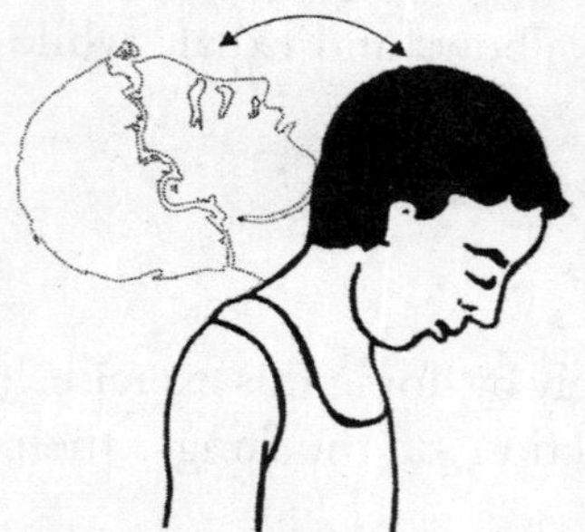

Exercise 17 a. Sit in any posture of Sukhasana. Make the gyana mudra with your fingers and keep them on your lap or on your knees. Now, slowly bend your head to touch the chin with the sternum. Then, bend it backwards. Come back to the original position. Repeat this 5-10 times.

Breathing: Exhale while bending forward and inhale while bending backward.

Exercise 17 b. Continue to sit in the same position. Now bend your head to the left so that the left ear touches the left shoulder. Slowly bring the head up and bend your head to the right in a similar manner. Repeat this 5-10 times.

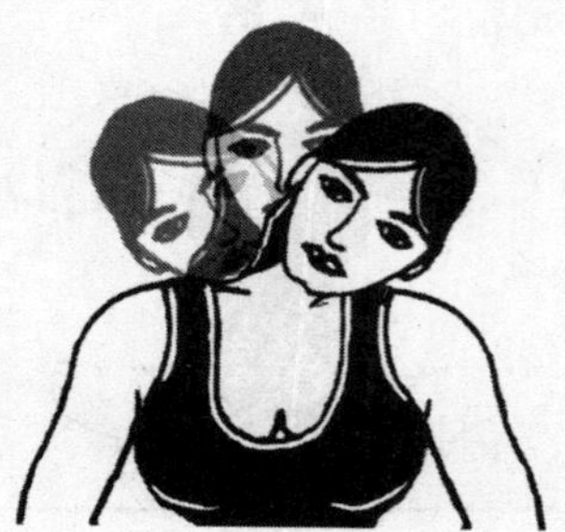

Breathing: Exhale while bending your head sideways. Inhale while bringing the head up.

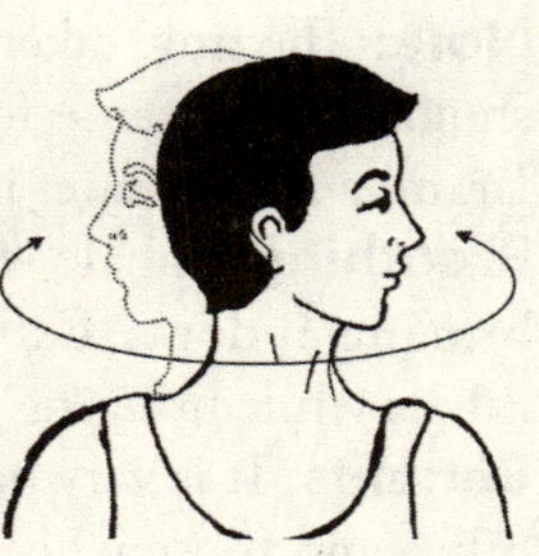

Exercise 17 c. Continue to sit in the same position. Now, without bending the head turn it to the left so that it comes in line with the left shoulder. Slowly bring the head back to the original position. Now, turn the head to the right to bring it in line with the right shoulder. This is one round. Repeat this 5-10 times.

Breathing: Exhale while turning your head to the left and right. Inhale while coming back to the original position.

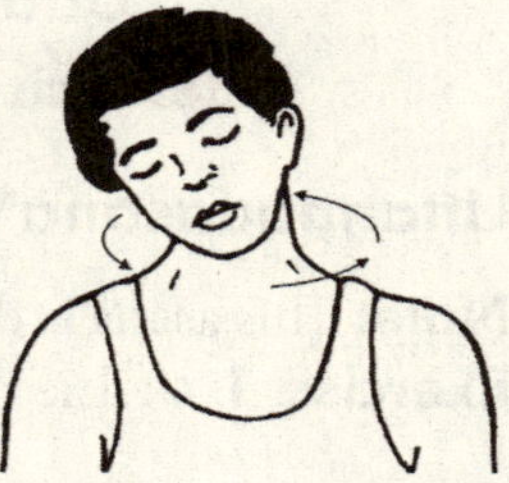

Exercise 17 d. Continue to sit in the same position. Keep your eyes closed. Now, move the head in circular motion. Bend your head forward and move it slowly from right to left in a circular motion. Do this at least 5-10 times. Now repeat this exercise in the opposite direction.

Breathing: Inhale while moving the head up and exhale while bring it down.

Precautions:

- If you start feeling giddy, stop immediately and open your eyes and relax.
- If you have any kind of pain in your neck or if you have any problem, consult a yoga guru.

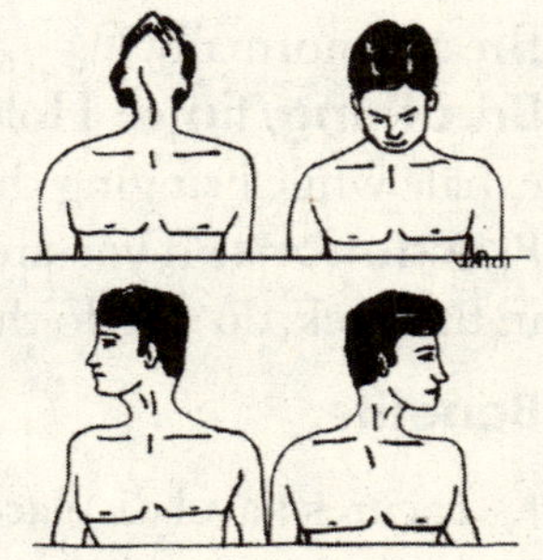

Exercise 17 e. Continue to sit in same position. Now, slowly bend your neck down. Hold the position for a while, then raise your head and slowly take it backwards. Hold the position for some time then, slowly straighten up. Again, hold the position for some time then, slowly turn it to the right. Hold the position for some time then, bring your head back to the original position. Hold it for some time and then, turn it to the left. Bring your head back in front after holding the position for some time. This is one round. Repeat this 5 times.

Note: The time taken to bend or move the head in one direction should be the same for all directions. To know more, read about Bramha Mudra later in the book.
Breathing: Inhale while moving your head up and exhale while bringing it down. Exhale while turning your head to the sides and inhale while bringing it in front.
Benefits: It is very beneficial for students, people working in the office and those who work long hours with their heads bent. It is also beneficial in curing all the disorders related to the neck.

Udar Pradesh Anga Kriyas
(Exercises for the Abdominal Area)

Uttanpadasana* (Raised leg pose)

Note: This asana is dedicated to Dhruv's father Uttanpada.
Exercise 1 a: Lie down on your back. Keep your hands beside your waist. Keep your palms firm on the ground. Inhale and exerting a slight pressure with the palms, raise both your leg up to an angle of 60 degrees. Keep the legs close together and point outwards with the feet. Hold this position for 1-2 minutes and then, slowly come back to the original position. Breathe normally.

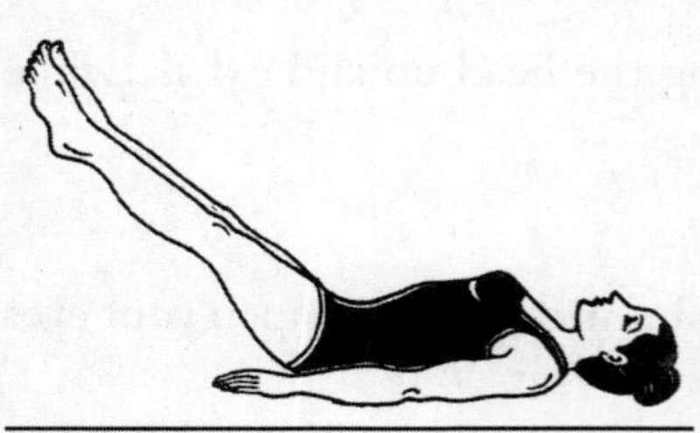

Breathing/time: Hold your breath while raising your legs and exhale while bringing them down. Repeat this 3-5 times.
Precautions: If you are suffering from severe pain in the spine or in the back, do not do this exercise.

Benefits:

- It cures navel displacement.
- Reduces fat around the abdomen.
- Definite cure for constipation.
- Strengthens the muscles of the back, waist and abdomen.
- Gives relief from disorders of the wind.

Gatimaya Uttanpadasana (Dynamic raised leg pose)

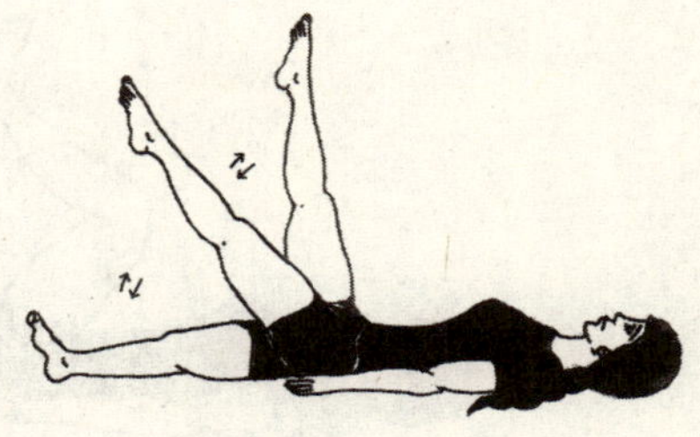

Exercise 1 b. Lie down on your back. Keep your hands on the sides. Inhale and raise your left leg to form a right angle with the body. Hold the position for some time and come back to the original position while exhaling. Do this 5-6 times. Repeat this kriya with the other leg. Then, do this with both the legs.

Benefits: Strengthens the abdominal region, digestive system, spinal cord, and the muscles of the lower back. It makes them supple and flexible.

Padvrittasana (Making a circle with the legs)

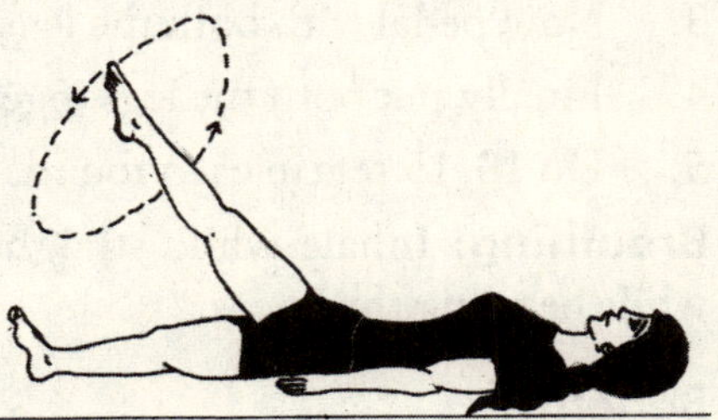

Exercise 2. Method: Lie down in Shavasana. First, raise your right leg and move it in circular motion from right to left. Repeat this 10-15 times. Then, move it from left to right. Do the same with the left leg. Then, do this exercise with both the legs together.

Breathing: Breathe normally while doing this exercise.

Benefits:

- It gives relief from lower-back pain.
- Buttocks become strong and shapely.
- Leg muscles benefit from this exercise.
- It is the best asan to get rid of obesity.

Note: You can keep both your hands under the hips in the beginning. When you feel tired, stop and relax.

Pad Sanchalan Kriya/Dvichakrika Asana (Cycling)

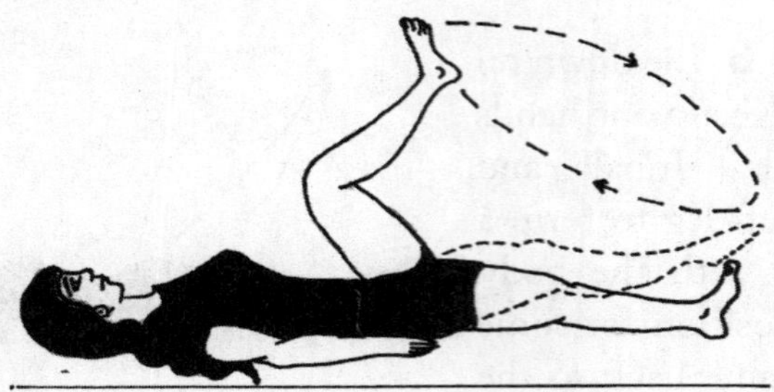

Exercise 3 a. Method: Lie down in Shavasana and imagine that you are cycling.

1. Raise one leg and move it forward and backward, up and down as you do while cycling. Do forward pedaling 10-15 times and then do pedaling in the opposite direction.
2. Do this exercise with the other leg.
3. Now, pedal with both the legs.
4. Finally, put both the legs together and pedal.
5. Do 10-15 sets in each round.

Breathing: Inhale while straightening up the legs and exhale while bending the knees.

Benefits:

- Benefits seen in the abdominal region.
- Its good for ankles, calves, knees, thighs, buttocks and waist.
- Opens up the joints and tones up the muscles.
- Relieves gas from the stomach.
- It is helpful in reducing obesity.

Note:

- Relax when you feel tired
- Do as per your convenience
- Take your legs back as far as possible
- You can also move your hands in similar fashion, along with your legs

Supt Pada Sanchalan Kriya (Reclined cycling position)

Exercise 3 b. Method: Lie down on our back. Keep your hands on your sides. Bend your left leg from the knee and try to touch your stomach with your thigh. Then, stretch and move your feet (two feet above the ground and then, place them down. Do this 5-10 times first with the left leg and then with the right leg. Now, do this kriya in reverse. First raise your left leg two feet above the ground, then bend your knee and your stomach with your thigh. Straighten your leg and bring it back to the ground. Do this with the right leg too.

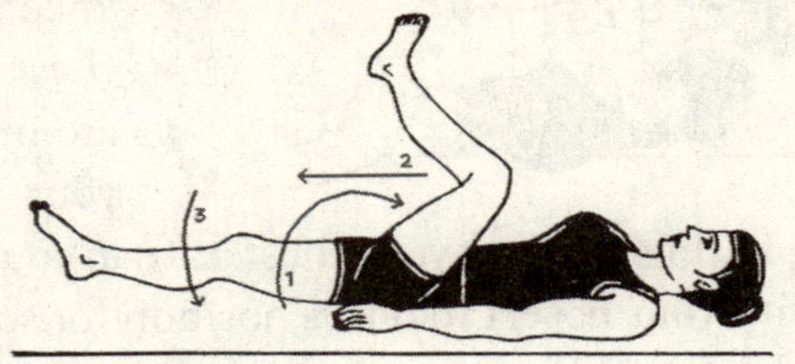

Finally, do this exercise with both the legs together. First, bend both the knees and bring the thighs close to the stomach. Straighten and move your feet two feet above the ground, then place them down. Do this kriya 5-10 times. Then, do it in reverse. Lift both your legs two feet above the ground, and then, bend them from the knees and bring them close to your stomach. Straighten your legs and bring them back on the ground.

Breathing/Time: Inhale while straightening your legs and exhale while bending your knees. Do all these exercises 5-10 times.

Benefits:

- Reduces the fat around the abdomen.
- Strengthens the digestive system and cures constipation.
- ures navel displacement.
- Increases blood circulation in knees, thighs and calves and strengthens them.
- Cures trembling of legs.

Variation: When this exercise is done in sitting position, it is called Uttan Janu Sanchalan kriya.

Supt Pavanmuktasana (Reclined air releaving pose)

Exercise 4 a. Variation 1: Lie down in Shavasana position. Bend your right leg from your knee and bring it close to your chest. Then, wrap your hands around the knee and interlock your fingers. Exhale and press your thigh against your chest. Lift up your head and touch your knee with your nose. Hold this position for some time. Inhale and come back to the Shavasan position. Be cautious of your breathing while doing this asana. Do this kriya 3-5 times. Repeat with the other leg.

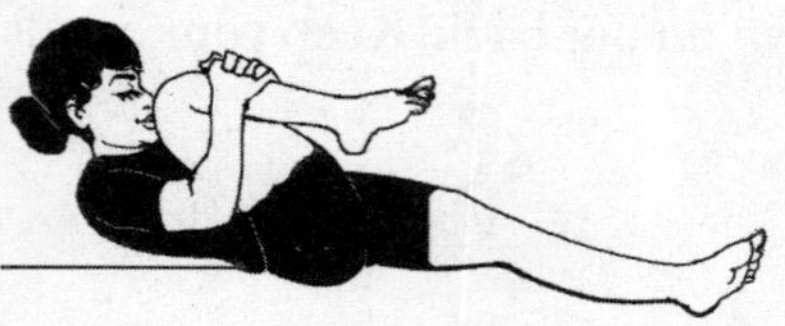

Supt Pavanmuktasana (Reclined air releaving pose)

Exercise 4 b. Variation 2: Lie down in Shavasana. Bend both your legs from the knees and bring your thighs close to the chest. Then, wrap your arms around your knees. Exhale and while pressing your knees with your arms, try to bring the thighs close to the chest. Lift your head and touch your knees with your nose. Hold this position for some time. Then, come back to Shavasana position. Do this exercise 8-10 times. This is also called Poorna Pavanmuktasana.

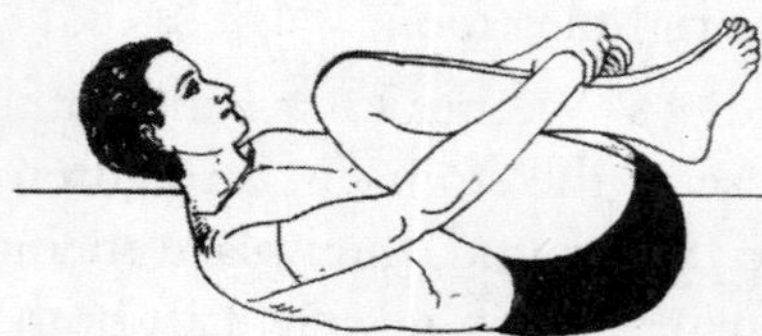

Poorna Pavanmuktasana Mein Ludhakna (Rolling in air releaving pose)

Exercise 5 a. Variation 3: You have to roll your body while being in Poorna Pavanmuktasana posture. First, roll to your left. You must try to touch your left ear, shoulder, knees and all the parts on the left side of your body to the ground. Then, roll in a similar manner to your right. Come back to the original position. This is one round. Do 10-15 such rounds.

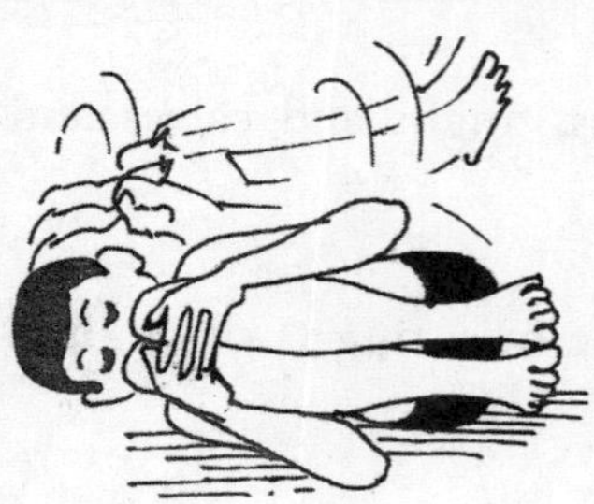

Gatimaya Pavanmuktasana (Momentum in air releasing pose)

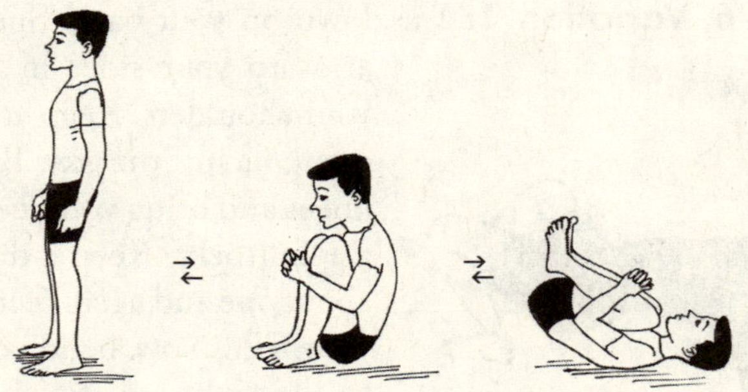

Exercise 5 b. Variation 4: To do Gatimaya Pavanmuktasana, first come to Poorna Pavanmuktasana position. Then, sit in the crow posture and then, release your hands and stand up (you can also raise your hands up). Come back to the crow posture and then, come the Pavanmuktasana posture. This is one round. Do this 5-10 times.

Precautions: Since there is a lot of stress on the spine during this entire exercise, you should be very cautious while doing it. Keep a blanket (folded into thick layers) under your back.

Breathing: Breathe normally.

Benefits:

- Pavanmuktasana is especially beneficial for people suffering from constipation. This asana is very beneficial in cases with problem in excretion, head aches due to disorders of the abdomen, excessive heat in the brain due to the upward movement of the gases, anxiety, etc.
- It expels the gases from the body; the body feels very light.
- It strengthens the spinal cord.
- It cures the disorders related to the heart. People with respiratory problems can also benefit from it.
- It enhances the glow and aura of the face.
- Stops the premature falling of hair.
- It is helpful in making the body slim.

Markatasana/Supt Udarakarshanasana (Monkey pose)

Exerise 6. Variation 1: Lie down on your back. Spread your arms to your sides in line with your shoulders. Keep your palms open, facing the sky. Bend your knees and bring your feet close to the buttocks. Keep a distance of about one and a half feet between your feet. Now, bend your knees to the right and touch them to the ground. In this position, the right knee will touch the ground and the left knee will touch the ground near the right foot. Turn your head to your left. Do this exercise on the left side too.

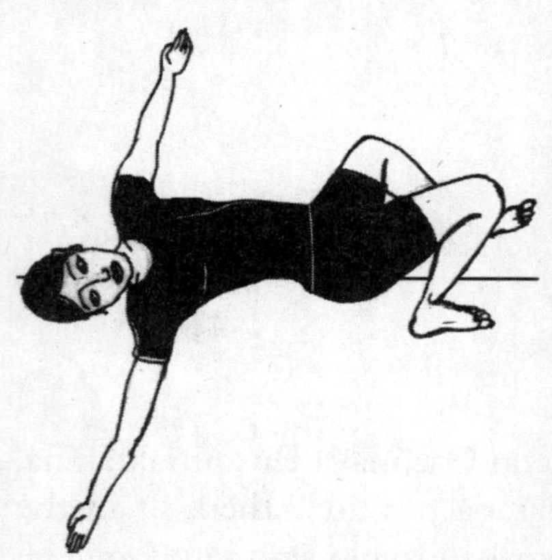

Exercise 6. Variation 2: Lie down on your back. The position of the hands will remain the same. Fold both the legs and bring them close to your buttocks. Keep the knees together. Now, bend your knees to the right and touch the ground. Your left knee should be placed on your right knee and the left foot on the right foot. Turn your head to your left. To complete this exercise, do it by bending the knees to the left and turning your head to the right.

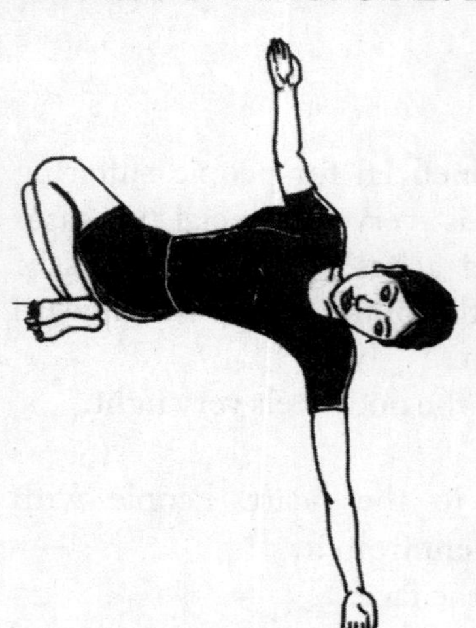

Exercise 6. Variation 3: Lie down on your back. Spread your arms to your sides in line with the shoulders. Now, lift up your right leg from your buttocks, making a right angle. Then, it on the ground on the left and hold the big toe with your left hand. Turn your head towards your right. Now do the same exercise in the opposite direction.

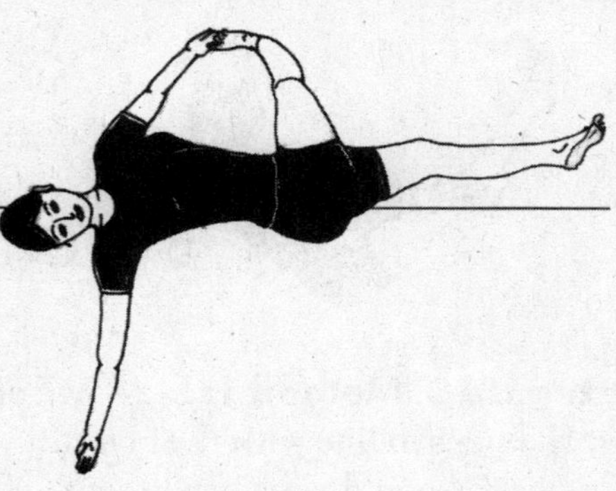

Benefits:

- It gives quick relief to people suffering from slip disc, back ache, sciatica and cervical spondilitis.
- It softens the stomach which means that it helps cure constipation and problem of gas.
- The spine and buttocks benefit from this exercise.

Note: Some yoga teachers call this asana **Kati Mardanasana.**

Yogabhyasa is not mere exercising, but a practical approach to providing physical and mental well-being and creating opportunities for the body and mind to work in harmony for newer manifestations.

–RJT

Naukasana (Boat pose)

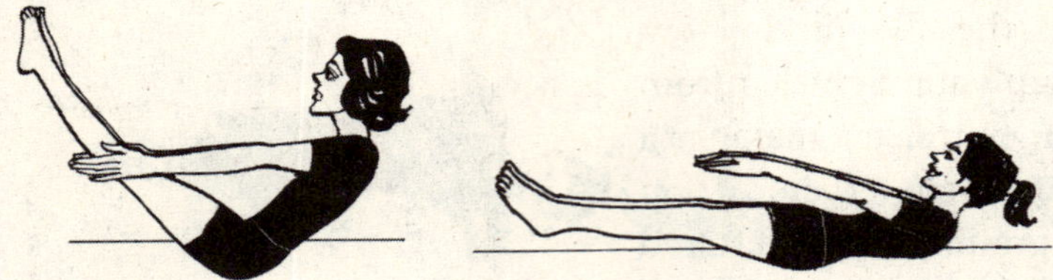

Exercise 8. Method 1: Lie down on your back. Keep your hands by the sides in line with the body. Inhale and slowly raise your legs, hands, torso and your head together. Remember the legs and the head should be almost at the same height. Hold this position for as long as you comfortably can. This is called Poorna Naukasan. Repeat this 5-6 times.

Method 2: In the second variation, keep your arms straight and raise your legs, shoulders, hands and head about one foot above the ground. This is called Ardha Naukasan.

Focus: On Svadhishthana, Manipura and Anahata Chakras.

Breathing: First, inhale and do Antah kumbhaka while rising up and holding the posture. Then exhale.

Benefits:

- The back becomes very strong by doing this exercise.
- It has a good impact on your intestines.
- Ardha Naukasan builds up the spleen, liver and bile duct.
- The spine becomes strong and firm.
- It kills worms in the stomach.
- The legs gain strength; the feet do not tremble in old age.
- It corrects navel displacement.
- By doing this exercise regularly, women can benefit in their gynae problems related to uterus, ovaries, post childbirth problems such as expanded uterus, womb and protruding abdomen.

Note: Some yoga teachers call the first method **Mukta Hasta Merudandasana.**

Kriyas of the Shakti Bandha
(Strengthening Exercises)

Pulling the Rope

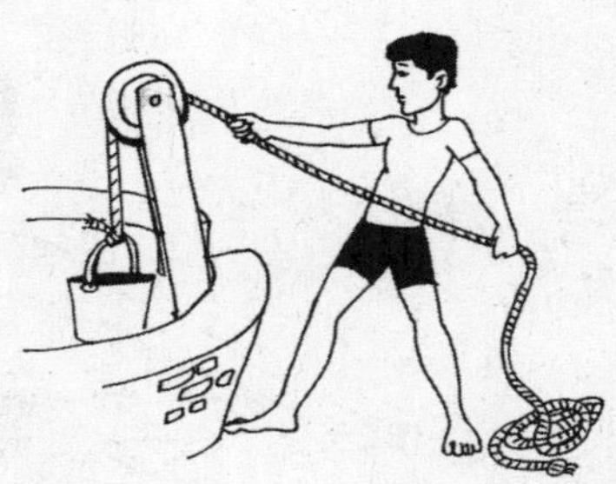

Exercise 1 a. The process of pulling the rope can be done in three ways. Imagine that you are drawing water from a well. Our actions should be exactly how people draw water from a well one foot ahead of the other, pulling the bucket out of the well first with one hand and then with another. First, do this exercise with one foot forward, and then do it with the other foot forward. Take your hands forward and backward as much as possible. Repeat this exercise 10-20 times.

Exercise 1 b. Do the same exercise in sitting position. Sit with your legs stretched in front and do the above mentioned exercise.

Churning the Curd

Exercise 1 c. Sit with your legs spread out in front and imagine that you are holding one end of two ropes with both your hands. Pull both the ropes with alternate hands one after another. Imagining another practitioner front of you, pulling the ropes towards themselves. Do this process 15-20 times. Take your hands as back as possible. This process is like churning curd.

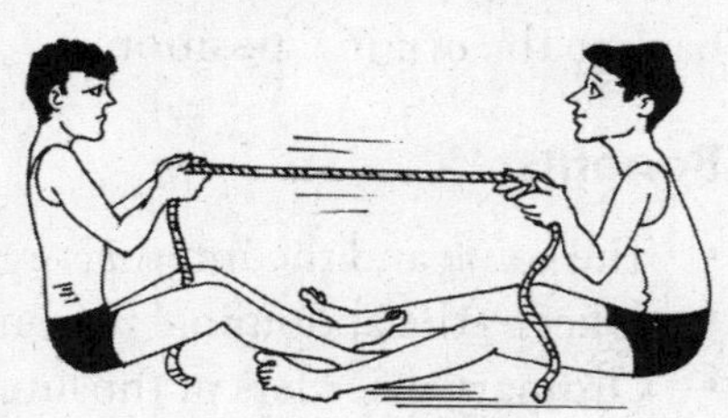

Breathing: Inhale while bringing your hands in front and exhale while taking them back.

Benefits:

- Fingers, elbows, arms and shoulders get a good exercise. They become strong and flexible. It develops breasts in women.
- Spine becomes flexible.

Gatimaya Meru Vakrasana (Dynamic spinal twist pose)

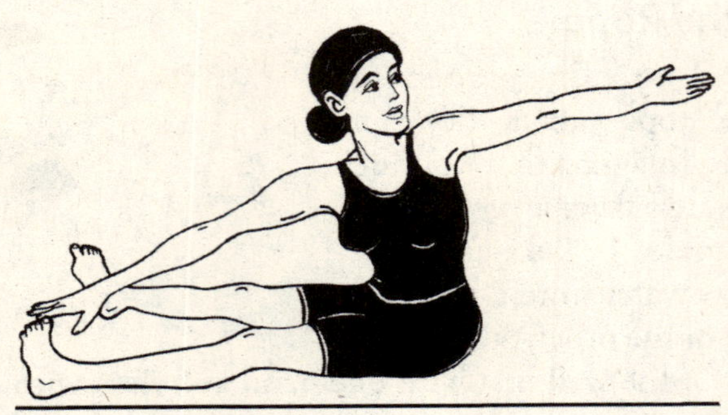

Exercise 2. Method: Sit on your mat with your legs wide apart. Bring the right hand to the left big toe. If possible, try to touch the toe with your hand. Now, bend your body above the waist to your left and take your left hand to the back. Turn and try to see your left hand. In this way, both the hands will be in one line. Similarly, do this on the other side too. This is one round. Repeat it 10-20 times. Once you get accustomed to it, you can increase your speed.

Breathing: Inhale when you turn and exhale when you come back to the original position.

Benefits:

- The spine and the internal organs of the back get massaged.
- It keeps the abdominal region disease free.
- Ordinary disorders of the lungs are cured.
- It is helpful in reducing the fat around the abdomen.

Chakki Chalana (Grinding the mill)

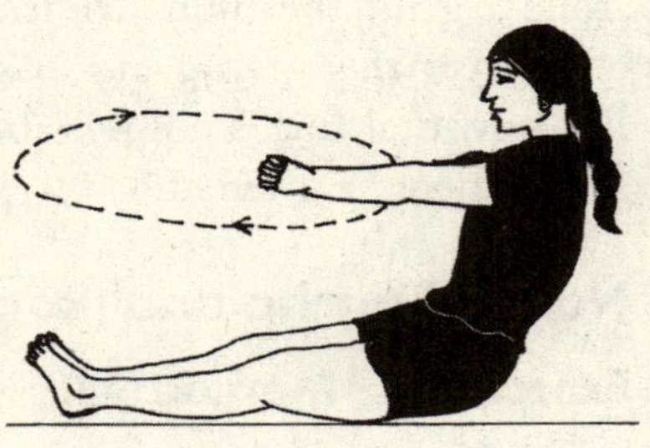

Exercise 3 a. Sit with your legs stretched in front. Stretch your arms in front and interlock your fingers. Imagine that you are grinding with a stone grinding mill. Move the upper part of your body from the waist in a circular motion. Bend forward and backward as much as you can. Then, do the same in the opposite direction – first move from right to left, and then from left to right. Repeat this exercise 10-15 times.

Breathing: Inhale while going back and exhale while bending in front.

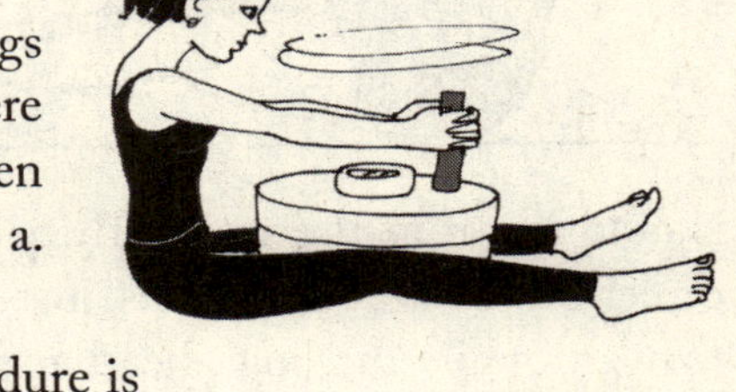

Exercise 3 b. Sit with your legs spread apart. Imagine that there is a grinding mill placed between your legs. Now, repeat exercise 3 a.

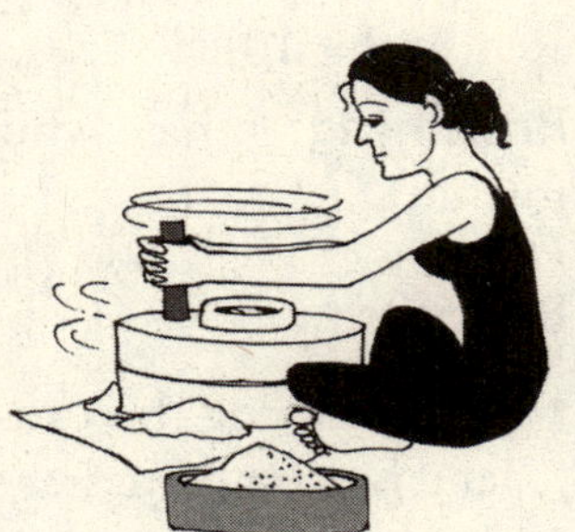

Exercise 3 c. The third procedure is also the same. But in this one you have to sit in Sukhasana and imagine that the grinding mill in kept in front of you and you are moving the mill. First, move from right to left and then from left to right. Repeat this 10-15 times.

Benefits:

- This is beneficial for people of all age groups. It massages all the internal parts of the abdomen.
- It is beneficial for those who have problem in passing motion.
- It gives relief from back ache.
- It helps get rid of menstrual problems.
- It helps reduce obesity.

Note: In the olden days, every house hold used to have a grinding stone to grind the grains. Men and women used to grind wheat and other everyday grains and unknowingly benefitted this exercise. But now that this is not possible, we can only do this exercise and get the benefits thereof.

Nauka Sanchalana (Rowing of a boat)

Exercise 4. Method: Sit in sukhasan. Stretch your legs in front. Image that you are rowing a boat. You have to do the actions accordingly. Bend forward and backward as much as you can. Keep your hands bent from the elbow and close to the waist. The maximum movement should be from the waist. Then, do the process in the opposite direction. Move your arms just as a boatman moves the oars forward while moving ahead and backward while moving back. Repeat this 10-15 times.

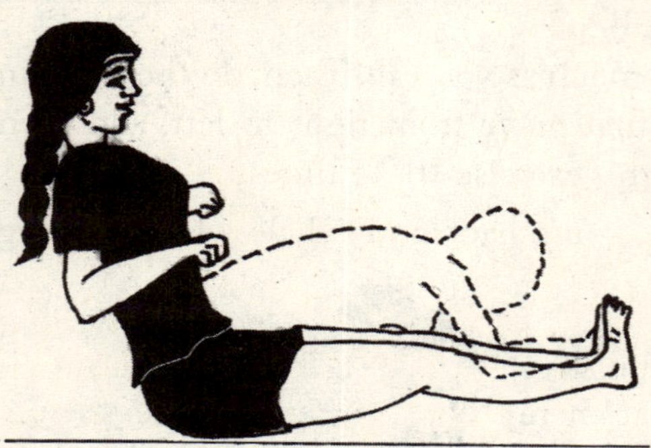

Breathing: Inhale while going back and exhale while bending forward.

Benefits:

- By practising this exercise, the waist, spine, legs, back, shoulder and hands get massaged and receive all the benefits.
- It removes the excessive fat from the body and makes it slim.
- The abdominal area benefit from it.

Mushtika Praghat Kriya (Chopping wood)

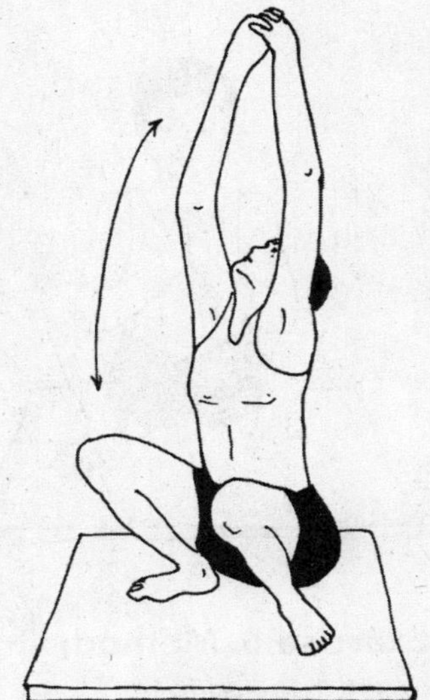

Exercise 5. Method: Sit on your haunches. Keep a distance of about 2 feet between your knees. Interlock your fingers and raise them straight up. Then, bring them down as if to hit something kept on the ground. In this process, try to take your hands back up as much as possible and try to look up at your hands.

Breathing: Inhale while taking your hands up and exhale while bringing them down. Repeat it for 5-10 rounds.

Benefits:

- It is especially beneficial for the uterus.
- The lungs gain stability and the shoulder joints also benefit from it.
- Women get greater benefit as it develops their breasts.
- The organs of the reproductory system benefit from it.

Note: Some yoga teachers call this **Kashtha Takshanasana.**

Supt Namaskaram (Sitting salutation)

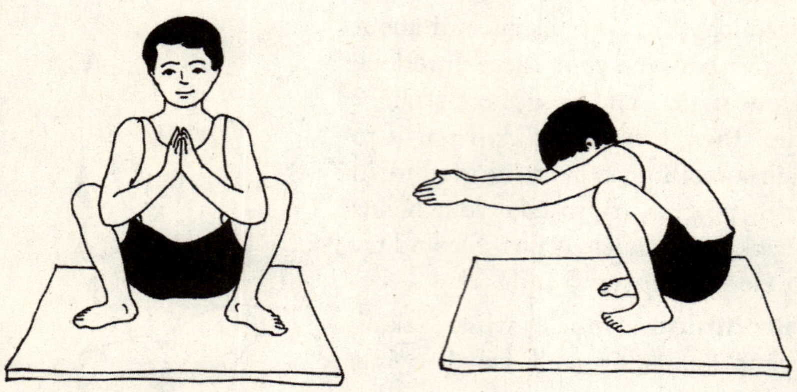

Exercise 6. Method: Sit on your haunches. Keep your feet wide apart. Join your hands in Namaskar Mudra and stretch them in front. Keeping both your hands between your knees, exert pressure on the hands with your knees. Inhale. Look up and bring your arms in a prayer posture, close to your chest. Exert pressure on your knees outwards with your hands. Exhale and come back to the original position. Repeat this 5-10 times.

Benefits:

- All the muscles of the legs benefit from it.
- One gets relief from ordinary pain in the shoulders and the back.
- It also beneficial for the entire pelvic region.

Vayu Nishkasana Kriya (Relieving gases from the body)

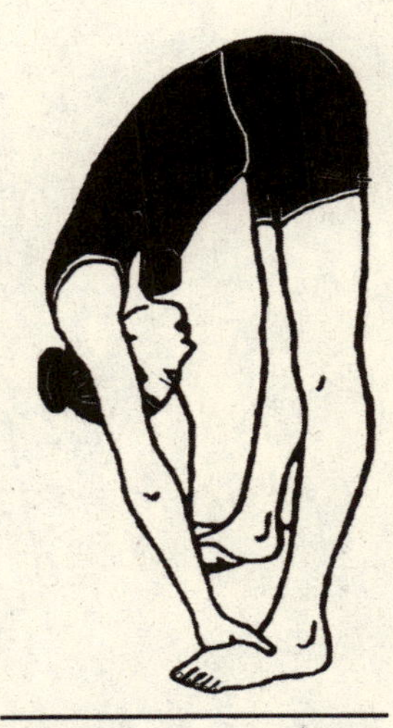

Exercise 7. Method: Sit on your haunches with some distance in between your feet. Keep your fingers under your feet. If you want, you can hold your feet with your fingers. Apply pressure on your elbows with your knees, inhale and look in front. Exhale, straighten up your knees and stand up with your buttocks out. Your head should be bent. Look at your knees and keep holding on to your feet. Keep your eyes open during this exercise. Bend your spine as much as possible. Hold your breath and remain in this posture for as long as you can comfortably hold this position. Inhale and come back to the original position. This is one round. Repeat for 5-10 such rounds.

Precautions: If you are suffering from high blood pressure, giddiness or stiff spine, then do this exercise very carefully.

Benefits:

- As the name suggests, it helps relieve the gases from the body.
- It gives relief to all the problems related to wind and helps keep the mind happy.
- It is beneficial for the entire shoulder area, ankle joints, knees and elbows and helps get rid of the air trapped in them thereby giving relief from the pain.
- It massages the calves, thighs, spine and the back and regulates blood circulation.

Variation: This exercise can be done by keeping the fingers under the feet in front as in Pad Hastasana.

Kauva Chalan Kriya (Walking crow)

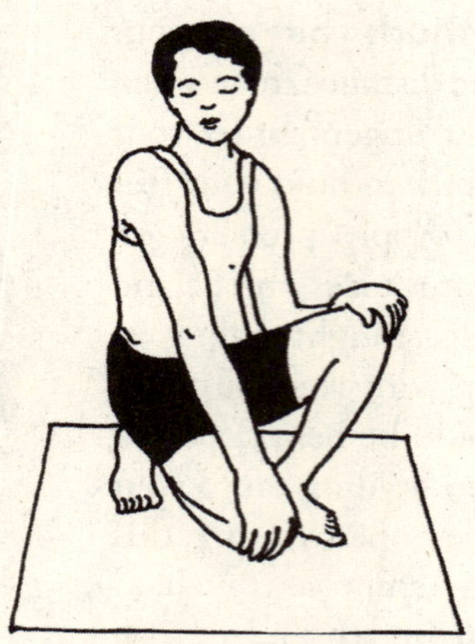

Exercise 8. Sit on the ground on your haunches. Place your palms on your knees and start moving forward by applying pressure on the interior part of the toes. When you move your left foot forward, your right knee should touch the ground and when you move your right foot forward, your left knee should touch the ground. Make at least 15-20 moves then come back to your place. Breathe normally.

Benefits:

- It increases the blood circulation in the legs and keep them healthy and disease free. It makes the muscles of the legs strong.
- It is also effective in curing disorders of the abdomen and waist.
- Those suffering from chronic constipation can do this exercise after drinking a glass of water.

Udarakarshanasana (Abdominal stretch pose)

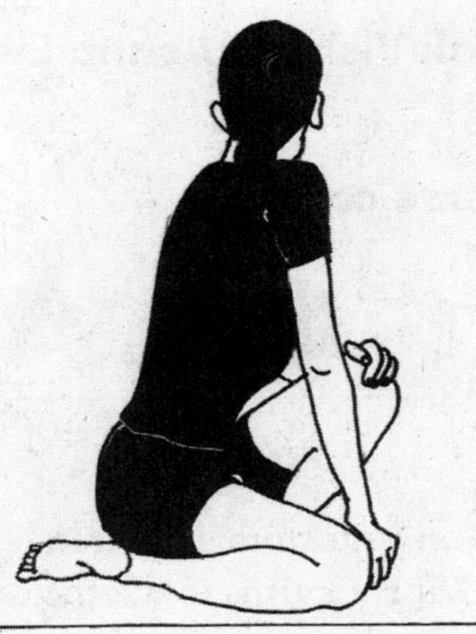

Exercise 9. Meaning: Udara means stomach and akarshana means to pull or stretch.

Method: This asana is used in the Shankh Prakshalana kriya. Sit on your haunches. Put all your body weight on your feet. Place both your palms on your knees. In this position, turn your torso to the right and try to look at the back. Bend your left knee to touch the ground. Exert pressure on your stomach with your right thigh. Hold for a moment then come back to the original position. Repeat the same process on the left side too. This is one round. Do this 8-10 times.

Breathing/time: Take a deep breath in the original position and then turn. Do Antahkumbhak for about 5 seconds then, exhale while coming back to the original position.

Benefits:

- It affects the entire abdominal region and cures the disorders.
- The digestive system gets a thorough internal massage, so it works efficiently.

Specific Exercises and Processes That Provide Energy

(Oorja Pradayak Vishesh Asana Evam Kriyayen)

Advasana (Reverse corpse)

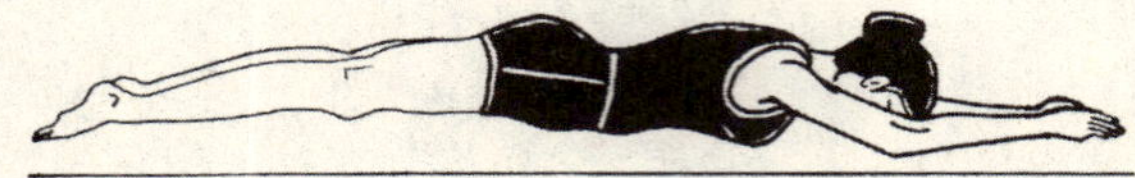

Method: Lie down on your stomach. Stretch both your hands in front in such a way that your arms touch the ears. Your palms and the back of your feet should also touch the ground. Similarly, your nose and forehead should also touch the ground. Relax your body in this position. Keep your breathing normal.

Gatimaya Advasan (Dynamic reverse corpse)

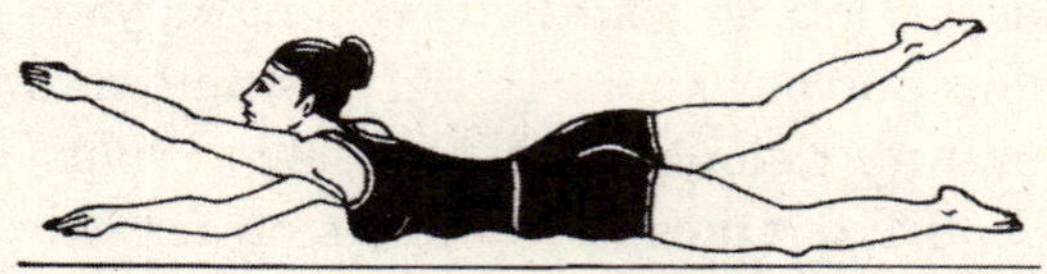

Variation 1. Lie down on your stomach. Stretch both your hands in front in such a way that your arms touch the ears. Raise your right arm and left leg up, simultaneously, as much as possible. Raise your head too. Remain in this position for some time then come back to the original position. Similarly raise the left arm and right leg. Come back to the original position. This is one round. Do about 10 rounds.

2. In the second variation, try to raise both the arms, both the legs and head simultaneously. Then come back to the original position. Repeat this process about 5-10 times.

Breathing/time: Breathe in while raising your body up and breathe out while coming back to the original position.

Benefits:

- It is very beneficial for the diseases related to the spine.
- It helps get rid of back ache, body ache and tension.
- It is ideal for relaxation.
- It gives freshness.

Gatimaya Gomukhasana (Dynamic cow face pose)

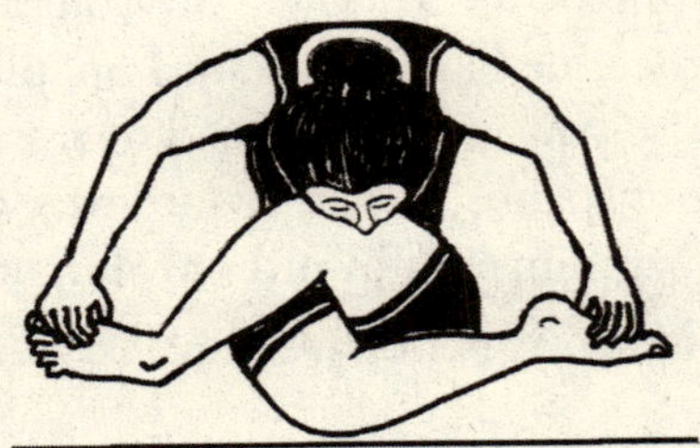

Method: Sit with your legs stretched in front. Bend your left leg from the knee and place it near the right buttock. Similarly bend your right leg from the knee and place it near the left buttock. In this way, the right knee will be on the left knee. Now hold the big toe of the left foot with your right hand and the big toe of the right foot with your left hand. This is the initial position of this asana. Then, exhale and slowly bend forward and try to touch your forehead to the ground. Remain in this position for some time. Inhale and rise up. This is one round. Do 5-10 such rounds.

Variation: You can do this exercise by bending towards your left and right foot.

Benefits:

- It is effective in curing back ache and the ordinary disorders of the spine.
- Due to the stretching of the back muscles, they receive sufficient blood circulation. The disorders of the back can be avoided.
- Makes the buttocks more flexible.
- Reduces the wrinkles of the face and gives freshness.
- Helps in curing the disorders caused by wind.

Makarasana (Crocodile pose)

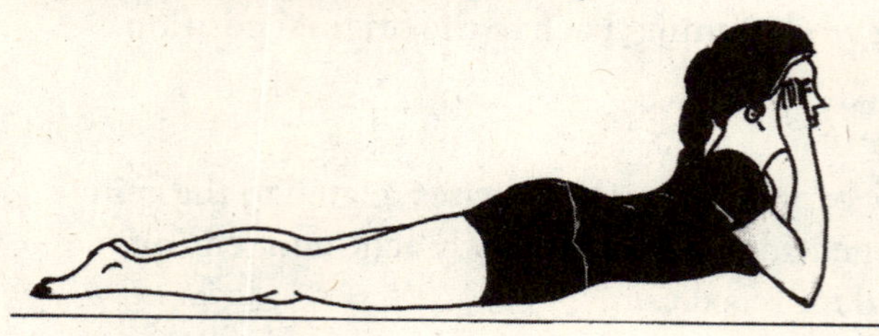

Meaning: This asana is called Makarasana because it resembles the posture of a crocodile formed.

Method: Lie down on your stomach. Since the head of the crocodile is always raised up, place your elbows on the floor and raise your neck and head to rest your cheeks and chin in between your palms. Close your eyes and try to relax completely by imagining an upward movement of the energy. Breathe normally.

Time: As per convenience.

Gatimaya Makarasana (Dynamic crocodile pose)

Note: In order to gain more benefit from Makarasana, we can add movements in the asana.

Variation 1. First come to the original posture of Makarasana. Then, slowly turn your head to your left and try to see your left heel and toe. Hold the posture for some time then come back to the original position. Now, do the same on the right-hand side. Come back to the original position. This is one round. Do 10 such rounds. Breathe normally.

Variation 2. First come to the original posture of Makarasana. Then, remaining in the same posture, slowly move your elbows forward. As the elbows move forward, the lower part of the neck will experience a slight strain. Hold the position for as long as you comfortably can. Bring your elbows close to your chest and come back to the original position. This is one round. Do 5-10 such rounds.

Variation 3. Remain in the Makarasana posture. First, bend one leg from the knees and place it on your buttocks. The other leg will remain firmly on the ground. Then, bring the first leg back on the ground and bend the other leg from the knee and place it on your buttocks. Do this repeatedly. You can do this exercise by increasing the speed. Also known as Supt Balasasana (Reclined child pose) by some yoga masters.

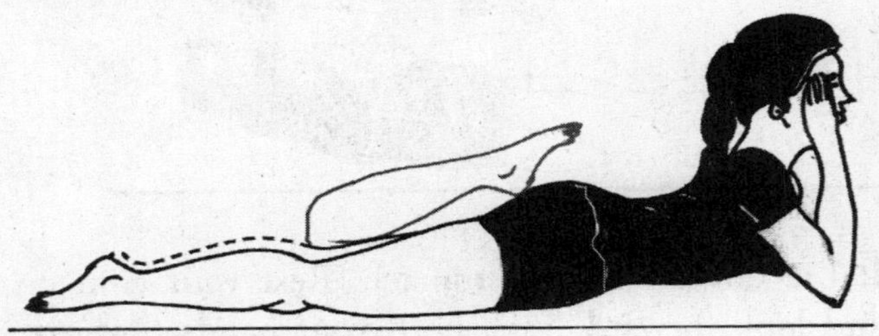

Variation 4. The same process can be done by bending both the legs together. Repeat for at least 10 times.

Variation 5. Lie down on your stomach. Spread your legs and maintain some distance. Fold both your arms and keep them under your head in such a way that right arm is on the left arm. Also, they must touch your ear. Change the position of your head after 10-20 seconds. (Close your eyes. This is also known as Makrasana/ Crocodile pose)

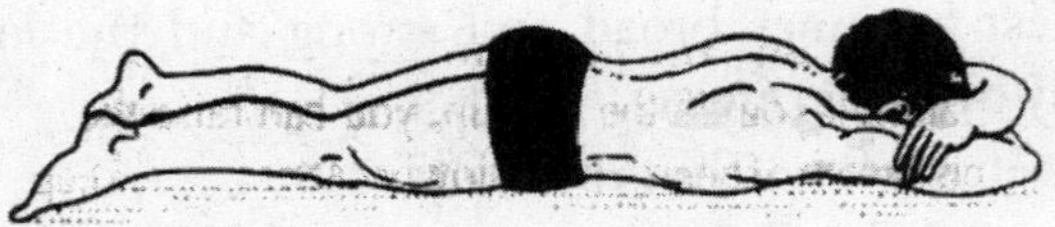

Benefits:

- It is highly beneficial for cervical problems, slip disc and spondylitis.
- It is also beneficial for the ordinary diseases of the neck.
- It provides a lot of freshness and swiftness.
- People suffering from asthma/lung diseases also benefit.
- You must do this asan after doing Sarvangasana, Halasana and Viparitkarni Mudra.

Sarpasana (Snake pose)

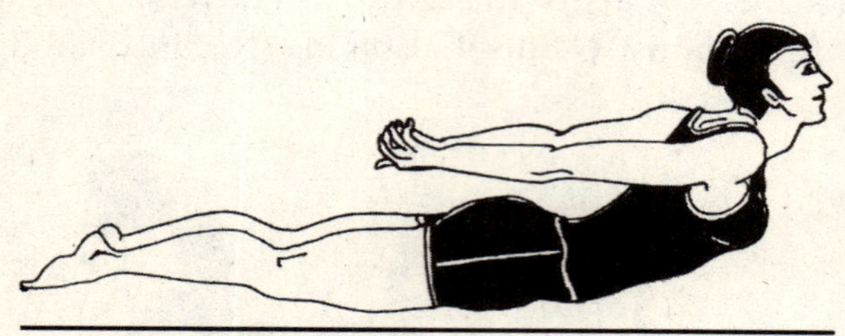

Method: Lie down on your stomach. Rest your chin on the ground and look forward. Take both your hands towards your back and interlock your fingers. Inhale slowly. Hold your breath and lift your body above the ground from your chest. Stretch your arms and try to raise them up as much as possible. You should get the feeling that someone is pulling your hands from the back.

Breathing/time: Hold the position according to your convenience and exhale while coming back to the original position. Do 5 such rounds.

Benefits:

- The chest becomes broad and strong and the lungs expand properly by this exercise.
- It is beneficial for asthma patients.
- The parts of the abdomen are massaged. Hence all the parts become disease free. Constipation is cured.

Precaution: Patients of high blood pressure and heart patients should not do this exercise with too much pressure.

Ardha Shalabhasana (Half locust pose)

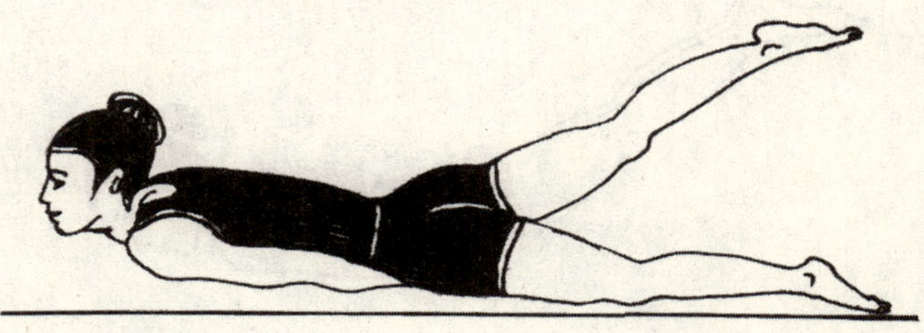

Method: Lie down on your stomach. Keep your hands under the thighs. Stretch your legs backward and pull your chin forward. Now, raise your left leg as high as possible. Keep your right leg relaxed. Hold as per convenience then, bring your leg down. Repeat with the right leg. Do 5-10 rounds.

Breathing: Raise your leg when you inhale. Hold your breath. Exhale when you bring your leg down.

Benefits:

- Cures constipation.
- All parts of the abdomen benefit from it.
- Those suffering from sciatica and slip disc can benefit from it.
- It is beneficial for back ache and pain in the waist.

Gatimaya Ardha Shalabhasana (Dynamic half locust pose)

Once you practice this asana well, you can increase the speed of your legs moving up and down. When your right leg goes up, the left leg comes down. Moving your legs in this way, bring about the speed in your legs.

Shalabhasana (Locust pose)

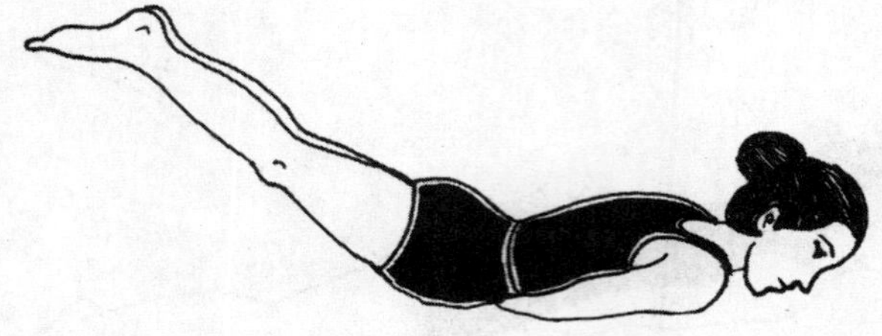

Method: Lie down on stomach. Make a half fist with your palms and place them under your thighs. Stretch your chin a little further and fix it on the ground. Relax your body, but be absolutely alert and aware.

Then, stretch both your legs, inhale and raise them together. Hold this position for as long as you can, then exhale and bring them down. Relax your body. Repeat this 5 times.

Focus: On the Vishuddhi chakra.

Precautions: Heart patients, people suffering from high blood pressure and hernia should do this asana with a lot of patience.

Those who are not suffering from the above mentioned ailments can do this asana in continuous movement. Since both the legs have to be raised together with balance, should be practised with absolute alertness.

Benefits:

- If this is practised regularly, one does not suffer from TB.
- It activates the clone glands, so it is beneficial for diabetic patients.
- It keeps the abdominal area disease free. Sciatica patients must do this asana.
- It keeps the liver and stomach active and functional.
- Slip disc patients soon get rid of the disease.

Note: Some yoga teacher call this **Ardha Shalabhasana**.

Vipareeta Naukasana (Reverse boat posture)

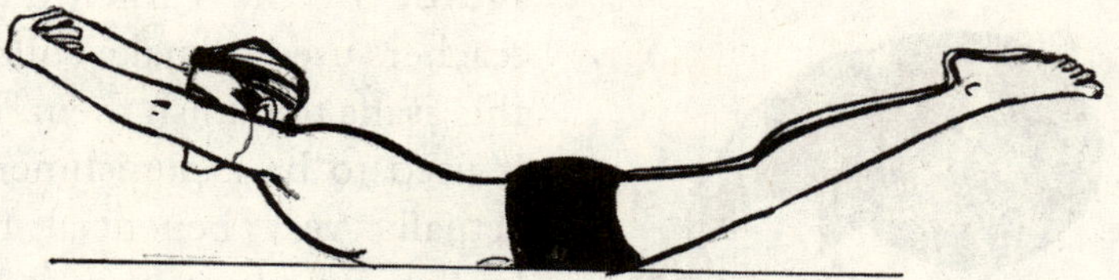

Meaning: Vipareeta means inverted.

Method: Lie down on your stomach. Bring your hands forward in such a way that they press your ears from the sides. Form a namaskar mudra. You can even interlock your fingers. Now, applying a little pressure, lift up your torso, head and legs. Breathe normally. Hold the position for as long as you comfortably can, then come back to the original position. Repeat this at least 5 times.

Focus: On the Vishuddhi chakra.

Benefits:

- It relaxes the entire body.
- Increases the heat in the body.
- It is very beneficial for the spine and the waist.
- It stretches the muscles of the legs and regularises the blood circulation.

Note: This is a variation of **Shalabhasana.**

If you are healthy and disease free, do yoga exercise
to always remain disease free, and if you are
suffering from any disease, you must do yogabhyasa
to get rid of the disease and become healthy
and beautiful.

–RJT

Murga Asanatmaka Kriya (Cock pose)

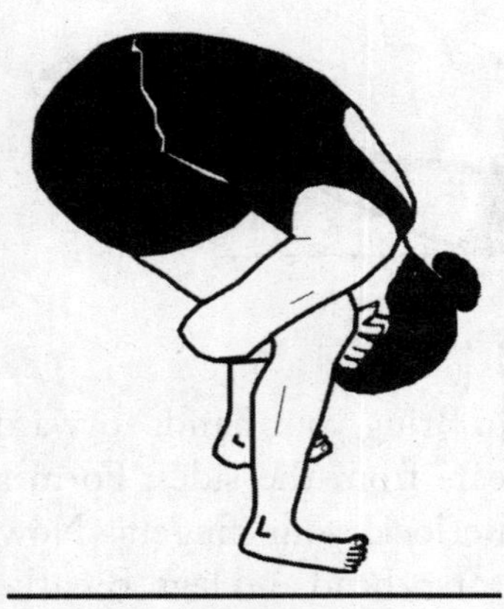

Note: In the earlier days, the teachers used to make children do this asana to punish them. Though it used to be a punishment, it is actually very beneficial for our bodies in many ways.

Method: Stand with your legs a little apart. Bend down, bend your knees a little and bring your hands from in between your legs to hold your ears. While doing this, slowly raise your hips up and bring your head down. Remain in this position for 5-10 seconds then come back to the original position. Repeat it 5-10 times.

Breathing: Exhale while bending forward and inhale while coming back to the original position.

Benefits:

- It is very good for expelling the wind.
- Since it increases the blood circulation in the face, the glow of the face is enhanced and wrinkles disappear.
- It enhances the memory.
- It is beneficial for the eyes. If this kriya is practised regularly, it helps in relieving migraine pain.
- It streaches the muscles of hips, thighs, back and spine. Hence, blood circulation improves and disorders are cured.

Precaution: Heart patients, patients of chronic back ache, high blood pessure and pregnant women should not do this exercise.

Trilokasana (Star pose)

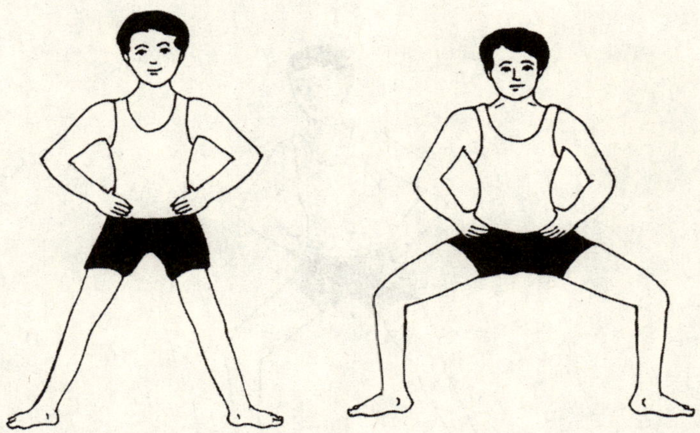

Meaning: Triloka means three worlds.

Method: Stand with your legs about three feet apart. Place your hands on your waist so that the thumbs are on the back and the four fingers are on your stomach. Your spine, neck and head should be in one line. Look in front, hold your breath and slowly try to sit down on the ground. Stay in this position for some time then come back to the original position. Try to come as close to the ground as possible with regular practice.

Breathing/time: Exhale while trying to sit and inhale while coming up. Repeat 4-5 times.

Note: Keep your feet pointed to the sides. In this position, with your hands on the waist, the elbows come in line with your feet.

Benefits:

- The calves and thighs are strengthened.
- Trembling in the feet is cured.
- Wind is relieved from the body.
- When this kriya is done regularly, excess fat from the thighs is removed. Helps in shaping thighs.
- The abdominal area benefits from it.

Gatimaya Trilokasana (Dynamic star pose)

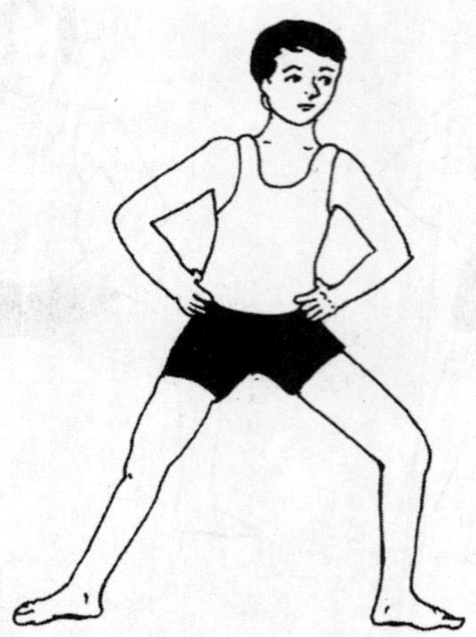

Method: Stand in the original position of Trilokasana. First, shift all your weight on the left thigh and slowly bend the left knee. Try to sit down by pressing the left foot on the ground. Keep the right leg straight. In this way, your left leg will be bent and the right leg will be stretched. Now, slowly exert pressure on your left leg and straighten up. Repeat with the right leg.

Breathing/time: Exhale while sitting down. Inhale while coming up. Do it 5 times with each leg.

Note:

- This is a little more difficult than the previous asana. So, do it slowly.
- It is easier to perform with the legs wide apart.

Benefit:

- It gives all the benefits of Trilokasana and strengthens the leg muscles.

Gatimaya Tiryak Prishtasana/Gatimaya Tiryak Trilokasana (Dynamic star bending pose)

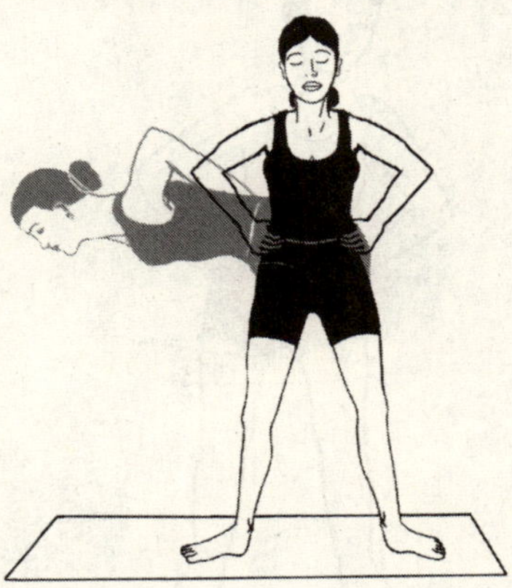

Method: Stand in the posture of Trilokasana, or stand with your legs about three feet apart. Keep your hands on your waist (thumbs resting on your back and the fingers resting on your stomach, and feet pointing outside). Twist your torso to your left and bend to form a right angle with the ground. Stay in this position for some time then bring your torso back to the original position. Repeat this on the right side too. Then, do the exercise in the opposite way. First bend forward, twist to the left, stay in the position, and then straighten up and look in front. Once you get enough practice, you can increase the speed of doing the exercise.

Breathing/time: Repeat this exercise 4-5 times on both the sides. Exhale while bending the body and inhale while coming back to the original position.

Benefits:

- Removes the disorders of the back and waist.
- Makes the body slim.
- Activates the digestive system.
- Removes excess air from the body.

Precautions: People with a stiff spine and severe back ache should not do this exercise.

Kati Vrittasana (Waist rotation)

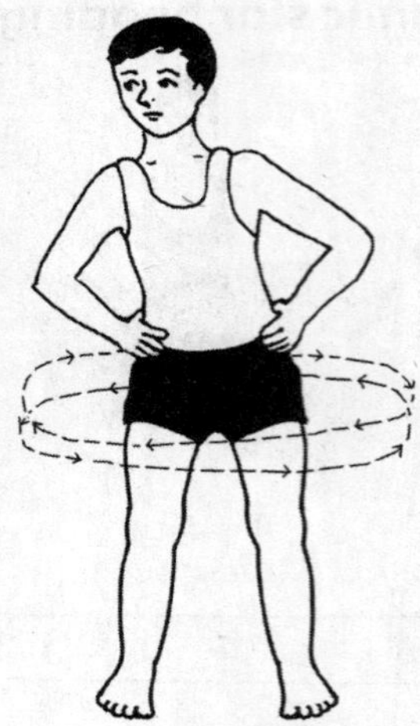

Method: Stand straight with your feet apart. Do not keep too much distance between your feet (only about 8-10 inches). Keep your hands on your waist. Move your waist in circular motion. To do this, bend your waist slightly forward and rotate it from right to left and bring it in front. Rotate from right to left at least 40-50 times and then from left to right at least 40-50 times.

Breathing: Inhale when the waist moves in front and exhale when it moves to the back.

Note: Move your waist forward and backwards as much as possible. While placing the hands on the waist, the thumbs can be kept towards the stomach.

Benefits:

- It cures constipation. It activates the digestive system and expels the gases out of the body.
- When done in abundance, this asana reduces excess fat around the abdomen.
- Slims down the waist and strengthens it.
- It is beneficial for women.

Kangaroo Kood (Kangaroo hop)

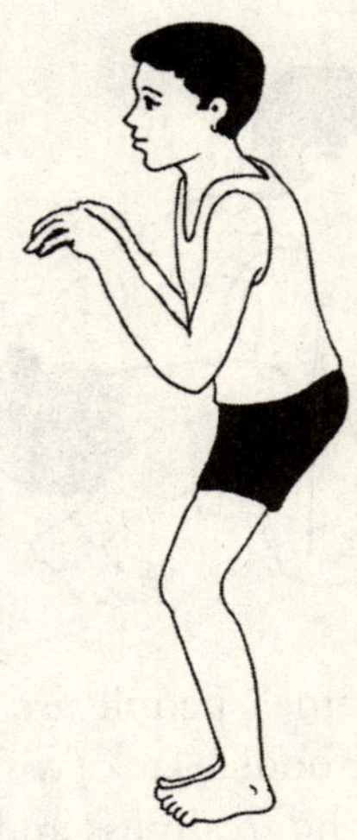

Method: In this asana, one has to hop like a kangaroo. So, stand as illustrated in the figure. Like a kangaroo, hop on your toes and keep hopping until you move at least ten steps ahead from where you are. Hop and come back to your original place. Do at least 2-3 rounds.

Breathing: Inhale while hopping and exhale while coming back to the final position.

Benefits:

- It puts an end to laziness and about swiftness and freshness in the body.
- Improves blood circulation.
- This exercise is very enjoyable.
- The abdominal region gets activated.

Note: Try to hop higher while going forward.

Precautions: Pregnant women and people who have undergone an operation in the lower part of the bodies should not do this exercise.

Mendhak Kood (Frog hop)

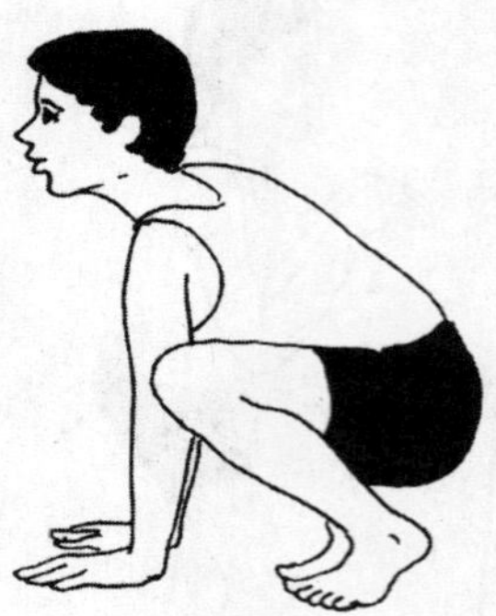

Note: In these modern times, people are becoming slaves of the machines. Therefore, their bodies lack swiftness. But these energy giving exercises enhance the freshness and swiftness of our body, giving us plenty of joy while doing them.

Method: Sit on your haunches like a frog (see illustration). Keep your knees wide apart. Spread your fingers. Keep your elbows close to the knees. Now exerting pressure with your feet and hands on the ground, hop like a frog and move forward. Repeat this kriya 10 times and then hop like a frog, while coming back to your original place.

Breathing/time: Hold your breath while hopping. Exhale while landing on the ground. In this way jump like a frog 20-40 times.

Benefits:

- The blood circulation of the entire body increases, and the nerves and veins open up.
- This exercise is very enjoyable.
- The muscles of the hands and legs become strong.
- The capacity of the lungs is enhanced.
- The digestive system is strengthened.

Precaution: Pregnant women and people who have undergone surgery in the lower parts of their bodies should not do this exercise.

Bal Hansi/Bal Machalan Kriya (Child's laughter exercise)

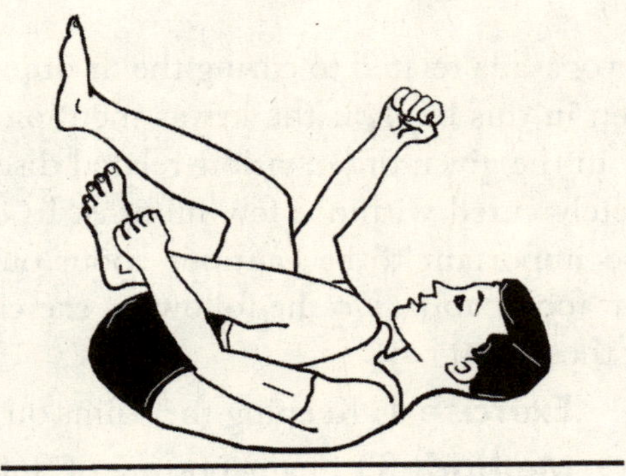

Method: Lie down on your back. Keep your body relaxed and tension free. Form a fist with your hands. Then, do just as a six-month-old child does with his/her hands while crying or laughing. To do this, bend your right knee and bring your left hand up from the sides of your chest. Similarly, do with the other leg and hand. Move your hands and legs in this manner quickly. Laugh like a little child.

Benefits:

- The hands and legs get a lot of relaxation. The blood circulation in the muscles of the spine and back and in the lungs is regularised.
- This is an enjoyable exercise.
- It removes mental stress.
- Ego mellows down.

Note: The main objective behind this exercise is to develop the feeling of affection and ingenuity in our hearts.

Yogic Exercises for the Eyes

Dhrishtivardhak Yogic Abhyasavali

Though many yogasana related to curing the disorders of the eyes have been given in this book, if the kriyas mentioned below are done everyday in the given order, vision-related disorders can be almost completely cured within a few months. In order to cure them, it is also important to be cautious about our day to day routine and our food habits. Do the following exercises and keep the diseases of the eyes at bay.

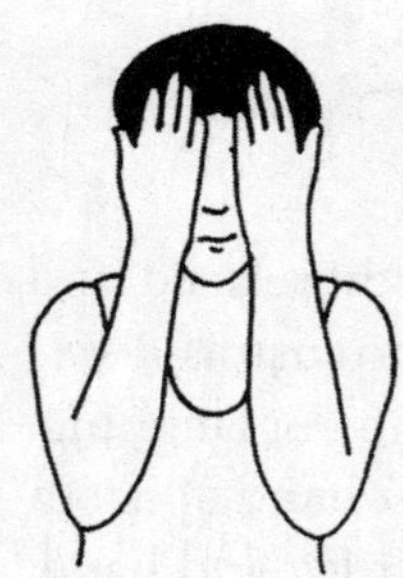

Exercise 1. Keeping the palms on the eyes

Method: Sit in any posture of Sukhasana. Rub your palms together till they become very warm. Close your eyes and place your palms on them. Feel the warmth of the palms on your eyes. When the palms cool down, rub them again and repeat the procedure. In this way, feel the energy being emitted from your palms on your eyes. Repeat this 3 times.

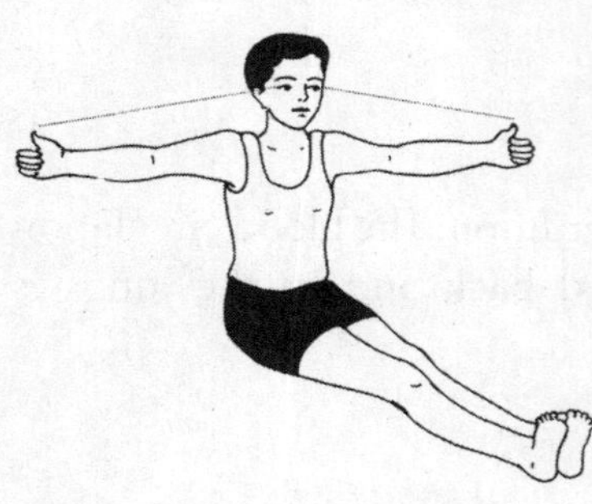

Exercise 2. Seeing right and left

Method: Sit in Sukhasana, or with your feet stretched in front. Spread your arms to the sides in line with the shoulders. Form a fist, but keep our thumbs out. Keep your head still. Then, without moving your head, shift your gaze and first look at the left thumb. Bring your gaze to the tip of your nose. Then, move your gaze to the right thumb and back to the tip of your nose. Repeat this 10-15 times or as per convenience, and then, rest your eyes for some time.

Breathing: Inhale while looking to the right and left and exhale while looking at the tip of your nose.

Exercise 3. Looking in front and right/left

Method: Sit as mentioned before. Spread your left arm in front, in line with the shoulder and spread your right arm to the side, parallel to the ground. Form a fist with the thumbs out at the shoulder level. Do not move your arms. Keeping your head still, look at the thumb in front and then at the right thumb. Repeat this 10-15 times. Then, change the position of your hands and bring the left hand to the side, in line with the left shoulder and right hand in front. Repeat this procedure 10-15 times. Rest your eyes for some time.

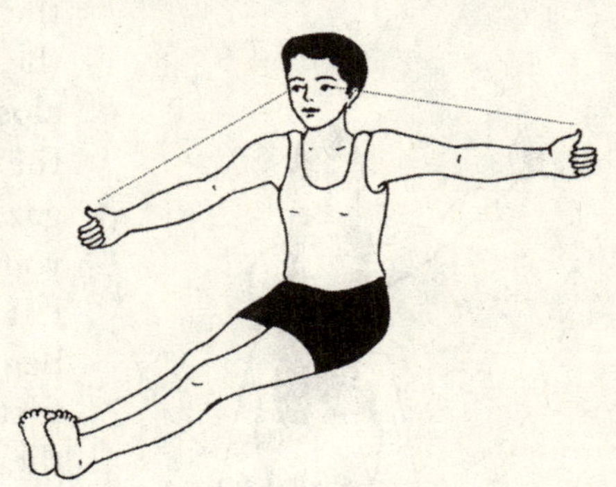

Breathing: Inhale while looking to the right and left and exhale while looking in front.

Exercise 4. Shifting the gaze right and left

Method: Sit as mentioned before. Bring your right hand up exactly in front of your eyes. Form a fist with your thumb out. Fix your gaze on the thumb. Now move your hand to the extreme right (keep your gaze fixed on the thumb). Then, take your arm to the left, and again fix your gaze on your thumb while keeping the arm still. In this way do this exercise 10-15 times. Rest your eyes after this for half a minute.

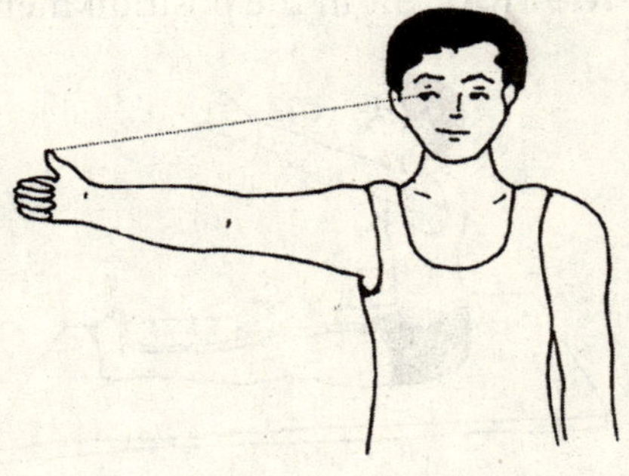

Breathing: Inhale while moving the arm to the right. Exhale while coming back. Do the same while moving your arm to the left.

Exercise 5. Moving the gaze in circular motion

Method: Sit in the same position as in the previous exercise. Keep the left hand on your thigh and the right hand raised in front (fist closed with the thumb out) and the head still. Now, keeping your gaze fixed on the thumb, move your right hand from right to left forming a big circle without bending the arm (move the arm first to the right, then up, and then to the left and then bring it in front).

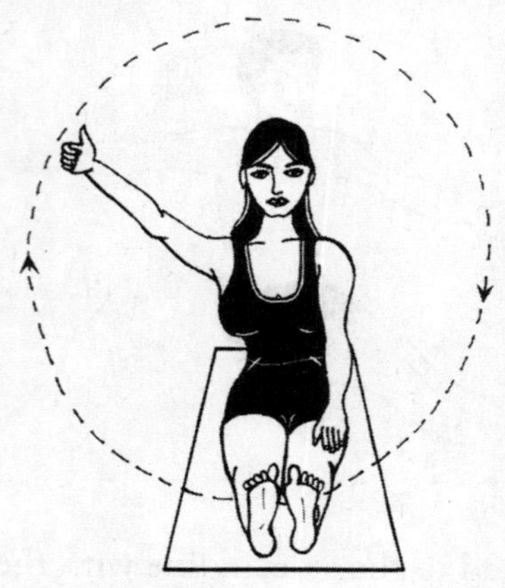

Do this kriya 5 times from right to left and 5 times from left to right. While making the circle, keep your head still, spine erect, and only move your gaze. Then, rest your eyes.

Breathing: Inhale while taking your hands up and exhale while bringing them down.

Exercise 6. Looking up and down

Method: Sit in the position mentioned above. Stretch both your hands in front. Form a fist and keep your thumbs out. Keep your spine erect and your head still. Fix your gaze on the thumb of the right fist and slowly move your hand up. Then, bring it back down (keep your gaze fixed on the thumb and shift it along with the movement of the thumb). Now repeat the same procedure with the left hand also. Repeat for this 5 times with each hand.

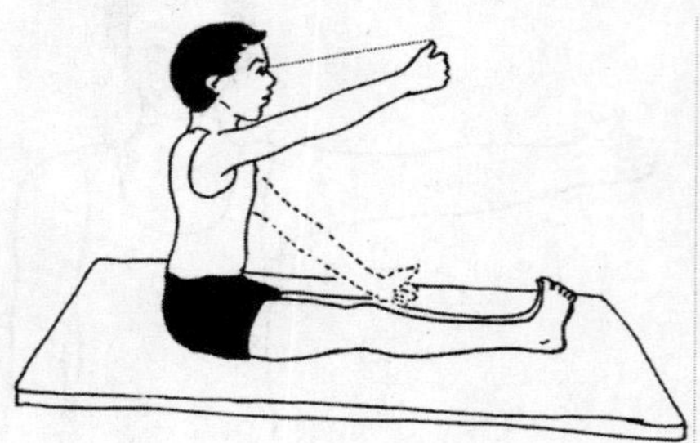

Breathing: Inhale while taking your hand up and exhale while bringing it down.

Exercise 7. Shifting the gaze far and near

Method: Sit in the same position as in the previous exercise. Stretch your right hand in front, in line with the shoulder. Form a fist and keep the thumb out. Fix your gaze on the thumb and slowly bring your thumb closer till it touches the tip of the nose and then slowly take it back to its original stretched position (keep your gaze fixed on the tip of the thumb). Again bring the thumb near the nose. Repeat this 5 times.

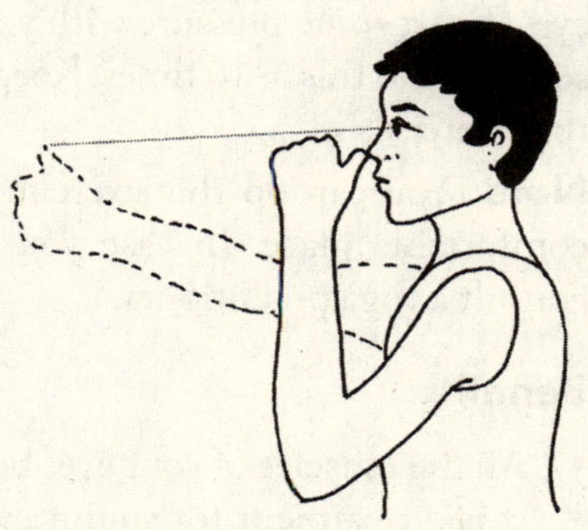

Breathing: Inhale while bringing the thumb near your nose and exhale while taking it back.

Exercise 8. Looking far and near

Method: We can do this exercise either in an open area or on the roof of our house. Fix your gaze on the tip of the nose for 5 seconds and then move it to a distant object either in the sky or anywhere else. Repeat this 5-10 times.

Breathing: Inhale while looking at the tip of the nose and exhale while looking at the distant object.

Notes:

- After each exercise, rub your palms and place them on your eyes.
- In the end, rest in Shavasana.
- Splash cold water on the eyes. Do not rub them.

Exercise 9. Closing and opening the eyes

Method: Keep your entire focus on the eyes. Quickly close your eyes. Exert some pressure with your eyes and open them after 1-2 seconds. Do this 5-10 times. Keep your teeth together while doing this exercise.

Note: You can do this exercise by sitting on a chair or in any comfortable place. In case you face any problem, immediately consult a yoga practitioner.

Benefits:

- All the muscles of your eyes benefit from it.
- It is a treatment for squint eyes, and practising it prevents its occurrence.
- For all those whose eyes are weak, who use spectacles or those whose with watery eyes, these exercises are very beneficial.
- Eyes become healthy and beautiful.
- Eyes remain disease free till old age.

We are returning back to our culture
through Yoga Kriyas.

–RJT

Asana for De-stressing and Relaxation

Shavasana/Mritasana/Poorna Vishramasana (Corpse pose)

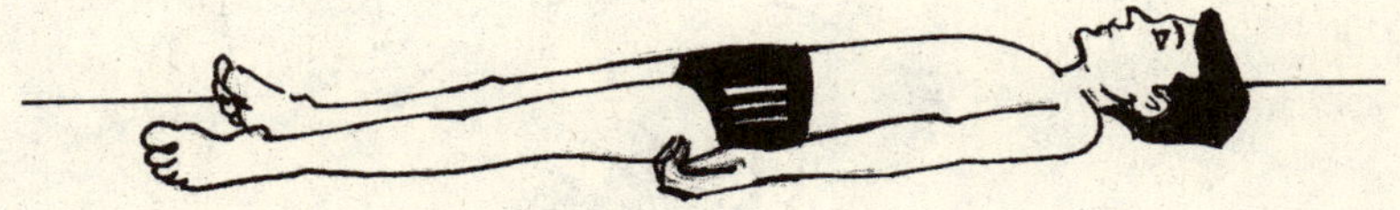

Meaning: Shava means a dead body. While doing this asana, your body becomes absolutely loose, as if it is dead. That is why it is called Mritasana.

Method: Lie down on your back. Keep your hands by the sides. Keep the palms partially open and facing the sky. The heels should be together but there should be some distance between the toes. Close your eyes and keep your tongue still. Slowly breathe in and out. Focus on your breath to enhance your concentration. After sometime, the nerves become inactive. The stillness within the practitioner starts increasing and he/she starts feeling light and happy. One can feel the flow of energy in the whole body. Remain in this position for 5-10 minutes.

Focus: Focus on the Mooladhara chakra and feel the energy rise up.

Benefits:

- People suffering from insomnia can gain total benefit from this asana.
- This asana provides extraordinary peace to people who are tensed or stressed.
- You can use this to enhance your mental and intellectual powers.
- People with high blood pressure should do this asana regularly.

Note: For more benefits, see the chapter on Yoga Nidra.

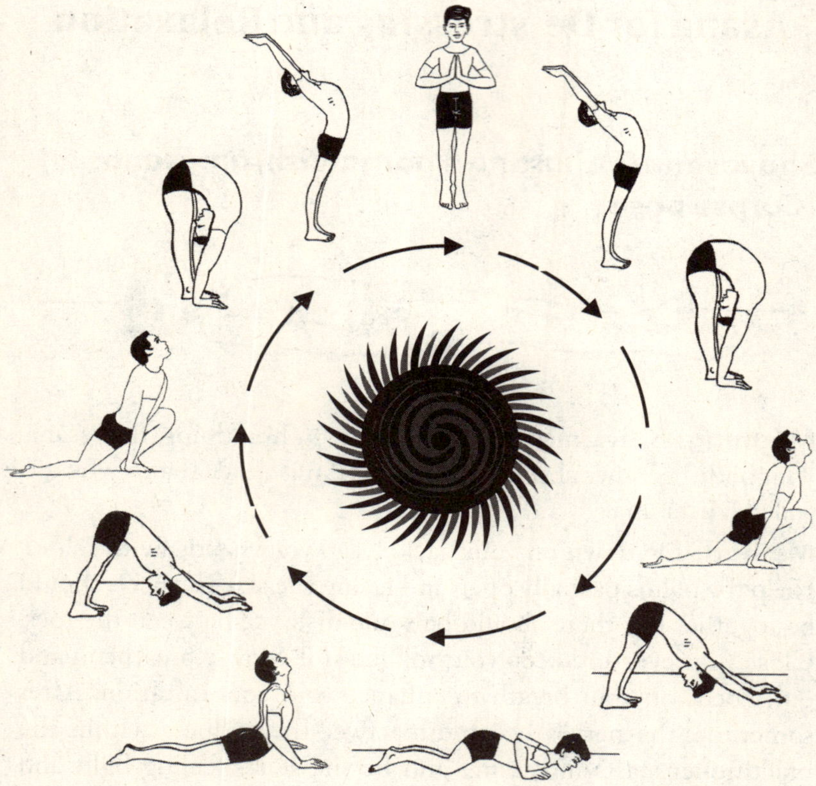

Surya Namaskara Phalshruti Mantra

आदित्यस्य नमस्कारान्, ये कुर्वन्ति दिने दिने।
आयुः प्रज्ञा बलंवीर्यं तेजस् तेषाञ् च जायते॥

Meaning: Those who do Surya Namaskara everyday are blessed with long life, good intellect, strength, virility and radiance.

आदिदेव नमस्तुभ्यं प्रसीद मम भास्कर।
दिवाकर नमस्तुभ्यं प्रभाकर नमोऽस्तु ते।।

Meaning : O'Heavenly God! Source of Cosmic Illumination! I bow to you. Please accept my prayer. O'King of the daytime! We salute to you, O'Radiant One! We pray to you.

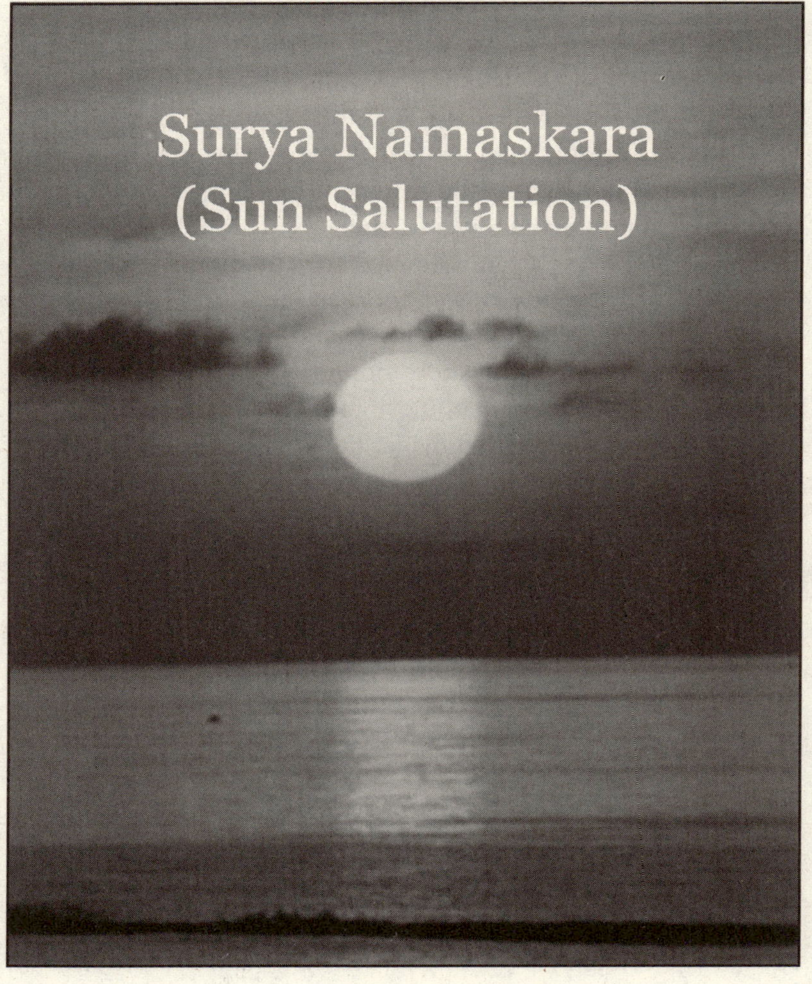

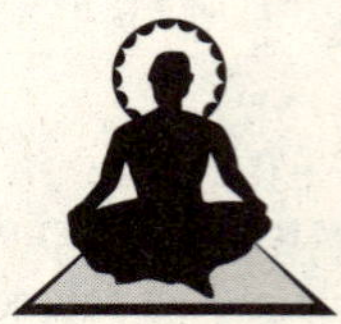

Surya Namaskara (Sun Salutation)

An Analysis

Since time immemorial, the significance of the Sun has been explained in our religious text. Even to this day, research is being done to understand the secrets of the Sun, yet it continues to remain a mystery. However, there is no doubt that it has always attracted our attention since ancient times. Whether we look back at the bygone eras or at the modern times, the Sun has always provided us with life giving energy. Modern scientists are struggling day and night to know more about the Sun; whereas our ancient saints and wise men knew about its divinity and how to put it to good use. The Sun provides life force with its invigorating energy to not only our physical body but to our subtle body as well. Modern scientists may choose to call it a ball of fire or a heavenly body, but our wise men of the yore had understood many of its secrets and helped make its utility accessible for the benefit of the common man. But today that knowledge has been almost lost. We would like to discuss a little about the secrets of the Sun, so that when we do Surya Namaskara, our hearts are filled with faith, perseverance and devotion, and we are able to gain maximum benefit from the asana.

The readers might already know about the great saint from Banaras Swami Vishuddhananda and his disciple Gopinath Kaviraj, Principal of Kashi Hindu Vishwavidyalaya. Since the story is a long one, we would only mention that he went to a remote cave in the Himalayas (Gyanganj Ashram) and did penance for twelve years. He came back to Banaras sometime around 1920 and astonished the entire world by narrating the miracles of the science of the Sun. People were wonder struck. He used to transform one object into another in the presence of thousands of disciple by using the science of the Sun. For example, he used to transform cotton into anything between a flower, stone, granite, diamond, to wood. In fact, once he even made a dead bird come alive. That ashram still exists in the Himalayas. This incident has been taken from Paul Brunton's book. The main objective behind narrating this incident is to enhance your curiosity and faith in the Sun, so that we can gain maximum benefit from it.

There are twelve positions in one round of Surya Namaskara. Every asana has a mantra. Every kriya has its own benefits. All we would say is that if you want to renew your life, you must do Surya Namaskara.

The daily practice of Surya Namaskara is more beneficial than doing any other exercise. Regarding the sun, no amount of words can be sufficient. Hence, now we will explain how to do Surya Namaskara.

The Ancient History of Surya Namaskara

The main reason behind doing Surya Namaskara is probably to get the life giving energy from the Sun and to express our gratitude towards it. The trend of offering prayers to the Sun has been in vogue since ancient times, when the first great ruler of India, king Bharat used to offer prayers to the numerous sun rays. Due to reasons unknown, this particular practice could not be propagated, but the ruler of the South imbibed this practice and kept it alive. Even when they went to religious places in other parts of India, they continued practising Surya Namaskara as a part of their daily routine. Other people observed them doing Surya Namaskara and followed the pattern. In this way, the propagation of Surya Namaskara began once again in India.

The Modern History of Surya Namaskara

There are many ways of doing Surya Namaskara, but Vedmurty

Shri Shripad Damodar Satavalekar of Surat (Gujarat) has designed twelve easy sequence of exercises, which are now being used all over India. Shivaji Maharaj's guru Samarth Ramdas taught him the right way of doing Surya Namaskara, which he practised and as a result his physique and character became unmatched in history. Shivaji Maharaj taught the way of doing Surya Namaskara to his soldiers, and in this way it became popular. The scientific significance of Surya Namaskara is enhanced because of the twelve unique Beej Mantras and kriyas included in it.

Surya Namaskara (Sun Salutation)

1. Prarthana Mudra/Namaskarasana/ Pranamasana (Prayer pose)

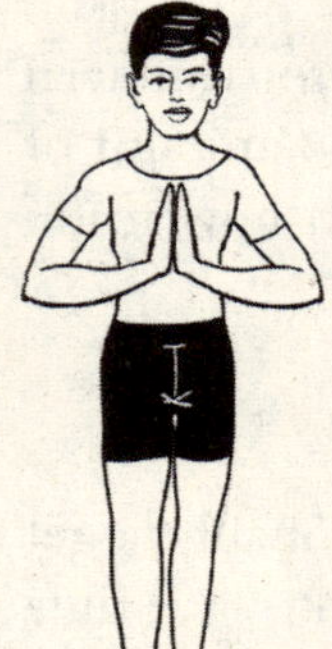

Method: Stand up straight with your feet together and hands joined in prayer, facing East. Keep your body relaxed and prepare it for the forthcoming postures.

Breathing: Normal.

Focus: On the Anahat chakra

Mantra: Om Mitraye Namah (ॐ मित्राय नमः)

Meaning: O' Sun God, Friend of the Universe! I salute thee.

Beej Mantra: Om Hraam (ॐ ह्रॉं।)

Benefits: It keeps the blood circulation normal and provides concentration and peace.

Note: This is also called Namaskar Mudra.

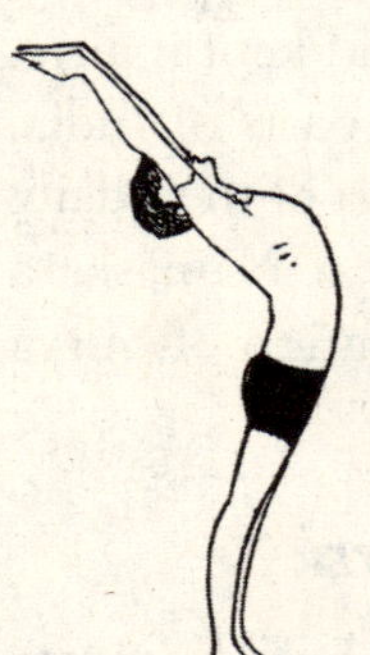

2. Hast Uttanasana (Raised arms pose)

Method: Raise both your hands up. Keep the distance between the arms equal to the width of your shoulders. Bend your head and torso backwards, as much as possible. Keep your arms in line with your ears.

Breathing: Inhale while taking your arms up.

Mantra: Om Ravaye Namah (ॐ रवये नमः)

Meaning: O' Sun God, Thou who brings about activity in the world! I salute thee.

Beej Mantra: Om Hreem (ॐ ह्रीं।)

Focus: On the Vishuddhi chakra

Benefits: It reduces excess fat around the abdomen. It improves the digestive system. Lungs become strong. Muscles of the arms and shoulders get exercised.

3. Padhastasana/Hastpadasana (Hand to feet pose/Standing forward bend pose)

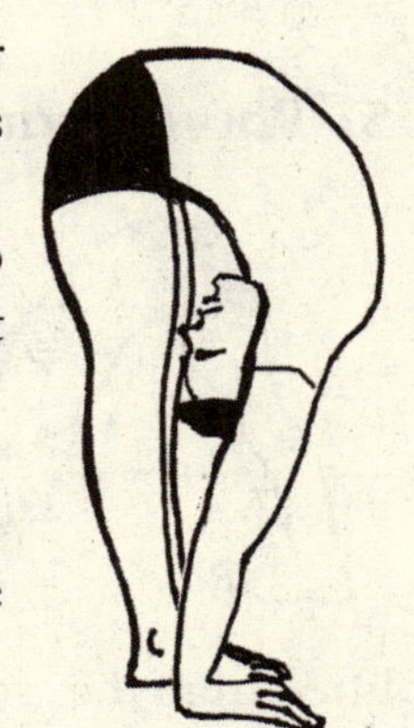

Method: Bend forward and place both your hands by the sides of your feet. Touch your knees with your forehead. Do not bend your knees.

Breathing: Exhale while bending forward. To expel maximum air out of your body, contract your stomach in the final position.

Focus: On Swadhishthana chakra

Mantra: Om Suryaye Namah (ॐ सूर्याय नमः)

Meaning: O' Sun God, Giver of Life to the World! I salute thee.

Beej Mantra: Om Hroom (ॐ ह्रूँ।)

Benefits: Reduces the fat from the abdomen. Prevents and cures the diseases of the stomach and intestine. It cures constipation. It makes the spine flexible and normalises the pressure of the nerves. It increases the blood circulation.

4. Ashva Sanchalana/Ek Pada Prasarasana (Equestrain pose)

Method: Now, take your left leg back, as much as possible and try to touch the ground with the left knee and the lower part of the left foot. Keep the right foot firm on the ground and bend the knee.

Arms should be firm and straight in their place. Keep the palms of the hands and the right foot in one line. In this kriya, the weight of the body will rest on the hands, left foot, left knee and on the upper part of the right foot. Now bend your head backward. Fix your gaze in front. The body will take the shape of a bow.

Breathing: Inhale while taking the left leg back.

Focus: On Aagya chakra.

Mantra: Om Bhanave Namah (ॐ भानवे नमः)

Meaning: O' Sun God, the Bright One! I salute thee.

Beej Mantra: Om Hraum (ॐ ह्रौं।)

Benefits: The spine becomes flexible. Due to slight pressure exerted on the abdominal region, the blood circulation increases in the digestive system, hence, it starts functioning effectively.

5. Parvatasana (Mountain pose)

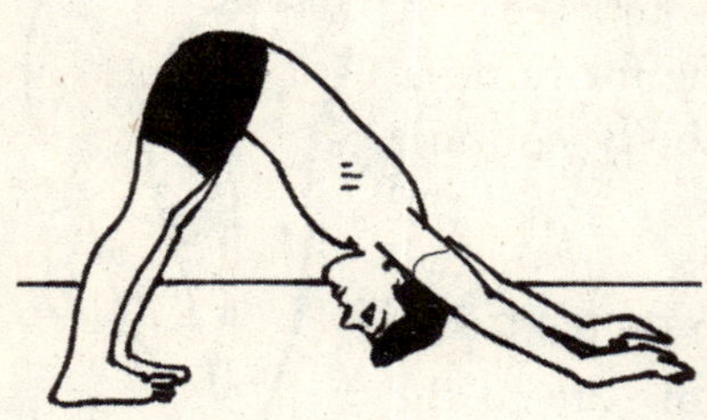

Method: Balance the weight of the entire body on both the hands and take the right leg back, next to the left leg. Lift up your buttocks and bring your head in between your hands. The heels should not be lifted from the ground. While looking at your knees, bring the feet and hands in one line.

Breathing: Exhale while taking your right leg back and lifting your buttocks up.

Focus: On Vishuddhi chakra

Mantra: Om Khagaye Namah (ॐ खगाय नमः)

Meaning: O' Sun God, Thou who moves in the sky! I salute thee.

Beej Mantra: Om Hram (ॐ ह्रं।)

Benefits: Since the head is bent forward in this exercise, the blood circulation in the head increases. Therefore, it brings about freshness on the face, and improves the eyesight. It keeps hair fall in check. The arms and legs get enough exercise. The nerves of the spine benefit from it, by becoming flexible. The spine becomes stronger.

6. Ashtanga Namaskarasana/Pranipatasana (Eight limbed pose)

Method: Bring your body down on the ground in a way that the back of both the legs, both the knees, both the forearms and the chin touch the ground. The buttocks and the abdomen should be slightly raised.

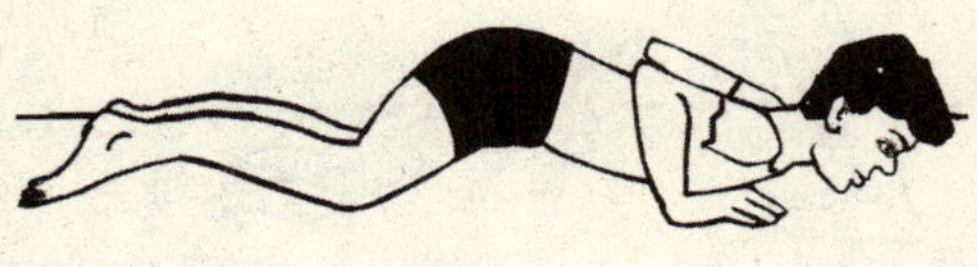

Breathing: Hold your breath

Focus: On Manipur chakra

Mantra: Om Pooshne Namah (ॐ पूष्णे नमः)

Meaning: O' Sun God, Thou who nourishes! I salute thee.

Beej Mantra: Om Hrah (ॐ ह्रः ।)

Benefits: It gives strength to the chest and lungs. It gives strength to the muscles of the hands and legs.

7. Bhujangasana (Cobra pose)

Method: Straighten your hands without shifting them. Lift up your torso – head, chest and waist – and bend your head and neck backwards.

Breathing: Inhale while bending your waist and chest like a bow.

Focus: On Swadhishthan chakra

Mantra: Om Hiranyagarbhaye Namah (ॐ हिरण्यगर्भाय नमः)

Meaning: O' Sun God, Thou with the brilliance of golden hue! I salute thee.

Beej Mantra: Om Hraam (ॐ ह्रां ।)

Benefits: It exerts pressure on your digestive system and increases blood circulation. Hence, the digestive system remains active. It removes constipation. It makes the lungs function well. It makes the spine flexible. It is beneficial for people suffering from asthma, bronchitis and cervical spondylitis.

8. Parvatasana/Bhoodharasana (Mountain pose)

Method: This is a repetition of posture 5. Raise your buttocks up and fix your feet on the ground. Try to take your waist and buttocks as high as possible in the final position. Keep your feet together. Keep your gaze on the navel.

Breathing: Exhale while raising your buttocks and upper body.

Focus: On Vishuddhi chakra

Mantra: Om Mareechaye Namah (ॐ मरीचये नमः)

Meaning: O' Sun God, Lord of infinite rays of light! I salute thee.

Beej Mantra: Om Hreem (ॐ ह्रीं ।।)

Benefits: It provides renewed energy to the muscles of the hands and legs. It makes the spine flexible. It gives all the benefits of posture 5.

Note: Some yoga teachers call this Adhomukha Shvanasana.

9. Ashva-sanchalanasana/ Ek Pada Prasaranasana (Equestrain pose)

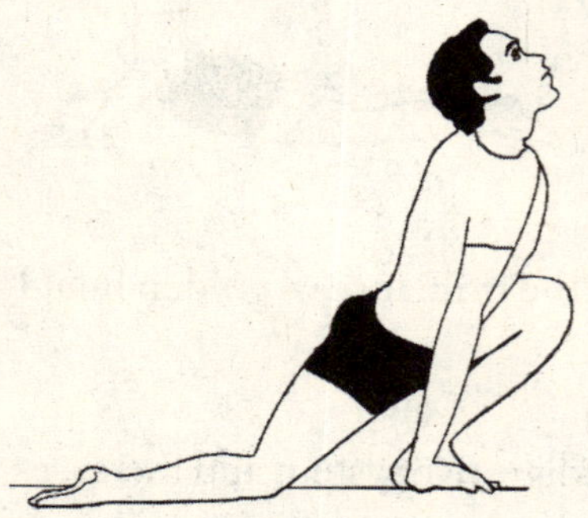

Note: This posture is a partial repetition of posture 4. In posture 4, the left leg goes back, whereas in this posture, the right leg goes back.

Keep the left leg forward between both the hands. Bend the knee and keep the foot firmly fixed on the ground. Then, take the right leg backward. Remember that the knee and the back of the foreleg should touch the ground. Do not bend your arms. The entire weight of the body will be on both the hands, left foot, back of the right foreleg and knee.

Breathing: Inhale while bringing the left foot forward.
Focus: On Agya chakra
Mantra: Om Adityaye Namah (ॐ आदित्याय नमः)
Meaning: O' Sun God, son of Aditi, I salute thee.
Beej Mantra: Om Hroom (ॐ ह्रूँ ।)
Benefits: Gives all the benefits of posture 4.

10. Pada Hastasana/Hast Padasana (Hand to feet pose/Standing forward bend pose)

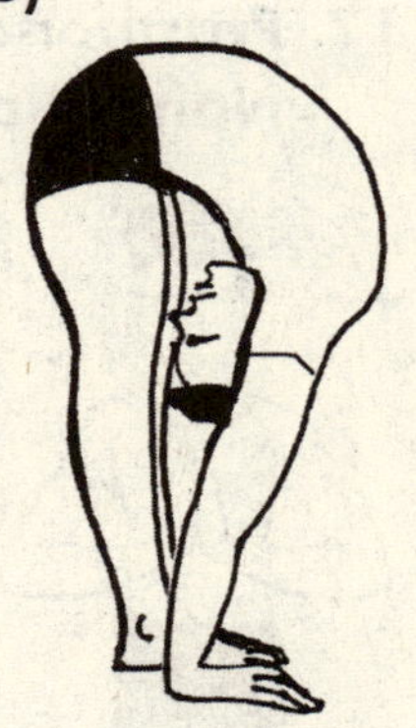

Note: This posture is the repetition of posture 3.

Method: Shift your weight on both your hands and bring your right foot forward, close the left foot. Straighten up your legs and touch your forehead to the knees. In this way, in the final position, the feet and the palms will be in one line.

Breathing: Exhale while bending forward. To expel maximum air from the body, contract your abdomen.
Focus: On Svadhishthan Chakra.
Mantra: Om Savitre Namah (ॐ सवित्रे नमः)
Meaning: O' Sun God, Thou responsible for life in the universe! I salute thee.
Beej Mantra: Om Hraum (ॐ ह्रौं ।)
Benefits: It gives all the benefits of posture 3.

11. Hast Uttanasanas (Raised arms pose)

Note: This posture is the repetition of posture 2.

Method: Raise your bent body up and take your hands above your head. Keep your arms apart at shoulder length. Then, bend your head and torso back as much as possible.

Breathing: Inhale while taking your hands up.

Focus: On Vishuddhi chakra

Mantra: Om Arkaye Namah (ॐ अर्काय नमः)

Meaning: O' Sun God, Thou who purifies and who is praise worthy! I salute thee.

Beej Mantra: Om Hram (ॐ ह्रं ।)

Benefits: It gives all the benefits of posture 2.

12. Prarthana Mudra/Pranamasana/ Namaskarasana (Prayer pose)

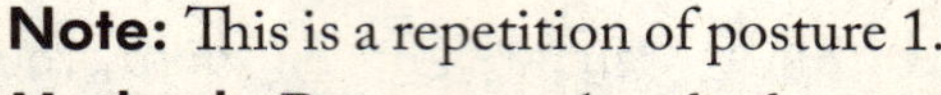

Note: This is a repetition of posture 1.

Method: Bring your hands down and join your palms in front of your chest in a prayer posture. Keep your feet together. Stand straight and relax your body.

Breathing: Exhale and then, breathe normally.

Focus: On Anahat chakra

Mantra: Om Bhaskaraye Namah (भास्कराय नमः)

Meaning: O' Sun God, Lord of Cosmic Illumination! I salute thee.

Beej Mantra: Om Hrah (ॐ ह्रः ।)

This is half a round of Surya Namaskar. In order to complete the round, we do the postures 4 and 9 by changing the legs. The leg which was taken back will now be brought forward. We first took the right leg back, now we will take the left leg back. In this way, a set of twenty four asanas is considered one complete round.

If you feel tired after doing half a round (twelve asanas), rest for a while and breathe normally. Be alert while doing every asana. Chant the mantras joyfully. If you are not able to do any asana properly, first practice it and then, incorporate it in Surya Namaskara.

Note: The practitioner should do two to three rounds according to his/her capability. The best time to do Surya Namaskara is at dawn. The practitioner should finish his daily morning routine then do this exercise with a joyful heart. One should wear loose and clean clothes while doing it. The atmosphere should be peaceful. That is why, early morning is the best time for doing this exercise as the air is pure in the morning and the ultraviolet rays of the Sun do not harm us. If one is unable to do Surya Namaskara in the morning due to any reason, it can be done in the evening on an empty stomach.

Precaution: All people above the age of eight years can do this asana. Those who are ill or suffering from diseases of the spine, high blood pressure, heart problems or hernia should do this asana under the guidance of a guru.

Complete benefits:

- It provides life force.
- It balances the energy at both physical as well as mental level.
- The entire body is exercised by practising Surya Namaskara.
- Since the spine is bent forward and backward alternately, along with being beneficial for the body, it is also significant in awakening the kundalini. Since the spine is the path of the sushumna, the energy starts flowing in the upward direction.
- Surya Namaskara gives mental peace. It enhances the memory. It also increases strength, virility and makes one glow.
- It is a staunch enemy of constipation. It keeps old age at bay.
- Women can maintain their bodies by practising it.
- Surya Namaskara cures all diseases. It makes us brilliant like the Sun.
- Students should practise Surya Namaskara to gain all these benefits.

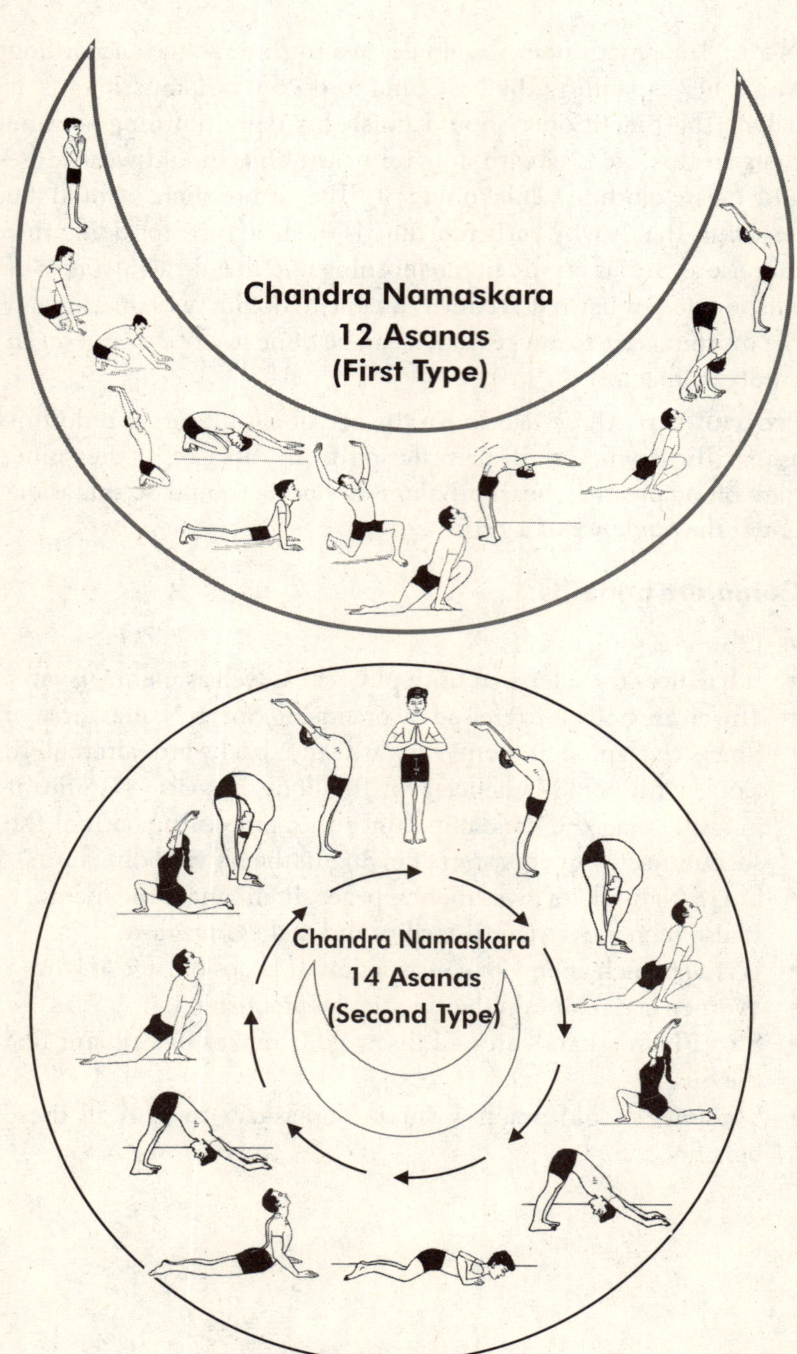
Chandra Namaskara
12 Asanas
(First Type)
Chandra Namaskara
14 Asanas
(Second Type)

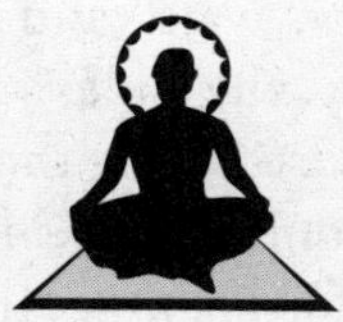

Chandra Namaskara

(Moon Salutation)

Just like Surya Namaskara, Chandra Namaskara is also very significant. This includes twelve kriyas which have their respective mantras (in some places, fourteen kriyas are mentioned). These mantras can be chanted with each asana. Though each asana has its own significance, when done in the mentioned order, the complete benefit can be achieved. Therefore, we must try to get the benefits from Chandra Namaskara.

Posture 1. Raised Arms Pose

Method: Face the Moon and stand in Tadasana posture. Raise both your arms and take them above your head. Bend your torso backwards from the waist, as much as possible. Keep your palms open towards the sky and chant 'Om Chandraye Namah' (ॐ चंद्राय नमः) in your heart.

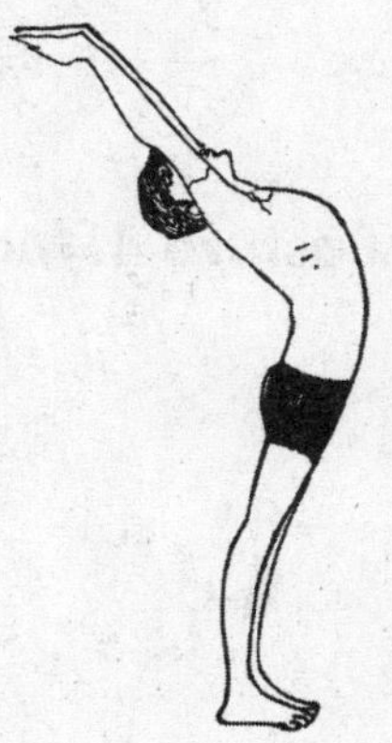

Posture 2. Hand to Feet Pose

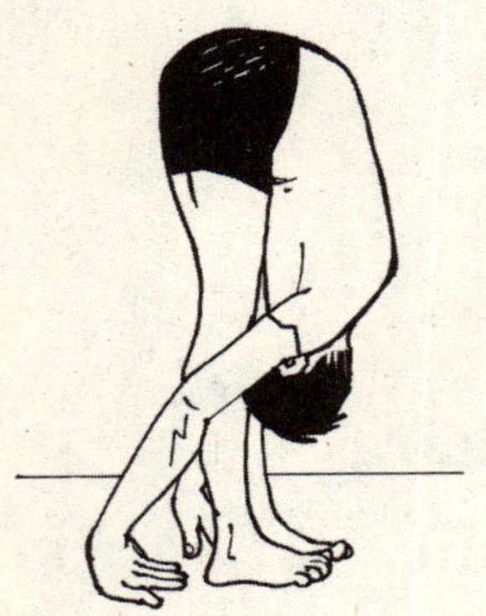

Method: Bend your body forward from the waist and bring your hands down by the sides of your feet. Make your nose touch the knees, but do not bend your knees. Chant 'Om Somaye Namah' (ॐ सोमाय नमः) in your heart.

Posture 3. Equestrain Pose

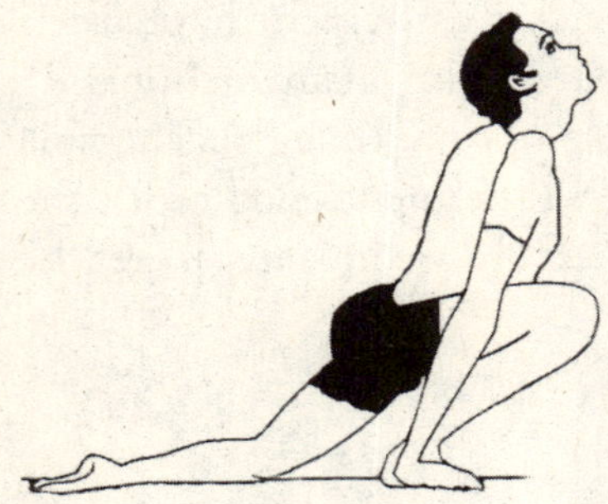

Method: After this, take your left back and keep it straight. Bend your right knee and shift the weight of your entire body on the right leg. Keep both your hands by the sides of your right feet and chant 'Om Indrave Namah' (ॐ इन्द्रवे नमः) in your heart.

Posture 4. Moon Pose

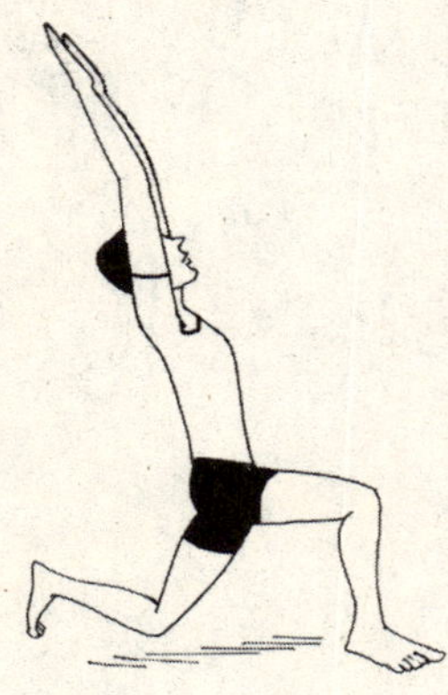

Method: Now keeping both your feet fixed in their respective places, raise your body in such a way that the left knee touches the ground and the right knee forms a right angle with the ground. Then, raise both your hands up and bend your body backwards from your waist. Chant 'Om Nishakaraye Namah' (ॐ निशाकराय नमः) in your heart.

Posture 5. Equestrain Pose

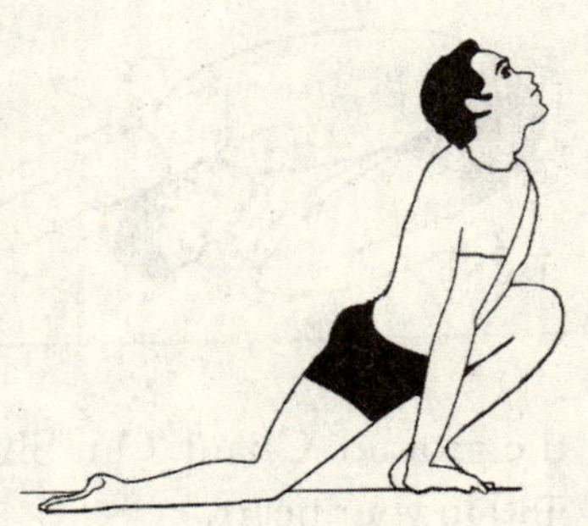

Method: Repeat posture 3, but instead of the right foot, shift your body weight on the left foot and take your right foot back. Bring the heel of the left foot and both the palms in one line and chant 'Om Kalabhritaye Namah' (ॐ कलाभृताय नमः) in your heart.

Posture 6. Extended Moon Pose

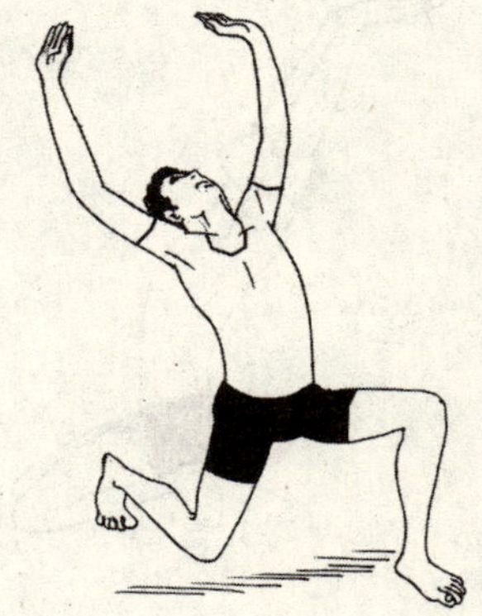

Method: As in posture 4, shift your weight on the left foot and stand in such a way that the right knee touches the ground. Stretch your hands up. Chant 'Om Sudhakaraye Namah' (ॐ सुधाधराय नमः) in your heart.

Posture 7. Cobra Pose

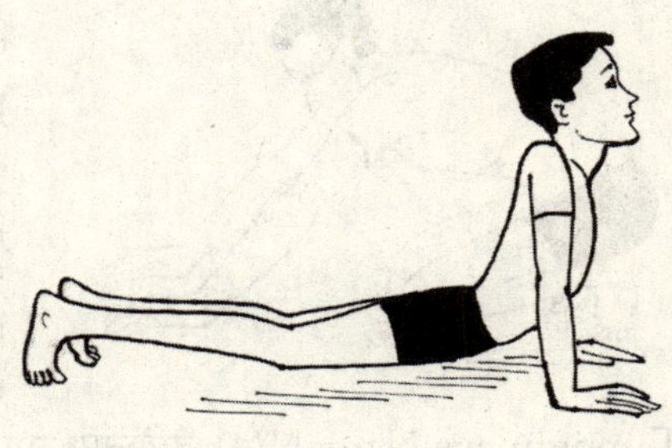

Method: Place both the palms firmly on the ground and take the left leg back, next to the right leg. Do one push up in this position and chant 'Om Nishapataye Namah' (ॐ निशापतये नमः) in your heart.

Posture 8. Child Pose

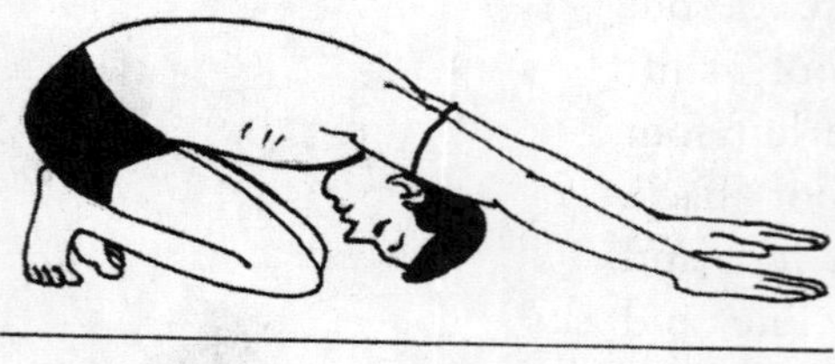

Method: After doing one push up, sit on your haunches, knees down, and without changing the position of the hands, bend forward and let your head touch the ground. Chant 'Om Shiv Shekharaye Namah' (ॐ शिव शेखराय नमः) in your heart.

Posture 9. Both Knees on the Floor Moon Pose

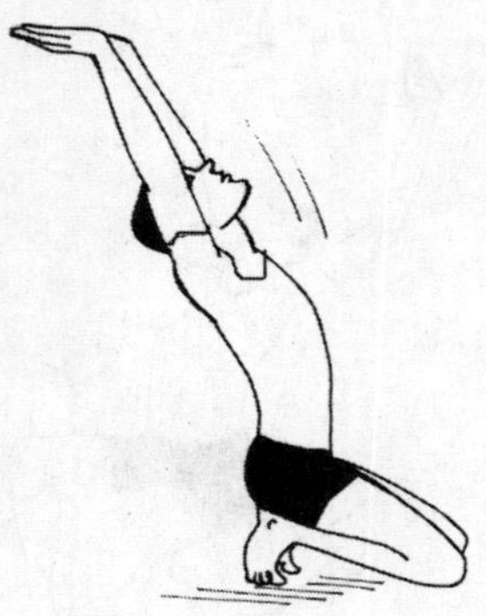

Method: Sit in the same position and take your hands and head up. Keep your body above the waist straight and bend it backward. Keep your hands towards the sky and sit on your haunches. Chant 'Om Amritdeedhitiye Namah' (ॐ अमृतदीधितये नमः) in your heart.

Posture 10. Caterpillar Pose

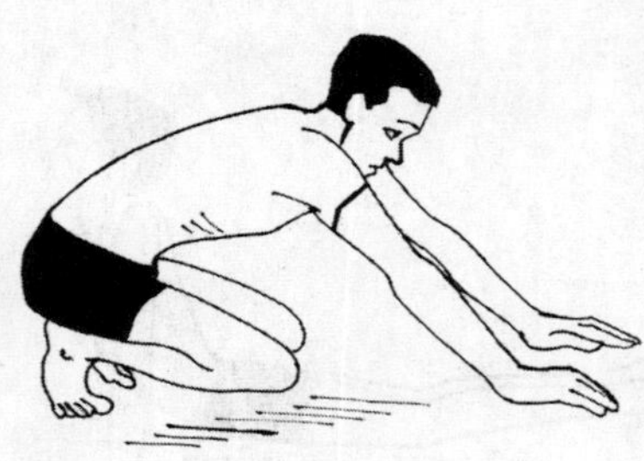

Method: Bring your hands down on the ground and place them one and a half feet apart. Do one push up in this position and then, balancing yourself on your toes and hands, raise your knees above the ground. Chant 'Om Tamoghnaye Namah' (ॐ तमोघ्नाय नमः) in your heart.

Posture 11. Squat

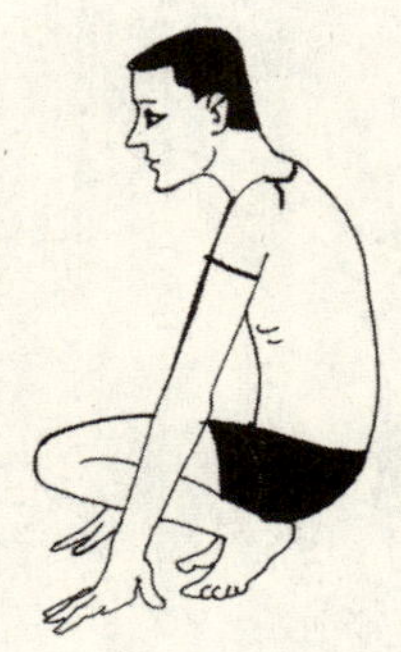

Method: After position 10, without changing the position of your hands, jump on your feet and bring them forward in between your hands. Sit on your toes. All the fingers of your hands should touch the ground. The weight of your buttocks should be on your heels. Chant 'Om Rajrajaye Namah' (ॐ राजराजाय नमः) in your heart.

Posture 12. Prayer Pose

Method: In the end, stand up straight, join your palms in a prayer posture and chant 'Om Shashank Devaye Namah' (ॐ शशांक देवाय नमः) in your heart.

This is one round. Do 5-6 such rounds. When you feel tired, rest in Shavasana.

Time: Just as Surya Namaskara is done specifically in the morning, similarly Chandra Namaskara should be done in the evening.

Benefits:

- Though each asana has its own significance and its own benefits, when the whole round is done, one can gain multiple benefits.
- The body becomes beautiful, strong and well-shaped. The abdominal region benefit from it. Constipation, indigestion, acidity, etc. are cured. The body gets a new aura and it glows. One achieves mental peace. One does not become lazy and lethargic. The whole body becomes healthy and disease free.

Note: In some yoga centres, Chandra Namaskara is taught differently.

Direction: Since we have to absorb the energy of the Moon to gain its benefits, we should choose to perform this exercise in the direction in which the Moon rises.

Yoga Vidya is not merely a set of exercises.
The entire Ashtanga Yoga enhances physical and mental health, builds a balanced perspective and motivates the soul to move towards self-development.

–RJT

Yoga is the positive approach to provide life with the highest form of opportunities.

–RJT

Yogasana

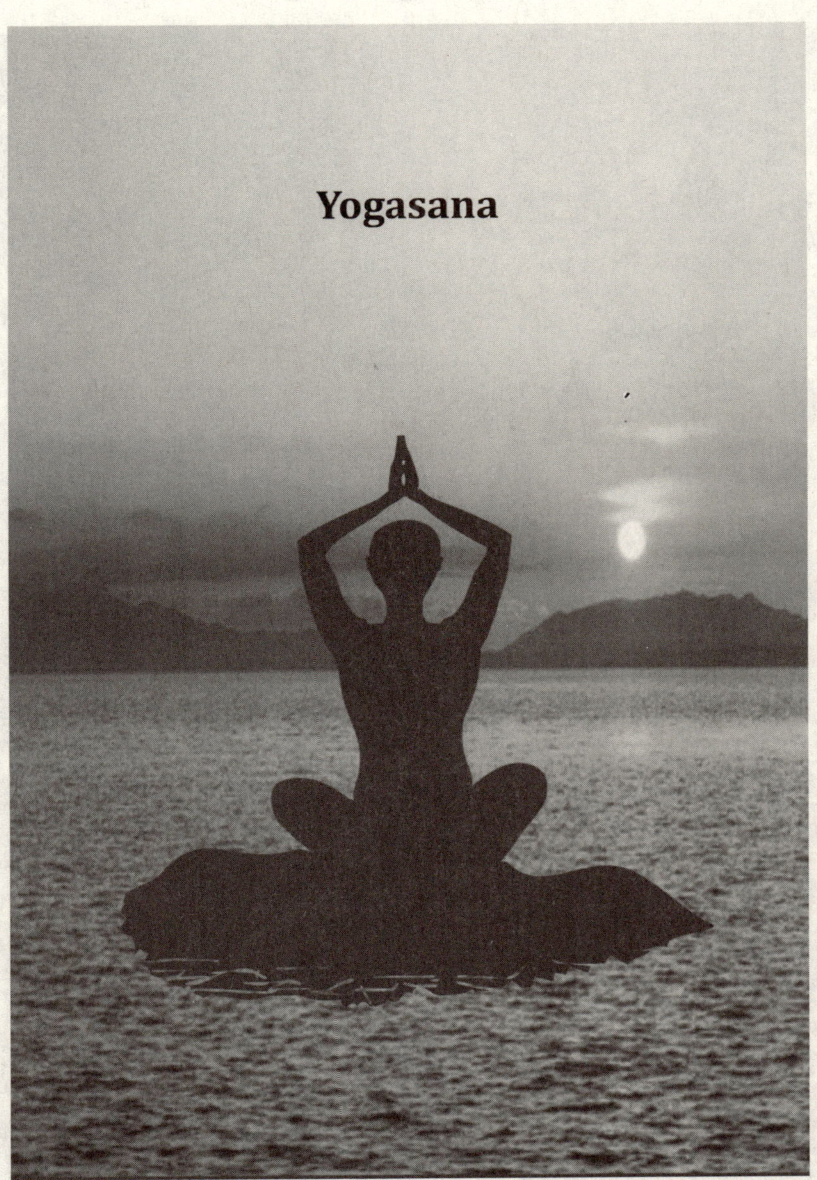

Ashtanga Yoga

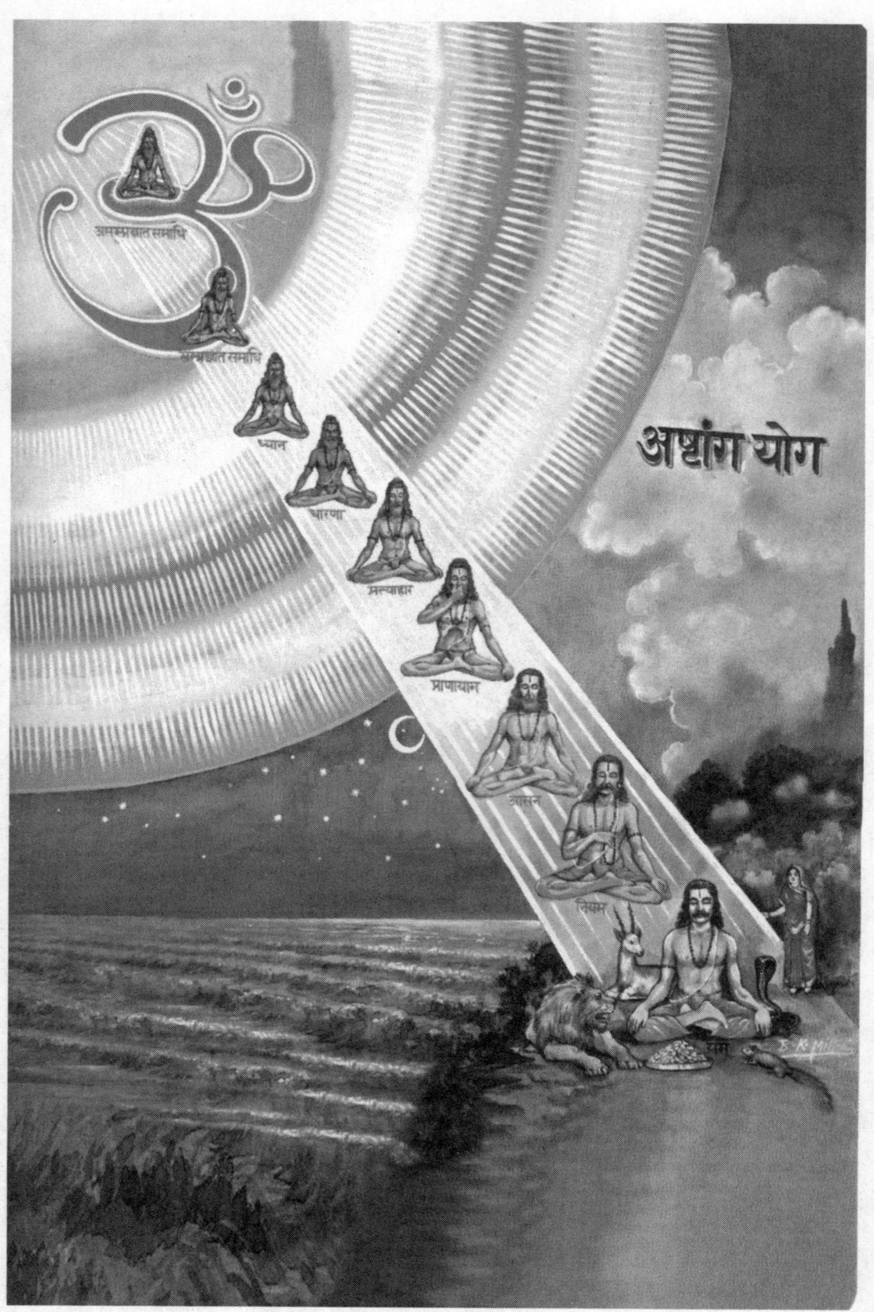

Padmasana (Lotus Position) and Other Asanas Related to Meditation

Sukhasana (Easy pose)

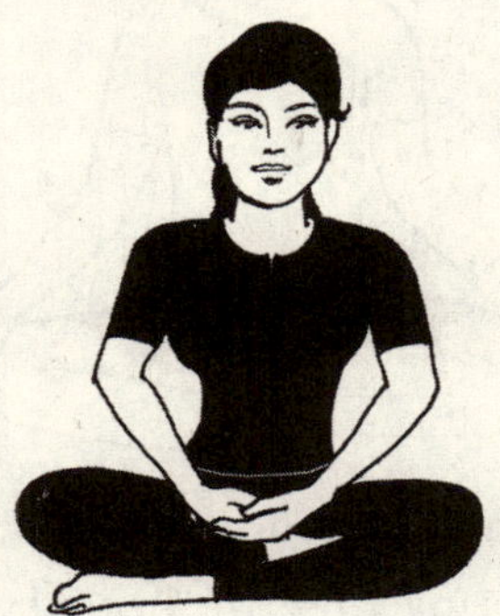

Meaning: 'Sukha' means happiness. Since we sit comfortably in the squatting position, this asana is called sukhasana. Even though any posture in which we are comfortable can also be called Sukhasana, since ancient times this posture is considered as Sukhasana.

Method: Sit down comfortably on the ground and bend your knees (see illustration). Keep both your hands in your lap, or on your knees. Keep the spine, neck and head straight.

Focus: Feel and experience the energy emitted from all the Chakras.

Breathing: As in Pranayam/as per convenience.

Direction: East or North (for spiritual benefits)

Benefits:

- This is a good posture for meditation
- It is beneficial to sit in this asana during meal
- Those who are not able to sit in Padmasana for meditation, can use this asana
- This asana is mostly used in prayers
- This asana is beneficial for the swiftness of the body, mental peace and for keeping the body disease free.

Guptasana

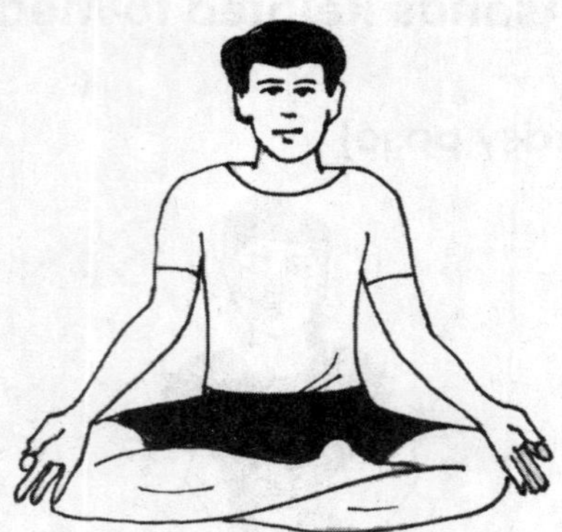

Meaning: 'Gupt' means hidden.

Method: Sit in sukhasana. Press the heel of your left leg along the Seevani Nadi or the peninium and place the right foot in between the thighs and calves of the left leg. Keep your hands on your knees in Gyana Mudra.

Focus: Meditate on all the chakras from the Mooladhar to the Sahasrar in their sequence of their placement.

Breathing: Breathe normally.

Time: Sit in this posture for as long as you comfortably can.

Direction: East or North (for spiritual benefits)

Benefits:

- It increases the strength and virility and enhances the glow of the face and makes one radiant.
- Improvement in eyesight.
- Nightfall and lust are cured and it develops the power of celibacy.
- If practised with a positive state of mind, it gradually removes all the disorders of the body.
- It purifies all the 72,000 nerves of the body.
- It keeps mental stress at bay.

Swastikasana (Auspicious pose)

Meaning: Everyone is familiar with the auspicious sign of Swastika (also called Satiya). This symbol is the provider of spiritual and materialistic happiness.

Method: Sit in Sukhasana. Place both the feet between your thighs and form an asana in the shape of a triangle. Keep your spine, neck and head erect. Fix your gaze between the brows.

According to Hathyoga Pradeepika:

जानूर्वोरन्तरे सम्यक् कृत्वा पादतले उभे।
ऋजुकायः समासीनः स्वस्तिकं तत् प्रचक्षते।।

Focus: On all the chakras in their sequential order for self-improvement.

Breathing: Breathe normally.

Time: As per your condition.

Direction: East or North (for spiritual benefits).

Chanting of Mantra: Chant 'OM' in a resounding voice.

Benefits: It gives all the benefits which are obtained from Guptasana and Sukhasana.

Yogasana

उत्तानौ चरणौ कृत्वा संस्थाप्य जानुनोपरि।
आसनोपरि संस्थाप्य उत्तानं करयुग्मकम्।।
पूरकैर्वायुमाकृष्य नासाग्रमवलोकयेत्।
योगासनं भवेदेतद् योगिनां योगसाधनम्।।

(Gherunda Samhita 44, 45)

Meaning: Lift your legs and place them on the thighs. Keep both the hands straight on the thighs. Then, pull the air up the body by doing Puraka Pranayama and fix your gaze on the tip of your nose. Hold the breath by doing Kumbhaka. This is called yogasana. Yogis should do this asana everyday.

Note: Breathing, time, benefits and **precautions** are the same as padmasana.

Ardha Padmasana (Half lotus pose)

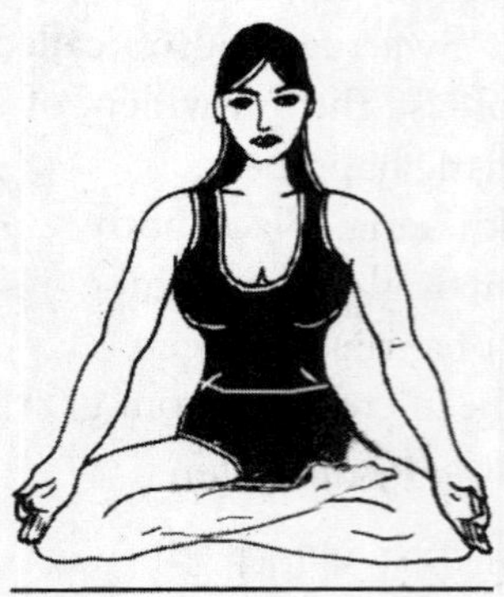

Meaning: 'Ardha' means half. It indicates not doing padmasana in its complete form.

Method: Sit down with a happy mind and spread your legs in front. Bend your left leg and place it under the right thigh. Bend the right leg and keep it on the left thigh. Keep both your hands on the knees. Keep your spine, neck and head straight. Remain in this position for some time and then switch the position of the legs.

Breathing: Breathe normally.

Focus: Meditate on all the chakras in their sequential order.

Direction: East or North (for spiritual reasons, if possible).

Time: As per convenience.

Benefits:

- Since the spine is kept erect, the whole body gets its benefit. This asana should be practised before doing Poorna Padmasana
- It enhances energy and awareness
- Any desired mantra, when chanted in this posture by focusing on inhalation and exhalation, gives stability to the mind.

Padmasana (Lotus pose)

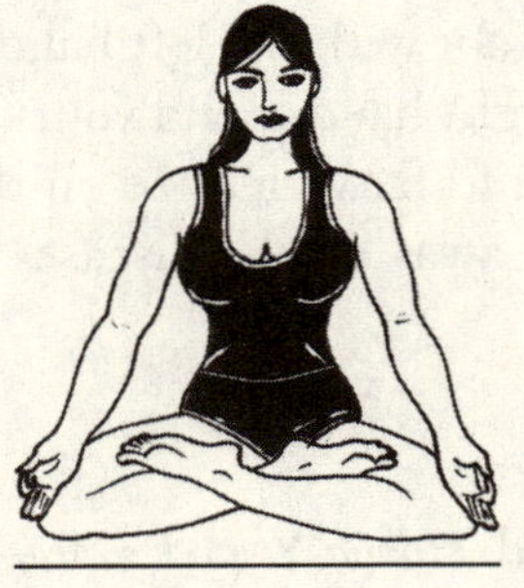
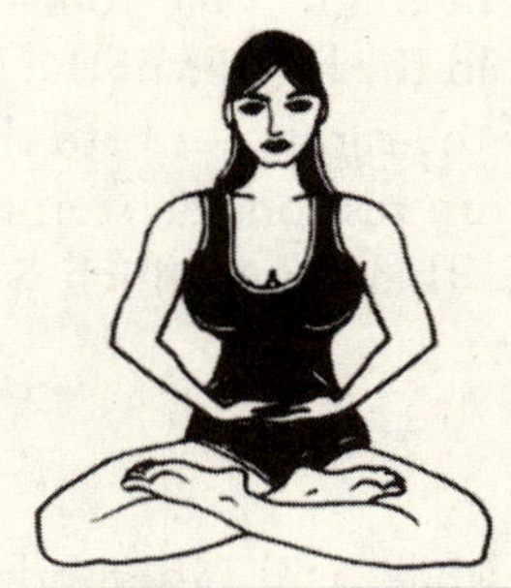

Meaning: 'Padma' means lotus.

Form: Like a lotus.

Direction: North or East (for spiritual reasons, if possible)

Note: Let us first understand the significance of this asana. This asana is one which grants all proficiencies or siddhis. It purifies all the 72,000 nerves of the body. This asana is the favourite of all spiritual practitioners. It is said to grant mastery over thousands of mantras. It is second to none in awakening the kundalini. When one meditates in this asana with a pure and concentrated mind, all sins are wiped out.

Method: To begin with, sit with your legs spread in front, or sit in Sukhasana. Then, place the left foot on the right thigh and the right foot on the left thigh. Let your spine remain erect. Both the knees should touch the ground. Keep your left palm on the soles of your feet and the right palm on the left palm in such a way that they touch your navel. Stay in this position for as long as you comfortably can. Breathe normally. In some places, it is suggested to keep the palms on the knees.

According to the Hath Yoga Pradeepika and Gherunda Samhita, Padmasana has been defined in different ways:

वामोरूपरि दक्षिणं हि चरणं संस्थाप्य वामं तथा,
दक्षोरूपरि पश्चिमेन विधिना धृत्वा कराभ्यां दृढम ।।
अङ्गुष्ठौ हृदये निधाय चिबुकं नासाग्रमालोकयेत्,
एतद्व्याधिविकारनाशनकरं पद्मासनं प्रोच्यते ।। (Gherunda Samhita 2/9)

Meaning: Place the right foot on the left thigh and the left foot on the right thigh. Take your hands to your back and cross them over to hold the big toe of the left foot with the left hand and the big toe of the right foot with the right hand. Bend your head and let your chin rest on the sternum and fix your gaze on the tip of your nose. This asana which wipes away all the diseases is called Padmasana.

Tips:

- Here, Maharishi Gherunda and *Hatha Yoga Pradeepika* have expounded the method of Baddha Padmasana as Padmasana. See Baddha Padmasana.
- In shloka number 44.45 in chapter two of Gherunda Samhita, the asana that is explained is like Padmasana.

Explanation: First, spread both your legs in front. Then, place the left foot on the right thigh and the right foot on the left thigh. Let the soles be turned up towards the sky. The heels must touch the abdomen and the knees should touch the ground. The back and the head should be straight. Bring your hands in front and hold the big toe of the left foot with the left hand and that of the right foot with the right hand. Bring your chin down to the sternum or in other words, do Jalandhar bandh and fix your gaze on the tip of the nose.

This asana, destroyer of all diseases, is called Padmasana.

According to Matsyendra Natha: Spread your legs in front and place the left foot on the right thigh and the right foot on the left thigh. Keep both your hands at the centre of your thighs and fix your gaze on the tip of your nose. Fix your tongue at the base of the jaw and place the chin at the sternum. Then, raise the air up, or in other words, do Moolbandh. This kriya destroys all diseases. Yogis call this kriya Padmasana.

According to Yogkundalyupanishada:

ऊर्वोरूपरि चेदद्यत्ते उभे पादतले यथा।
पद्मासनं भवेदेतत्सर्वपाप प्रणाशनम्।।

Meaning: When the soles of both the legs are placed on the opposite thigh, the asana so formed is called Padmasana. It is the destroyer of all sins.

It is mentioned in *Hatha Yoga Pradeepika*:

कृत्वासंपुटितौ करौ दृढ़तरं बद्धवा तु पद्यमासनं,
गाढं वक्षसि सन्निधाय चिबुकं ध्यायंश्च तच्चेतसि।
वारंवारमपानमूर्ध्वमनिलं प्रोत्सारयन्पूरितं,
न्यंचन्प्राणमुपैति बोधमतुलं शक्तिप्रभावान्नरः ।।

Explanation: According to the writer of *Hatha Yoga Pradeepika* you should place both the hands on your lap and sit firmly in Padmasana. Fix your chin firmly on your sternum, or in other words, do Jalandhara bandha and meditate on Bramha (God). Then, contract your anal muscles repeatedly and raise the Apana upwards and do Puraka and lower the Prana Vayu. In other words, merge the Prana and Apana together. In this way, the Kundalini is awakened and the practitioner gains unparalleled strength and knowledge.

Focus: Meditate on all the chakras and believe that all your chakras are being awakened; your soul is being purified, or you can chant the mantras given to you by your guru.

Precautions:

- Do not do this asana forcefully beyond your capacity.
- If you have pain in your knees, first do the kriyas related to Pavana Muktasana.
- Those who are suffering from sciatica and severe pain in the knee should do this very gradually.
- Whenever you do this asana, keep your spine, neck and head straight.
- You must change the position of your legs, so that the development of the body happens in a balanced manner.

Benefits:

- By doing this asana, the Prana Vayu merges with the Apana.
- This asana opens up all the nerves of the body.
- The Prana starts flowing through the Sushumna. As a result, one receives life giving energy.
- It destroys lust and balances the sexual power.
- It enhances energy and awareness.
- It enhances the glow on the face.
- It gradually decreases the diseases of the body and finally makes the body disease free.
- It helps lessen the fluctuations in the mind and provides mental peace.
- When this asana is done regularly, it destroys all the sins.
- It is especially helpful in awakening the kundalini.
- If one meditates in this asana for 10-15 minutes, it rectifies the displaced navel.
- By regular practice of this asana, all the 72,000 nerves of the body get purified.
- By doing this asana, the blood circulation decreases in the legs, and as a result, it improves in the abdomen and the waist. So, one gets benefit in these parts of the body.

Note: Some yoga teachers call this asana **Kamalasana, Shri Asana, Aadi Asana, Bramha Asana** and **Muktpadmasana.**

Variation: Lie down on your stomach in Padmasana posture and take your hands and join them in **Namaskara Mudra**. This posture is called **Gupta Padmasana**. Some yoga teachers call it **Patanga Asana** as well.

Baddha Padmasana (Locked lotus pose)

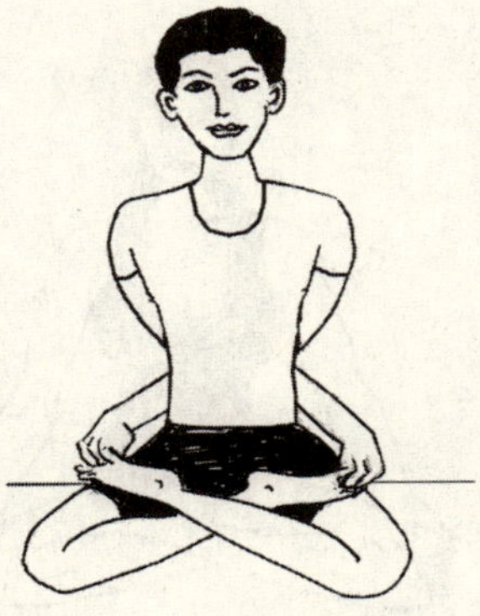

Meaning: 'Baddha' means tied or held.

Method: Sit in Padmasana. Exhale and taking both your hands back, cross them over and bring them in front. Then, hold the big toe of the right foot with your right hand and that of the left foot with the left hand. If you find it difficult to reach your toe, try to bend forward and then hold it. Place your chin on the sternum and fix your gaze at the tip of your nose. Come back to the original position. Breathe normally.

Focus: On Swadhishthana chakra and Anahata chakra

Breathing/time: Practice doing this asana for 2-5 minutes. Breathe normally or do Pranayama.

Benefits:

- Lifts up the chest and makes it strong.
- It strengthens the muscles of the hands, shoulders, knees and legs.
- The disorders related to stomach are cured. The power to digest becomes strong. Constipation is cured and hunger is enhanced.
- It enhances the capacity of the heart, lungs and kidneys and makes them active.
- It enhances the beauty of the breasts in women.

Note: It is not necessary that you will be able to get hold of the big toe in the first attempt itself. So try to only reach till the legs. After a few days, you will be able to hold the big toe.

Precautions: People with sciatica and severe pain in the spine should do this asana very carefully.

Comments:

- You can do Yoga Mudrasana (Psychic union pose) in this posture.
- It is more beneficial if Jalandhara bandha and Moolbandha are practised in this asana (see chapter on Bandha).

Siddhasana/Vijayasana (Accomplished pose)

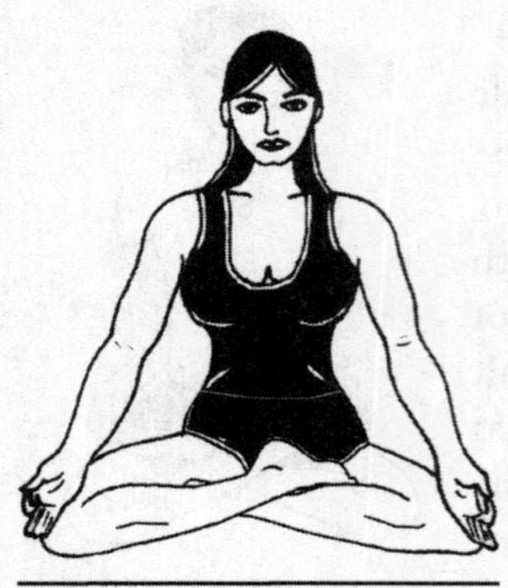

Form: Similar to Padmasana, it is helpful in acquiring Siddhis, that is why it is called siddhasana.

Focus: On all the chakras

Method: Sit down in Sukhasana. Place the sole of your left foot close to the right thigh in such a way that the heels touch the area in between your anus and the ovaries. Then, place the heel of the right foot close to the genitals or the testicles. Let the toes of the right foot be in between the calves and thighs of the left leg. Make sure that the knees touch the ground. Body should remain erect. Place your hands on the knees in Gyana Mudra. Keep your chin on the sternum. Fix your gaze in between the brows and sit in this position without feeling any stress. Then, change the position of the legs.

Direction: East or North (for spiritual benefits)

Breathing: Do this asana with Pranayama/as per convenience.

Time: For as long as you can comfortably sit.

Mantra: Chant the mantra given to you by your guru or chant 'Om Namah Siddhebhyaha'.

Note: The benefits of Padmasana and Siddhasana are almost similar. This asana is ideal to make the energy and awareness move in the upward direction, therefore, all practitioners and celebs (Bramhacharis) should do this asana without fail. This asana must be done to gain the benefits of Pranayama and meditation.

Benefits:

- By doing this asana, one is able to develop strong willpower.
- The spine becomes strong and firm.
- Disorders related to the anus are cured and lust is destroyed.
- By doing Siddhasana everyday for 48 minutes, one can attain Siddhis.

- The back does not bend even in old age.
- If Trataka is done in this asana, one can develop the power to hypnotise people.
- The abdominal region gets optimum benefits through this asana.

Precautions: If you are suffering from sciatica or severe pain in the back and knees, do this asana very carefully and with a lot of patience.

Parvatasana/Viyogasana (Mountain pose)

Meaning: The general meaning of 'Parvata' is a mountain. Parvatasana is also called Viyogasana.

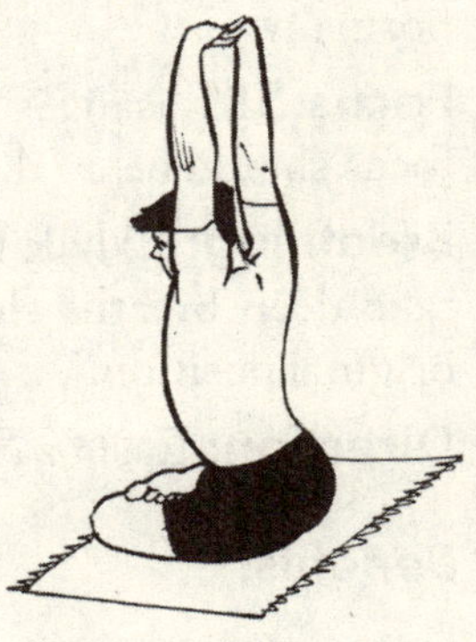

Method: Sit down in Padmasana. Raise your arms above the head in Namaskara Mudra, and then interlock the fingers and stretch your hands upwards. The hands should be absolutely stretched. Hold this position for as long as you comfortably can.

Focus: On Agya chakra

Breathing: Inhale while taking your hands up and exhale while bringing them down.

Time: This kriya should be repeated 5-6 times/do it for 1-2 minutes.

Benefits:

- It stops the trembling of hands and strengthens then hand muscles.
- The lungs become stronger. It has a salutary effect on the spine.
- It has some effect on hernia as well.
- It gives good shape to the breasts in women.

Notes:

- This is also done by standing on the knees (see **Gorakshasana**).
- The posture no. 5 in Surya Namaskara is also called **Parvatasana.**

Yoga Mudrasana (Psychic union pose)

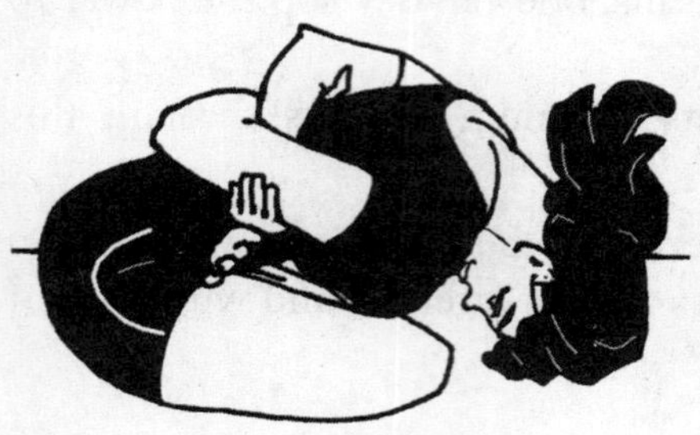

Method: Sit in Padmasana with your eyes closed and mind at peace. Take your hands to your back and hold one wrist with the other hand. Exhale and bend forward from your waist. Try to touch your head to the ground. Remain in this position for 10-15 seconds. Breathe normally.

Focus: This asana is ideal to awaken all the chakras. But the main focus should be on the Mooladhara and Agya chakra.

Breathing: Exhale while bending forward. In the final position, take deep breaths slowly and inhale while coming back to the original position.

Direction: East or North (for spiritual reasons)

Benefits:

- It activates the functioning of the digestive system.
- It removes constipation.
- It improves the contraction of the lungs.
- It is beneficial for spiritual reasons.
- The spine gets complete benefit.
- It is helpful in awakening the kundalini.

Precautions: People suffering from high blood pressure, sciatica, heart diseases and pregnant women should not do this asana.

Notes:

- To do this asana perfectly, try to hold the toes of your feet and bend forward gradually. If you have any problem while doing this, interlock your arms at the back.
- To know more, see Padmasana and Baddha Padmasana.

Vajrasana and Related Asanas

Vajrasana (Thunderbolt pose)

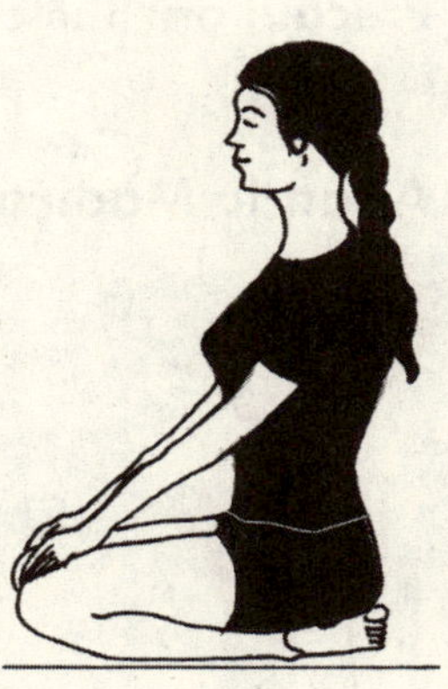

Meaning: 'Vajra' means firm or stern. This asana makes us firm.

Method: Bend your knees and sit in a manner so that your buttocks rest in between your soles and the genitals are placed in between your heels. The big toes of both the feet should touch each other. Place both your hands on the knees and form Gyana mudra or sit in a normal posture. Remember to keep your spine, back and neck absolutely straight, to gain more benefits from this asana.

Note: Though this asana is very easy to perform, it is like a wish granting tree.

Breathing: You can do Pranayama in this posture. If you do it after your meals, breathe from your right nostril.

Focus: On all the chakras, but mainly on the Manipura chakra.

Mantra: You can chant the mantra given to you by your guru, or you can meditate on your God, or chant 'Om Namah Siddhebhyaha' in your mind.

Benefits:

- Those who practice Vajrasana regularly will be strong and firm even in old age.
- It is beneficial for self-realisation.
- It opens up the path for Sushumna.
- It is beneficial in hernia and piles.
- One must do this asana for 10-15 minutes after meals.
- This asana is very beneficial for diseases related to the wind.
- It gives happiness when done while facing east or north.
- It removes the irregularities of the menstrual cycles in women and keeps them disease free.
- It is best for headaches caused due to wind disorders.
- It cures constipation and poor digestion.

Note: Some yoga teachers ask to place one big toe on the other while doing this asana.

Precaution: Those suffering from knee pain should not do this asana.

Ananda Madirasana (Intoxicating bliss pose)

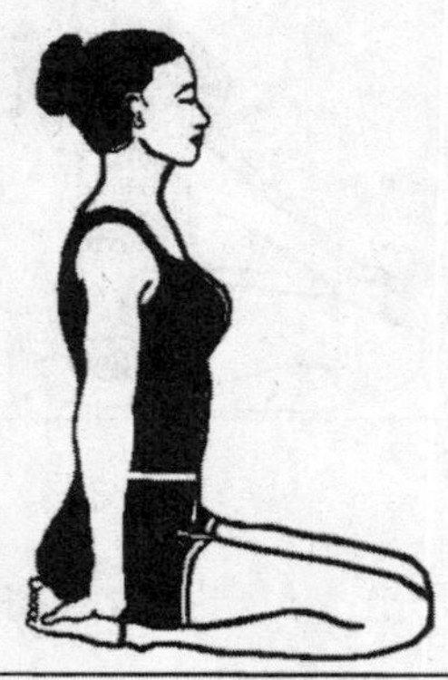

Variation 1. Sit in Vajrasana and place your hands on your feet in such a way that the thumbs are on the soles and the fingers of both the hands face each other. This posture is called Ananda Madirasana.

Note: Focus, benefits and precautions same as Vajrasana.

Padadirasana (Breath balancing pose)

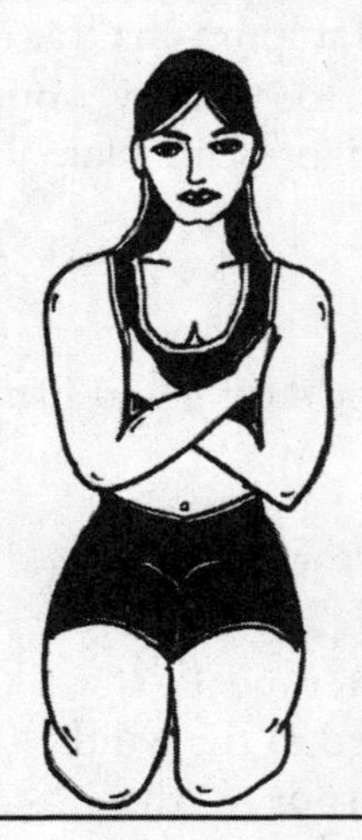

Variation 2. Sit in Vajrasana and cross your arms over your chest. Place your right palm under the left armpit and the left palm under the right armpit in such a way that the fingers are in and the thumbs are out, turned up. Then, forcefully press the part between the fingers and the thumb. Close your eyes and focus on your breathing.

Benefits: This asana removes the obstacles faced while breathing

Note: This asana can be practised to bring about ease in doing Pranayam. If your right nostril is blocked, press the armpit of the opposite side with the right hand. The breathing will be normalised in a short while. If both the nostrils are blocked, then press both the armpits.

Shashakasana (Rabbit pose)/ Shashankasana (Reclined moon pose)

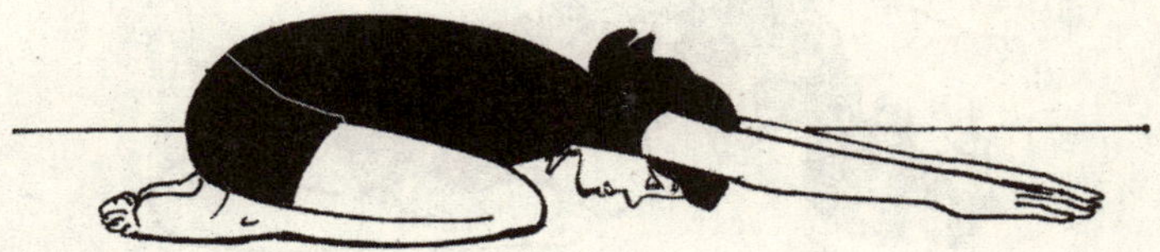

Meaning: 'Shash' means rabbit. It also means the blot seen in the Moon. Since this asana resembles a rabbit in a sitting posture, it is called Shashakasana. Shash + ank = Shashank which means Moon.

Method: Sit in Vajrasana. Inhale and take your hands up, arms touching the ears. Inhale and bend forward to touch your head and both the hands to the ground. Do Bahya kumbhaka. Then, inhale and raise your arms and body together. Exhale and come back to the original position. Be cautious of your breathing.

Breathing: Already mentioned in the method.

Time: Repeat this kriya 10-15 times.

Benefits:

- This asana helps get rid of all the disorders related to the abdomen.
- The disorders of the spine are cured.
- It benefits the urinary bladder in women.
- It regularises the blood circulation.
- It cures mental disorders.
- It cures wind-related disorders.
- It cures the disorders of the reproductive organs.

Precaution: People with very high blood pressure should not do this asana.

Supta Vajrasana (Reclined thunderbolt)

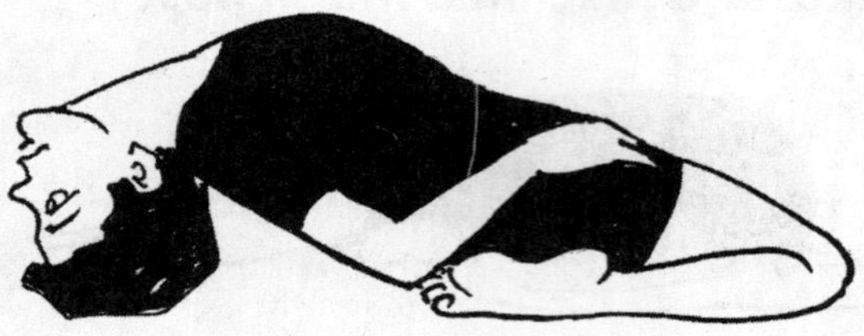

Method: Sit in Vajrasana. Place your elbows one at a time on the sides. Supporting your body on the elbows, lie down on the ground. Then, lift your back and place the top of your head on the ground by raising your neck. Keep your hands either on your chest or on the thighs. Do this asana according to your capacity.

Focus: From Svadhishthana to Vishuddhi chakras.

Breathing: Exhale while bending backwards. Take slow deep breaths in the final posture. Inhale while coming back to the original position.

Time: 2-3 minutes

Benefits:

- Cures constipation and brings glow on the face.
- This asana strengthens the calves, thighs, chest and the backbone.
- This asana gives complete benefit to the abdominal region, spine and chest.

Precautions:

- Only after coming back to the original position (in Vajrasana), unfold your knees and spread your legs, otherwise the joints of the knees may get dislocated.
- People suffering from sciatica, back ache, knee pain and slip disc should do this asana carefully, with a lot of patience.

Note: By doing this asana, one can obtain almost all the benefits of **Vajrasana, Matsyasana, Paryankasana** and **Uttana Mandookasana (Variation 2)**.

Paryankasana (Couch pose) Variation 1

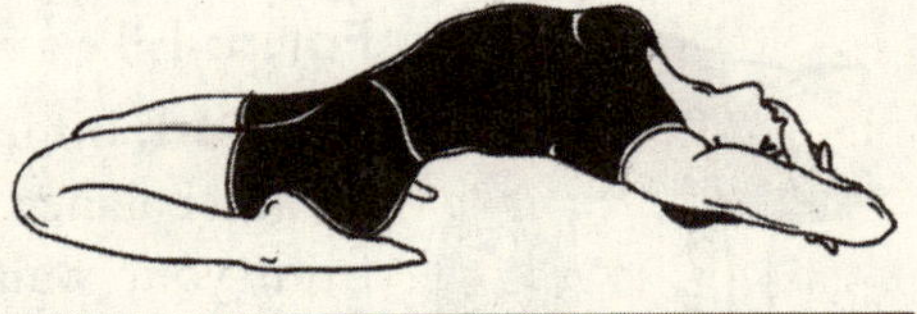

Meaning: 'Paryanka' means bed.

Method: Sit down in Vajrasana. Bend backward. In this asana, only the upper part of your head should touch the ground. Lift your back and neck to resemble a bridge. Take your hands beyond your head and interlock them. Hold the left elbow with the right hand and the right elbow with the left hand (see illustration). Breathe normally. Hold this position for 50-60 seconds. Unfold your hands and come back to the Vajrasana position. Then, unfold your knees one by one and straighten your legs. Relax in Shavasana.

Breathing: Exhale while forming the position of the asana. When you reach the final position, take slow deep breaths. Inhale while coming back to the original position.

Time: Once you get used to it, you may increase the time of this asana from 50 seconds to 3 minutes. Repeat it 2-3 times.

Benefits:

- It gives all the benefits of **Vajrasana, Supta Vajrasana** and **Matsyasana.**
- All the parts of the back expand completely, which gives a chance to the lungs to expand. Hence, people who have breathing problems benefit from it.
- The nerves of the neck get stretched and the thyroid glands get activated. Hence, they start functioning well.
- It cures thyroid.

Precautions: Observe all the precautions which are to be observed for Supta Vajrasana.

Note: Some yoga instructors consider this asana similar to Supta Vajrasana. The second variation of Paryankasana is given in later pages under the section 'Exercises of advanced order and balance'.

Special: In the book Maranya Kandika, Padmasana has been called Paryankasana. This text was written in 940 AD (is about 1080 years old) and is available today as well.

Ushtrasana (Camel pose)

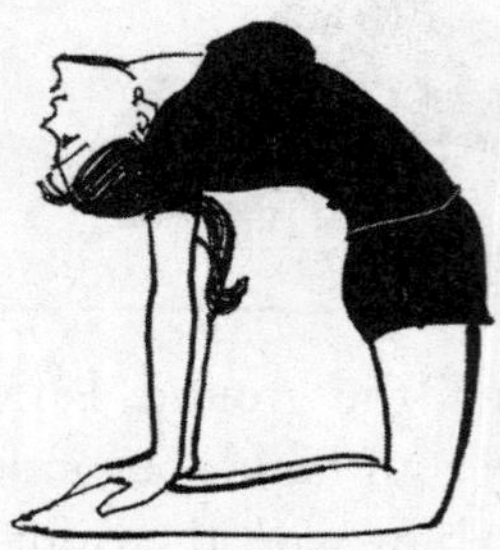

Form: Like a camel; 'Ushtra' means camel.

Method: Sit in Vajrasana. Raise your body up and balance it on your knees. Bend back from your waist and hold the right heel with the right hand and the left heel with the left hand. Bend your head backwards. Lift up your abdominal region, navel and the genital area. Bend your head and spine backwards as much as possible and remain in this position for about 10-15 seconds.

Breathing: Inhale while holding the heels. Breathe normally in the final position.

Time: 10-15 seconds

Focus: On Svadhishthana chakra and Vishuddhi chakra

Special note: Keep your focus on the Mooladhara chakra and pull the anus inward.

Benefits:

- It reduces obesity and makes the body slim.
- Asthma patients should definitely do this asana. By doing this asana, the respiratory system gets strengthened.
- It strengthens the lungs.
- It destroys diabetes.
- It is a sure shot remedy for constipation. People with constipation should do this asana everyday.
- It cures all diseases related to the stomach.
- It cures back ache and pain in the waist. It removes all the diseases of the reproductive organs.
- This asana is very beneficial for many ailments in women.
- It enhances the power of the eye.
- It keeps the vocal chords in order.

Precaution: If you are suffering from any chronic or major disease of the spine, back or hip, you should do this asana very cautiously.

Note: To do **Poorna Ushtrasana,** touch your hands to the ground.

Koormasana (Tortoise pose) Variation 1

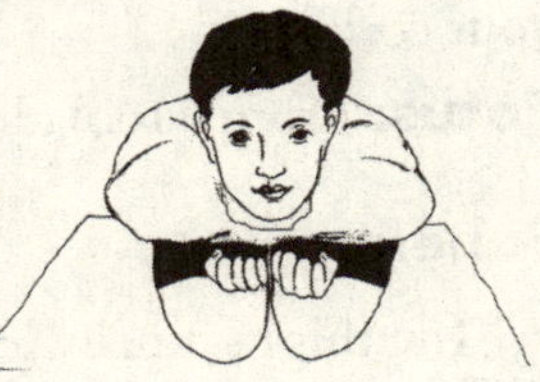

Method: According to Gherunda Samhita, 'Keep your heels in inverted order under the Sivni Nadi and sit with your body, head and neck straight in one line'. This is called Koormasana. After sitting in this posture, join your elbows and place them on your navel. Form partial fist with your hands and exhale while bending forward. Try to look in front.

Breathing: Breathe normally in the final posture.

Time: 1-2 minutes

Benefits:

- The objective of this asana is to withdraw our body inwards like a tortoise, or in other words, the practitioner should not let his sense organs go astray towards materialistic things, but win over them through self-control, meditation and sacrifice.
- The abdominal region benefits from it and the digestive system becomes strong.

Precautions: People suffering from hernia should not do this asana. Those with chronic stomach disorders should also not do it.

Note: The second variation of Koormasana is given under 'Exercises of advanced order and balance'.

Bhadrasana (Gracious pose)

Meaning: 'Bhadra' means modest or well-mannered.

Method: Sit in Vajrasana. Slowly spread your knees and bring the fingers of your feet close to each other. (Spread your knees as much as possible). Let your buttocks touch the ground. Place your hands on your knees in Gyana Mudra. According to Gherunda Samhita– keep both the heels in an inverted posture under the Seevani Nadi. Then, move your hands to your back and hold the toes of your feet. Do Jalandhara bandha and fix your gaze at the tip of your nose. This asana is the destroyer of all diseases.

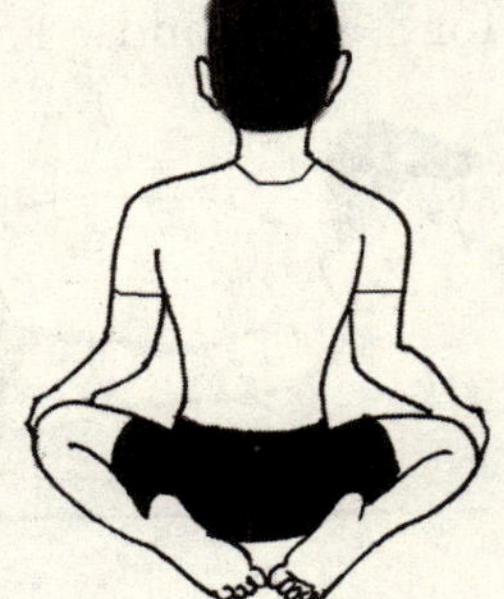

Breathing/time: Breathe normally. Hold the posture as per your comfort.

Focus: From Mooladhara to Agya chakra

Benefits:

- The thighs, knees, legs and heels become firm and strong.
- Lust is destroyed. Therefore, it is beneficial for spiritual progress.
- It cures diseases such as piles, diabetes, enlargement of the scrotum and fistula.
- By doing this asana, one can automatically get all the benefits of Vajrasana.
- It is helpful in the development of Mooladhara chakra.

Precaution: People with severe back ache should do this asana very slowly.

Mandookasana/Bhekasana (Frog pose)

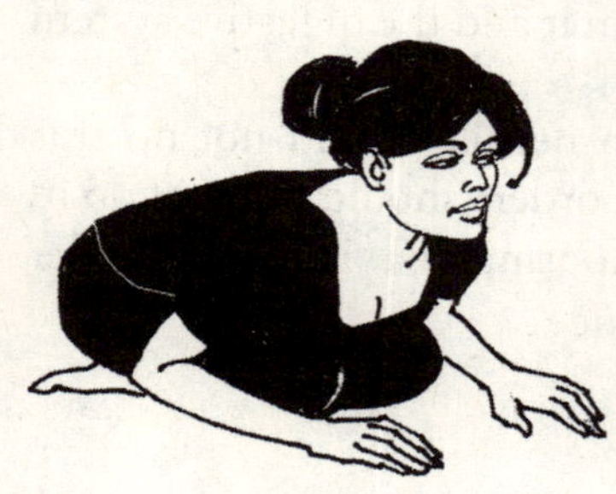

Meaning: 'Mandooka' means frog. When we do this asana, our body resembles a frog. That is why it is called Mandookasana.

Method 1: Sit in Vajrasana. Slowly move your knees apart and come in a position where both the toes touch each other. Keep your palms flat on the ground either in front of the knees or by their sides. Bend forward from your waist while keeping your spine straight. Keep your head up. Breathe normally. Hold this posture for 8-10 seconds.

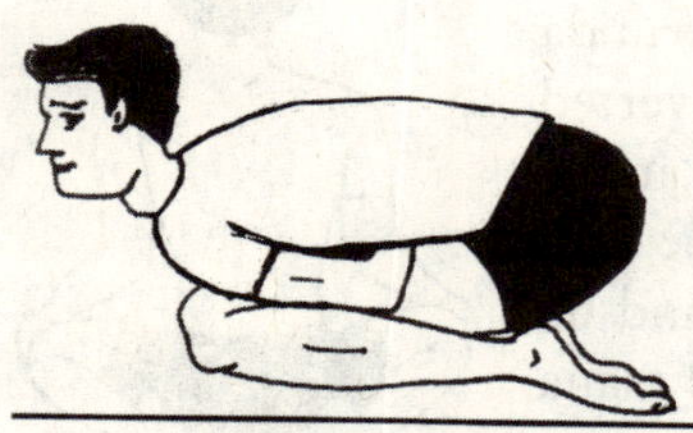

Method 2: In the same position, instead of keeping your hands by the side of your knees, form a fist and place them near your navel, then, press them against your stomach. Bend forward and look straight ahead.

Breathing: Exhale while bending forward. Inhale while coming back to the original posture.

Focus: On Swadhishthana chakra

Benefits:

- It regulates the digestive system and destroys bad odour and diseases caused due to its malfunctioning.
- It prevents the back from bending in old age.
- It is very beneficial for women. It affects their reproductive organs.
- It reduces extra fat from the thighs, buttocks and the abdomen area.

Note: Both the above mentioned methods are very popular. That is why they have been mentioned here. The first method is called Mandooki asana in some places.

Caution: Pregnant women should not do this asana.

Uttana Mandookasana (Extended frog pose) (2 type)

Meaning: 'Uttana' means severe or stretch, and Mandooka means 'frog'.

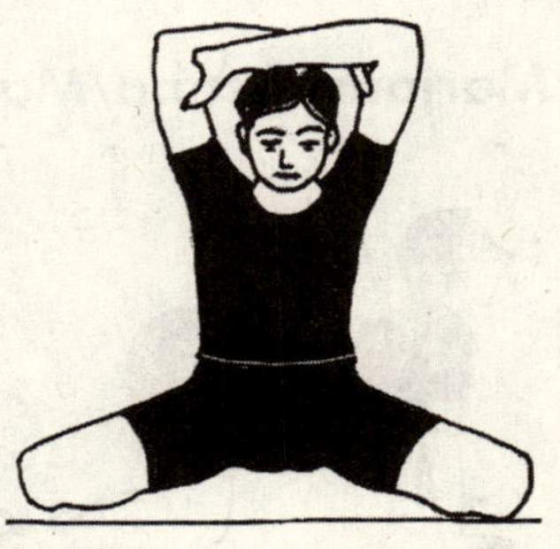

Variation 1: This posture is same as Mandookasana, only the position of the hands must change. The hands are taken over the head and interlocked. The right elbow is held with the left hand and the left elbow is held with the right hand. Inhale and broaden your chest. Look straight ahead. Do this as per your comfort.

Benefits:

- When this asana is done while doing Kumbhaka, the power of the lungs is enhanced.
- The impurities of the blood are removed and the energy is kept under control by this asana.

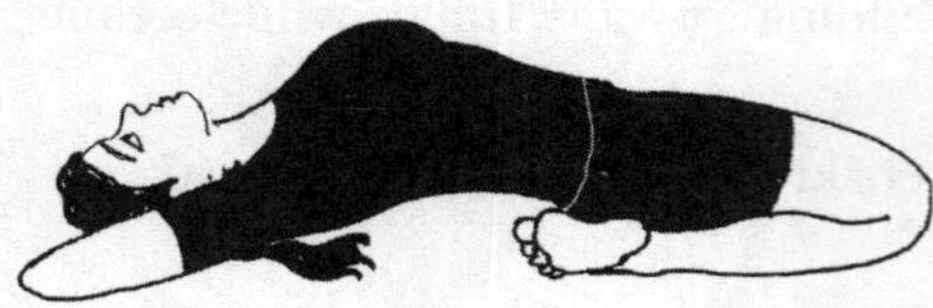

Variation 2: Sit in Vajrasana. Slowly bend your body backwards and let the head touch the ground. Take your hands back and let your head rest on your elbows. For extra information, see Supta Vajrasana and Paryankasana. The benefits of this asana are also similar to those asanas.

Focus: Concentrate on Svadhishthana, Manipuraka and Anahata chakra.

Breathing: When you reach the final position, breathe normally. Inhale while coming back to the original position.

Time: For about 2-3 minutes, 2-3 times.

Benefits: All the benefits of this asana are similar to those of Paryankasana and Supta Vajrasana.

Note: Both the above mentioned methods are given here because they are very popular.

Marjaari Asana/Marjaara Asana (Cat pose)

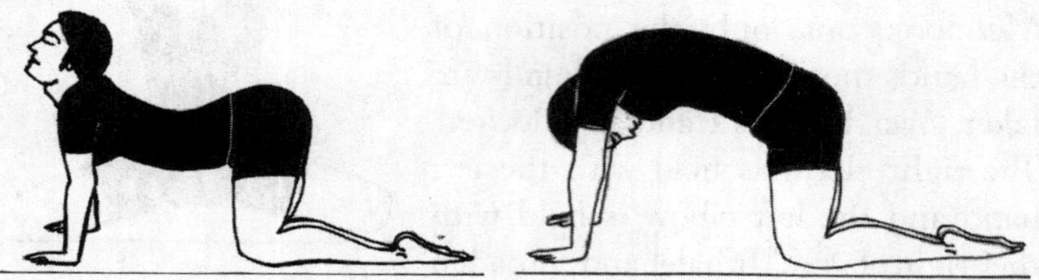

Meaning: 'Marjaari' means cat.

Method: To start with, sit in Vajrasana. Raise yourself on your knees and keep your hands on the ground in such a way that the fingers point towards the front. The elbows should not be bent. The position of the legs should be as shown in the illustration. This is the preparatory position to begin this asana.

Then, inhale and bend your spine downwards, as if someone is pressing down your back, and slightly lift your neck up. Then, exhale and lift up your spine and bend your neck down to touch the chest. For special benefits, exhale and contract your stomach. This is one round.

Breathing/time: Be very cautious of the pattern of breathing in and out. Repeat this kriya 8-10 times.

Benefits:

- Cures constipation.
- It fortifies the waist, spine and the neck and keeps them disease free.
- It is extremely effective for women.
- It is also beneficial for the lungs .

Precaution: People suffering from severe pain in the spine and waist/hips should do this asana very slowly.

Veerasana (Warrior pose)

Meaning: 'Veer' means Kshatriya, warrior and brave.

Note: There are many popular methods of doing this asana.

Variation 1: Sit in Vajrasana, but with your buttocks touching the ground from in between your heels. Your heels should be by the sides of your buttocks. The distance between your heels should be about one and a half feet. Place your hands on your knees in Gyana Mudra. Keep your back straight. Take deep breaths and remain in this position for as long as you comfortably can. Then, join both your hands and raise them straight above your head. Take deep breaths and remain in this position for some time. Then, loosen your hands and bring them down on your soles. Bend forward. Fix your gaze on the tip of your nose. Breathe normally. Exhale and get up to straighten up your legs and relax.

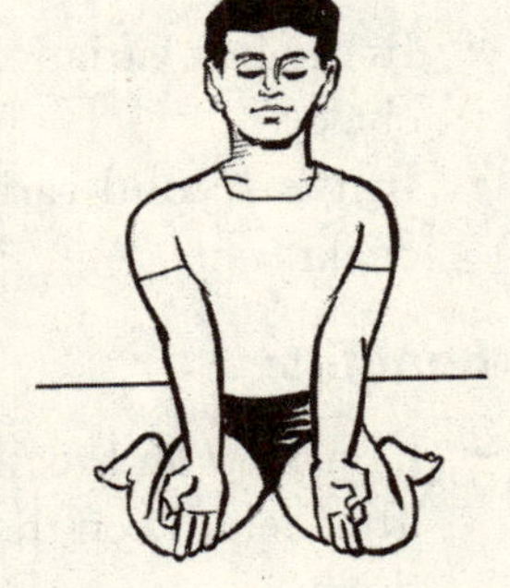

Benefits:

- Since this is a variation of Vajrasana, it can be done after meals. It helps normalise the digestive power and removes the heaviness caused by eating meals (If you do this asana after meals, do not bend forward).
- It removes common pain in the knees caused due to wind. It also cures gout.
- It gives relief from pain in the ankles.
- It destroys the disorders caused due to wind.
- The body becomes light and the mind becomes happy.

Variation 2: In this second variation, sit in Vajrasana. Bend one leg (place the heel flat on the ground and raise the folded knee) and place it next to the other knee. Join your palms together and take them above your head, or keep them as shown in the illustration. Breathe normally. Then, do this asana by changing the legs. Stay in this position for at least 8-10 seconds. Do this kriya 4-6 times. Some yoga masters also called it Heros Pose.

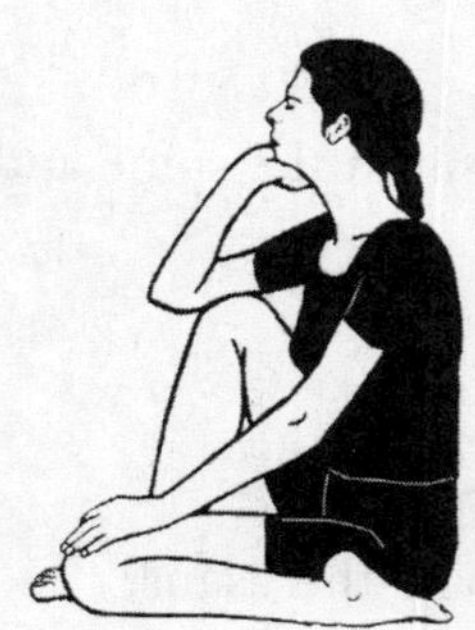

Focus:

- In the first variation, the focus should be on the Svadhishthana chakra.
- In the second variation, the focus should be on Mooladhara chakra.

Benefits:

- Control your breath while focusing on the Mooladhara chakra. This helps keep the breath in Kumbhaka situation for a longer time.
- All the chakras get benefit from it.
- It helps in increasing concentration.
- It makes the nervous system sensitive.
- It activates and helps in the efficient functioning of the liver, stomach, kidney and the reproductive organs.

Variation 3: Make the Vajrasana posture with one leg and place the foot of the other leg on the thigh of the first leg. Those who are new in the practice can take the support of their hands to stand on their knees and then maintaining balance. They should take their hands above their head and join the palms in the prayer posture. Remain in this position for some time and then come back to the original position. Change the legs and repeat the posture. Keep your gaze fixed on the tip of the nose or look in front.

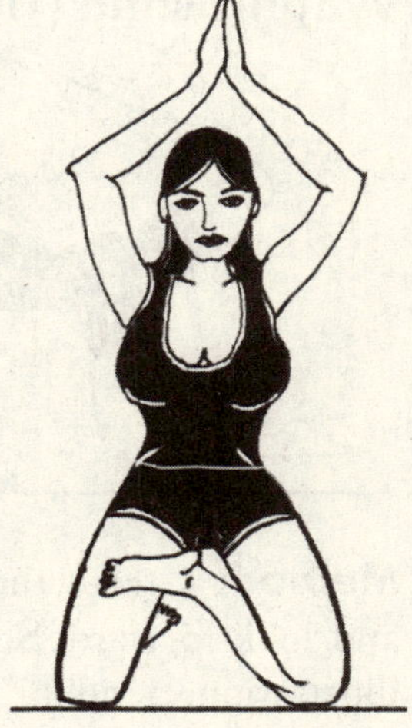

Breathing: Inhale while raising your body up. When in the final posture, breathe normally. Exhale while coming back to the original position.

Benefits:

- It benefits the abdominal region.
- It eliminates laziness.
- It brings stability to your vision.
- Eye sight becomes sharper.

Note: Some Yoga teachers teach this asana according to the first variation. Some yogacharyas call the first method **Bramhacharya asana**. The second variation is according to the Gherunda Samhita. There are other variations of this asana as well.

Yoga exercise was as much needed by humankind yesterday as it is needed today, and will be needed tomorrow as well.

–RJT

Vyaghrasana (Tiger pose) Variation 1

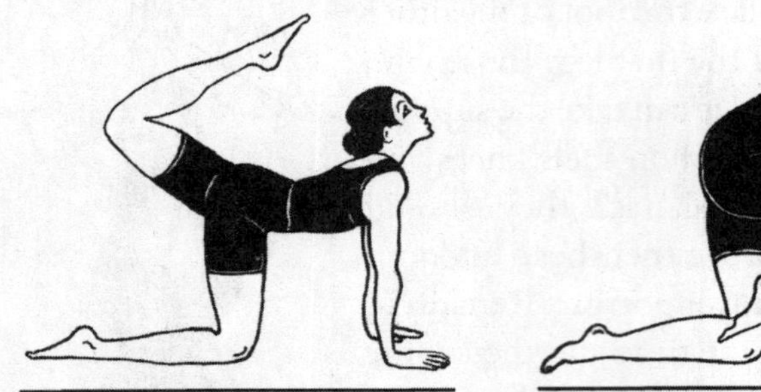

Method: Create the Marjaari asana posture. Raise your head and look forward. Straighten up your right leg as shown in the illustration. Bend it from the knee and bring it towards your head.

Then, bring down the same leg and bring it forward close to the chest, touching your nose with the knees. While doing this, the spine should be raised. Repeat the above mentioned process with the other leg.

Breathing/time: Repeat this kriya at least 3-5 times. Inhale while stretching your leg back. Hold your breath while bending your knee and taking it up, and exhale while bending the knee towards the chest.

Note: While bringing the knee close to the chest, do not let the feet touch the ground.

Benefits:

- It is very beneficial for women. It tones up their reproductive organs. A few months after pregnancy women can do this asana and gain benefits.
- Those who are suffering from sciatica can do this asana and become disease free.
- It makes the spine flexible and helps the digestive system function effectively.
- It makes the abdomen, thighs and buttocks well-shaped.

Note: The second variation is given later under 'Exercises of the Advanced Order and Balance'.

Asanas Done by Standing and Bending

Tadasana (Palm tree pose with raised bound hands)

Method: Stand absolutely straight with your legs together (in Samavastha), but keep the big toes and the heels a little apart, in one line. Put pressure on the toes and lift your heels and body up; interlock your fingers and stretch your arms straight up. In this position, the muscles of the knees and thighs should either be pulled up or left loose. Contract your stomach as much as possible. Bring your chest out in front. Keep your spine and neck straight. The entire weight of the body should be balanced only on the toes. Remain in this position for some time.

Breathing: Inhale while raising the body up and exhale while coming back to the original position.

Time: Repeat it 5-6 times/do it for 2-4 minutes.

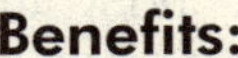

Benefits:

- This is the best exercise to increase the height.
- It gives stability to the body.
- It makes the muscles strong.
- Those who are suffering from slip disc must do this asana.
- It is beneficial for women, specially during the first few months of pregnancy.
- It ensures that the child is born healthy.
- It is an important part of the Shankha Prakshalana kriya.

Precautions: Put pressure on your toes together and balance your weight on them. Be mindful of your balance. After doing this, do any asana related to Sheershasana.

Note: When you are in the final position, look up and imagine that an object is kept at a height and you are trying to get hold of it. By doing this, you will automatically get several benefits.

Tiryaka Tadasana/Urdhva Hastottanasana (Swaying palm tree pose)

Meaning: 'Tiryaka' means crooked, bent, or something which is not straight. Tada is a tree (palm tree) which is very tall.

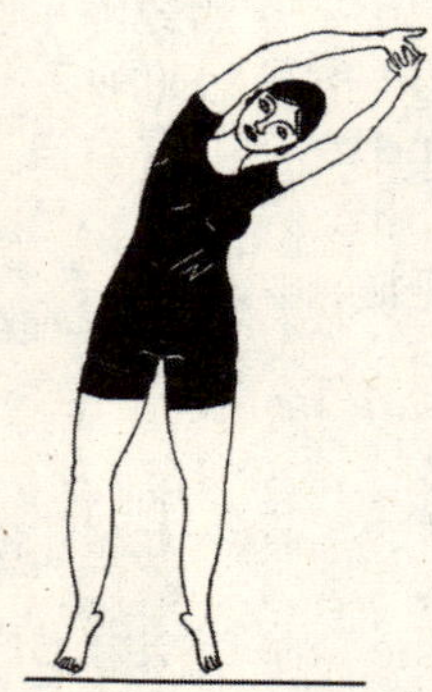

Method: Stand in Tadasana. Lift up your body, balance it on your toes and twist it right and left 10 times each. If you find it difficult to stand on your toes, you can do this exercise without lifting your heels.

Breathing: Inhale while raising up your body. Exhale while twisting your body to the right and to the left. Inhale while coming back to the original position.

Kati Chakrasan (Standing Spinal Twist)

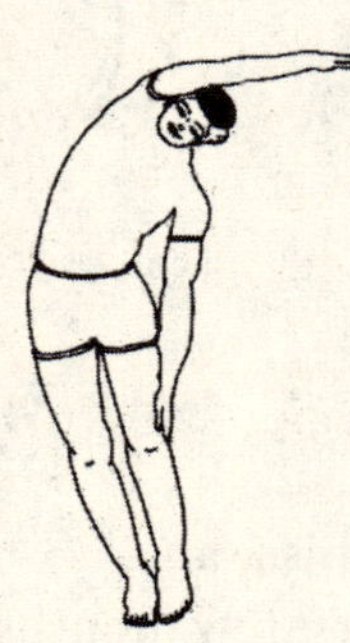

Method. Stand in the attention position. Now stretch your right hand up in such a way that your arm touches the ears. Try to bend your body so much that the left palm touches your knee. Repeat this exercise with your left hand. Breathe out while bending and breathe in while returning to normal position.

Benefits:

- You will automatically get all the benefits of Tadasana.
- This asana is excellent for the Shankha Prakshalana kriya.
- It destroys all the disorders of the stomach. It cures all problems of passing the motion.
- It reduces fat around the belly. The waist becomes slim and flexible.

Note: Some yoga teachers teach this asana by changing the position of the legs.

Gatimaya Samkonasana (Dynamic straight angle pose)

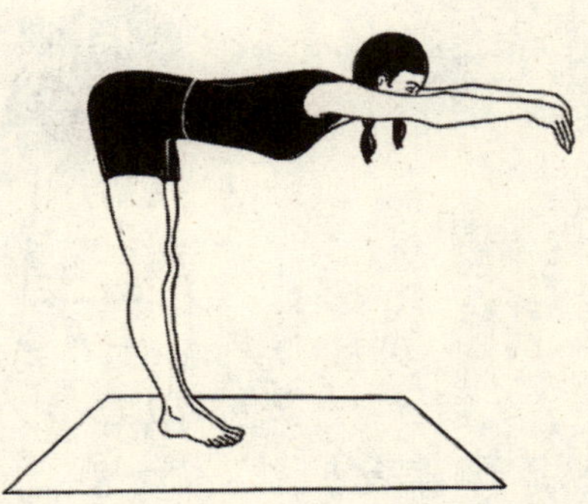

Method: Stand in Samavastha. Raise both your hands and join them above the head in the prayer posture. The arms should touch the ears. Slightly bend your back and take your buttocks a little back. Then, bend your body from the waist and bring your head, chest and hands forward to form a right angle between the legs, the waist and the head. In other words, form a right angle with the upper body and the ground. Hold this position for 5-10 seconds then, come back to the original position. After practising, you can increase the speed of doing this asana.

Breathing/time: Exhale while bending forward and inhale while coming back to the original position.

Benefits:

- The disorders of the spine are cured.
- Since it is effective for the back of the neck, it cures ordinary disorders and is also beneficial in curing many diseases.

Precaution: People with a stiff spine, cervical problems and sciatica should not do this asana.

Gatimaya Dolasana (Dynamic pendulum pose)

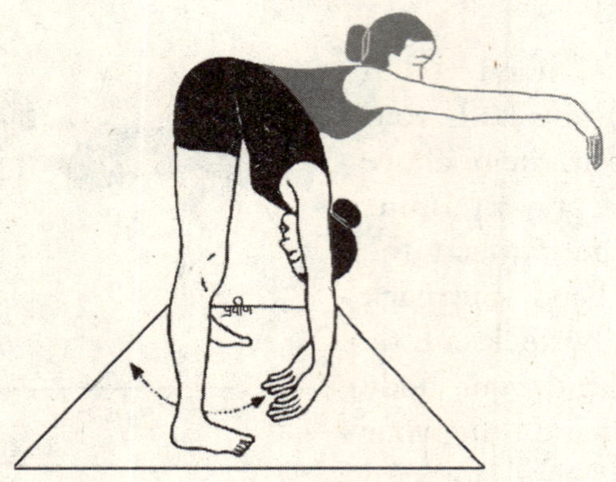

Method: Stand in the posture of Trilokasana, which means that stand with your feet apart. Raise your arms straight up and let your arms touch your ears. Either join the fingers of your hands or leave them open. Then, bend your body from the waist to form a right angle with the ground. Let your body loose and let it swing down like a pendulum. Come back to the right angle posture and then, to the original position.

Breathing/time: Swing your body in between your legs in the final position at least 4-5 times. Breathe out from your mouth to completely empty your lungs. Inhale while coming back to the original position.

Benefits:

- The lungs get toned up. Gradually, all their disorders are removed and their capacity to receive oxygen increases.
- The nerves at the back of the knees and those at the back of our body receive are stretched, as a result the blood circulation in these areas is regularised.
- The face and the head receive abundant blood supply, and as a result many disorders automatically get cured.

Precaution: People with high blood pressure, giddiness, back ache and pain in the waist/hips should not do this asana.

Sakatasana/Sankatasana (Difficult pose)

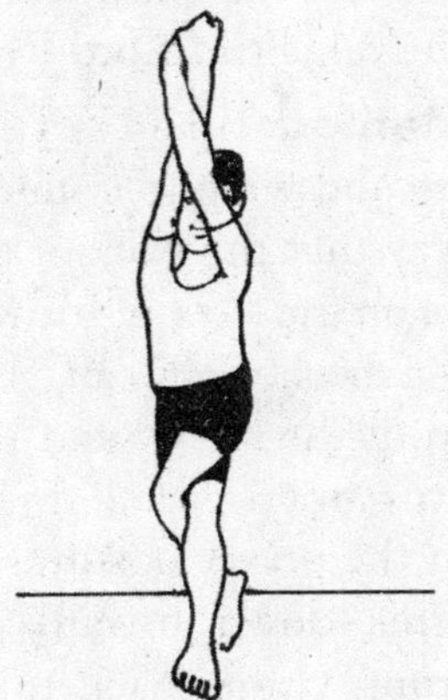

Meaning: 'Sankata' means trouble or problem, and 'Sakata' or 'Shakhota' is the name of a tree.

Method: Stand in Tadasana. Wrap your left leg over the right leg. Take your hands above your head and intertwine your left hand around the right hand (some yoga teachers suggest keeping the hands on the knees). Breathe normally. Then, change the position of the legs and hands and repeat the exercise. Keep your body straight.

Breathing/time: Breathe normally. Do it for a time period as per your convenience.

Benefits:

- It makes the legs strong. By regular and constant practice, the trembling in the legs can be cured.
- The hands gain strength.
- It is beneficial for hip pain, back and in cases of hernia.

Note: Garudasana is quite similar to this asana.

Precaution: People with ailments like arthritis should do this asana very carefully.

Garudasana (Eagle pose)

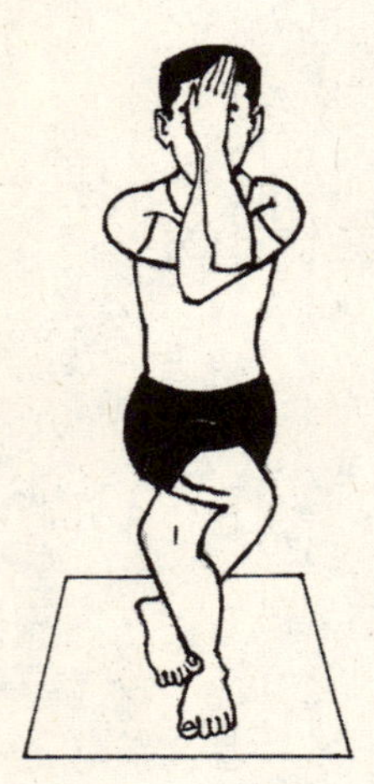

Meaning: 'Garuda' means the king of birds, the vehicle of Lord Vishnu.

Method: Stand in Tadasana. Lift your right leg and wrap it around the left leg in such a way that the back of the right thigh should be on the left thigh and the right foot should touch the left calf. Then, bend your arms from the elbow and intertwine them, right arm around the left. The palms should join in the prayer posture. Pull your intertwined arms down towards the chest. Look in front. Come back to the original position (Tadasana). Switch the legs and hands and repeat the posture. Hold it for the same duration of time. Repeat this kriya 2-5 times.

Breathing: Take slow deep breath in the final position.

Time: Hold this position for about 15-20 seconds.

Focus: On Agya chakra

Note: After thorough practice, bend forward and try to touch the ground with your hands.

Benefits:

- The ankles develop well by doing this asana.
- This asana increases concentration. It also helps practice the act of balancing the body.
- This is very beneficial in preventing sciatica and the cramps in the muscles of the calves.
- It strengthens the hands and legs and makes them flexible.
- It removes the disorders of the reproductive organs.

Precautions: People with ailments like Arthritis should do this asana very carefully.

Vrikshasana (Tree pose)/ Eka Pada Namaskarasana/ Urdhva Haststhita Eka Pada Virama Asana

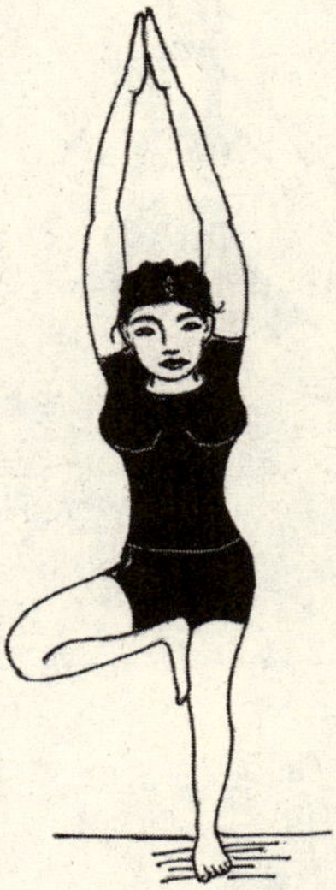

Form: Since the body takes the form of a tree, it is called Vrikshasana.

Method: To start with, stand in Samavastha. Then, balancing your body on the left leg, bend your right leg from the knee and place the foot on the base of the left thigh. Remember that the toes of the right foot should face downwards. Now, join your palms and raise your hands straight above the head. Do not bend the elbows.

Focus: On Agya chakra

Breathing: Inhale while raising both the hands. In the final posture, breathe normally. Exhale while bringing the hands down.

Time: Stay in this position for 5-10 seconds. Come back to Tadasana position. Repeat this exercise by balancing the body on the right leg. Do this exercise 4-5 times.

Direction: East or North. (If possible)

Benefits:

- Since the focus in this exercise is on the Agya chakra, the memory power is enhanced. The eye sight also improves.
- The trembling in the hands and legs is reduced and the arms and calves become firm. It provides balance to the body.
- Some yogacharyas teach Vrikshasana with the head down and the legs up, body balanced on the hands.

Special note: The same asana, when done with hands joined in front in the prayer posture is called **Namaskarasana.**

Dhruva Asana/Bhageeratha Asana (Advanced tree pose)

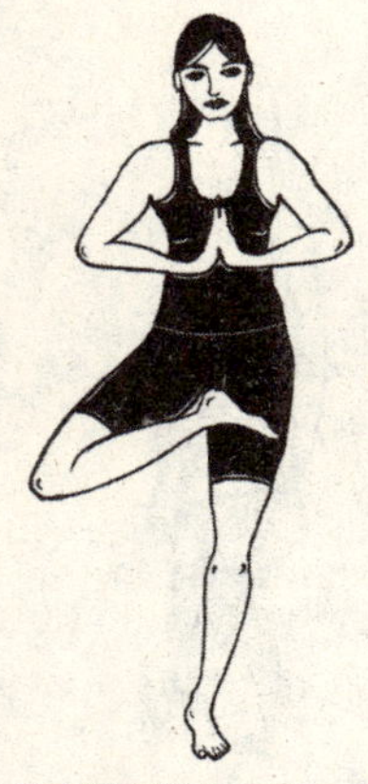

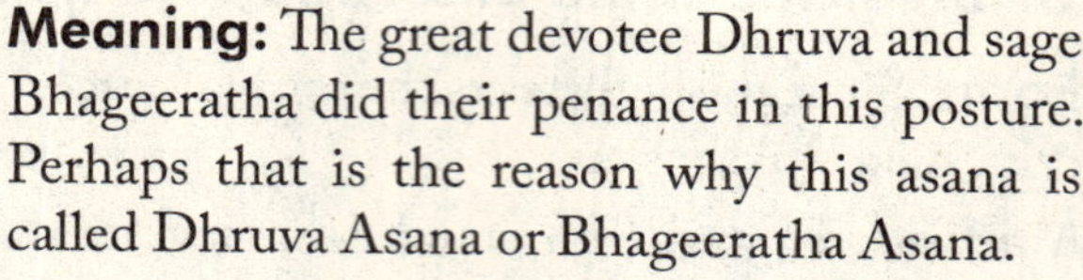

Meaning: The great devotee Dhruva and sage Bhageeratha did their penance in this posture. Perhaps that is the reason why this asana is called Dhruva Asana or Bhageeratha Asana.

There are two methods of doing this asana.

Method 1: Stand in Samavastha. Bend the right leg from the knee and place the foot on the base of the left thigh. Then, join both the palms in the prayer posture in front of your chest. Balance your body by keeping the left leg fixed firmly on the ground. Repeat with the other leg. Breathe normally in the final posture.

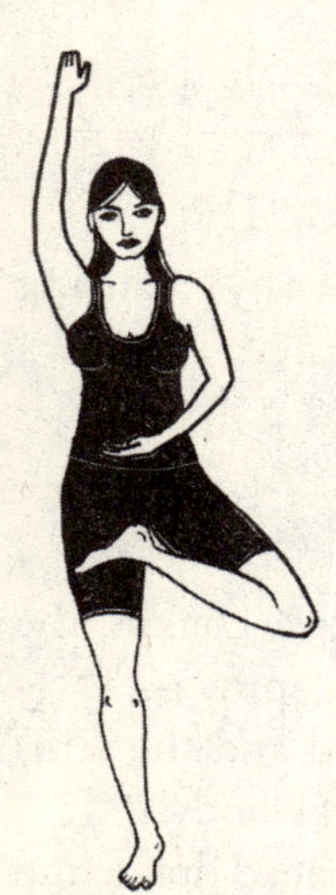

Method 2: Stand in Samavastha. As mentioned in the above method, bend the right leg from the knee and place it on the base of the left thigh. Then, keep your left palm near the navel. The palm should face up. Hold your breath (do Kumbhaka) and take your right hand straight above your head. Hold this position as long as you comfortably can. Come back to the original position and repeat the entire procedure with the other leg.

Breathing: Breathe normally in the final posture.

Time: As per convenience

Benefits:

- Legs become firm and the trembling of the legs is cured by this asana.
- Laziness disappears and life becomes balanced.
- Mooladhara chakra is awakened and a new energy is generated.
- It is helpful in mastering Sadhana.

Utthita Hasta Padangushthasana (Hand-to-big-toe pose)

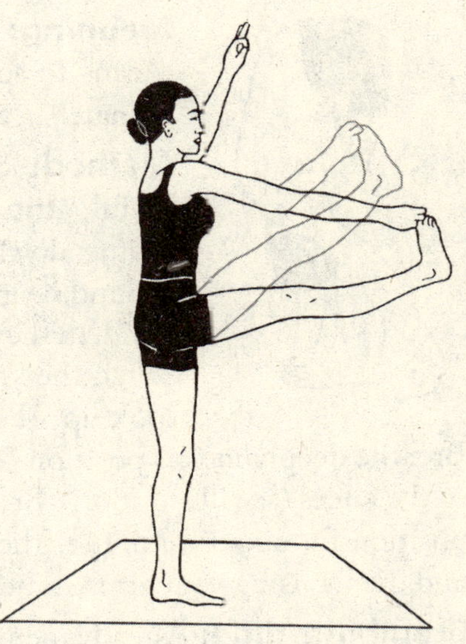

Method: Stand in Samavastha. Let both your feet be close to each other. Look in front. Bend the right leg from the knee and hold the big toe with your right hand. Hold it in such a way that the right hand is inwards, touching the stomach. Then, slowly start straightening up your leg and take it up. Keep your left hand either on your waist, or if you cannot keep the balance, raise it in front or above your head.

Note: After enough practice, try to raise your leg to such a height that your thigh should touch your chin. For this, hold your leg with both the hands and raise it up. Repeat with the other leg.

Breathing/time: Hold this position as per your convenience or for 5-10 seconds. Do five rounds with each leg. Inhale while raising your leg and do Kumbhaka while completing the asana. Exhale while bringing the leg down.

Benefits:

- The muscles of the legs and the buttocks become strong.
- The buttocks and thighs get toned and become well-shaped.
- It brings about control over both mind and body.

Precaution: People suffering from sciatica and severe pain in the back and hip should not do this asana.

Uttanasana (Bending forward while standing)

Variation 1

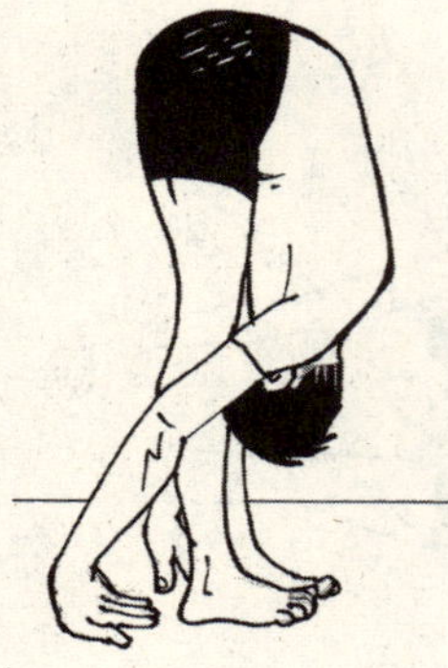

Meaning: 'Ut' is a Sanskrit prefix. 'Tana' means to spread, stretch or increase. In this asana, the spine is forcefully stretched.

Method: Stand straight on the mat in a joyful attitude. Exhale and bend forward. Come down and place your palms on the ground near the heels. Do not let your knees bend. In the final posture, do not let your head touch the knee, rather stretch your neck and look up. The spine should also be stretched. Breathe deeply in this position. Then, exhale and bring your head to the knees (see illustration). Breathe normally and remain in this position for about a minute. Then, first lift up your head, inhale, and then, raising your arms come back to the original position.

Breathing/time: Already mentioned in the method above.

Benefits:

- It reduces the abdominal pain caused by menstruation.
- This asana is very beneficial for those who get exited very soon, those who get irritated very soon and those who are very impulsive and short tempered, as it calms down the muscles of the brain and removes the negativity from the mind.
- It cures stomach ache.
- It benefits the liver, spleen and kidneys.
- It tones and strengthens the heart.
- It makes the spine flexible and benefits the spine.

Note: Padangushthasana and **Pada Hastasana** are similar to the above mentioned asana. According to many yogacharyas, there are other variations of these asanas as well. Yet another variation of this asana is mentioned in the next page.

Hence, practitioners are suggested to use their wisdom while adopting the procedure.

Precautions: People suffering from high blood pressure and those with a rigid spine should do this asana very carefully and cautiously.

Uttanasana (Squat and rise pose) Variation 2

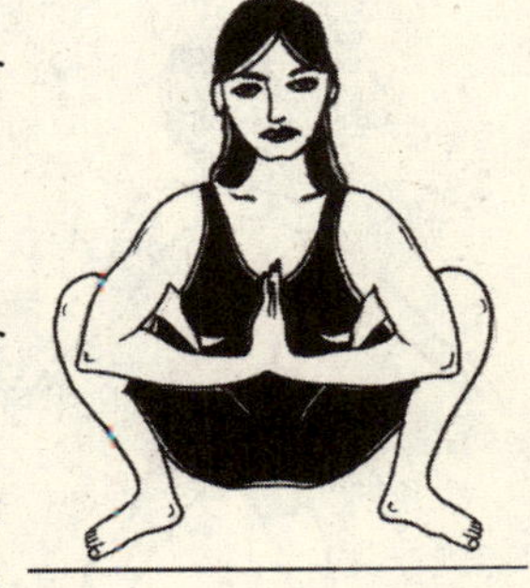

Method: Stand with your feet apart. Keep a distance of about two to two and a half feet between your feet. Your toes should point outwards. Let your hands be straight in front of your stomach. Interlock your fingers, or you may keep them in front of your chest in the prayer posture.

Exhale and slowly start sitting down. Let the knees be on the outside just above the feet. Inhale and come back to the original position. In this exercise, try to go down as much as possible. Keep your spine straight and look in front. Repeat 5-10 times.

Notes:

- The knees should be bent towards the outside while sitting down.
- If you are not able sit down completely in the first instance, go down up to one foot. Then, increase to one and a half feet gradually. When you have practised enough, you can try sitting down completely.

Benefits:

- It cures the disorders of the reproductive organs.
- It gives strength to the muscles of the legs.
- It strengthens the thighs, knees and calves.
- It regularises the flow of the life force. The urinary bladder and the uterus gain benefit from it.
- The ordinary disorders of the back are removed through this asana.
- It benefits the joints of your ankles, knees and hips.

Precautions:

- Do not try to sit down completely at the first instance itself.
- Keep your spine and head straight. Do not bend forward.
- If you are pregnant, do not sit down completely and do not do this asana after three months of pregnancy.

Kaala Bhairavasana (Shiva the destroyer) Variation 1

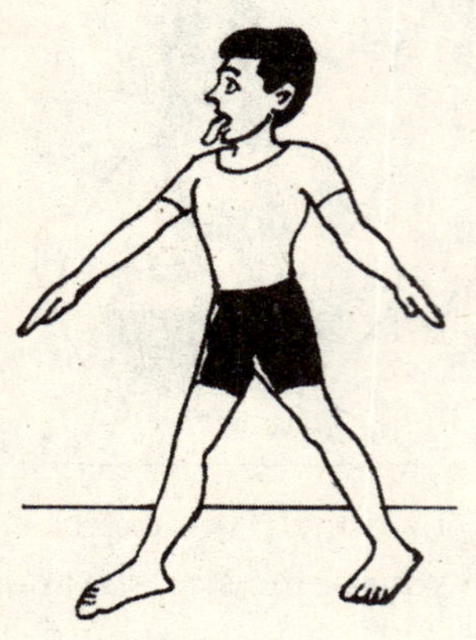

Meaning: 'Kaala' means destruction or time. 'Bhairava' means dreadful or violent. This is one of the eight forms of Lord Shiva.

Note: As is evident from the name, this asana is dedicated to Kaala Bhairava. There are many methods of doing this asana. In India, we find many statues of Kaala Bhairava in various postures.

Methods: This asana adopts a posture as shown in the illustration. To begin with, stand straight. Keep a distance of about one foot in between your feet. Your feet should be in such a position that one foot is behind the other. Keep your hands either raised up or in the front and back respectively. Keep your gaze fixed in front without blinking and your tongue protruded out a little.

Time: 3-5 minutes

Focus: Focus on your breathing and believe that all the anger is being driven out of you and spiritual bliss is being taken in.

Benefits:

- The body becomes firm.
- Eye sight becomes sharper.
- The practitioner becomes fearless and bold.
- The chest becomes broad and strong.

Note: The second variation of Kaala Bhairava Asana is given given later in the book under 'Exercises of Advanced Order and Balance'.

Pada Hastasana (Hands under feet)

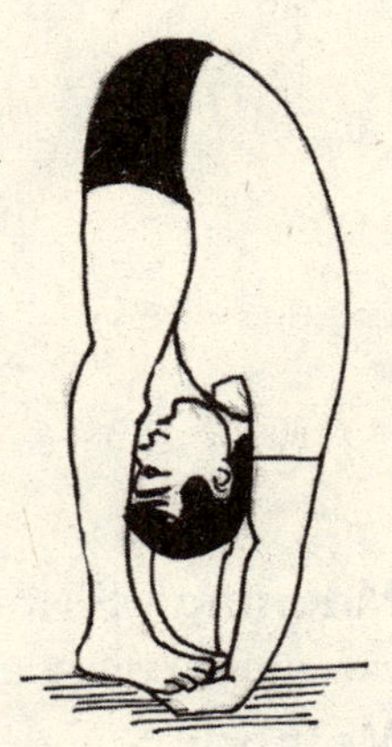

Meaning: 'Pada' means feet and 'Hasta' means hands. It means standing while resting your feet on your hands.

Method: Stand in Tadasana posture. Keep a distance of about half to one foot between your feet. Exhale and slowly bend forward and place your palms under the soles of your feet. While doing this, do not bend your knees. Bend your head and bring it in between the knees.

Breathing/time: Hold this position for 5-10 seconds. Breathe normally. Inhale and lift up your head, and come back to the original position.

Focus: On Mooladhara and Svadhishthana chakras

Benefits:

- This asana is very beneficial in ailments such as excessive gas in the stomach, headache due to gas, or bloating of the stomach.
- This asana gives the benefits of Pashchimottanasana too.
- It reduces excessive fat.

Precautions: Those suffering from high blood pressure, pain in the hips/back, heart patients and those who have giddiness should do this asana very cautiously and carefully.

Note: **Padangushthasana** (Variation 1) and **Uttanasana** (Variation 1) are very similar to this asana.

Shuturmurga Asana (Ostrich pose)

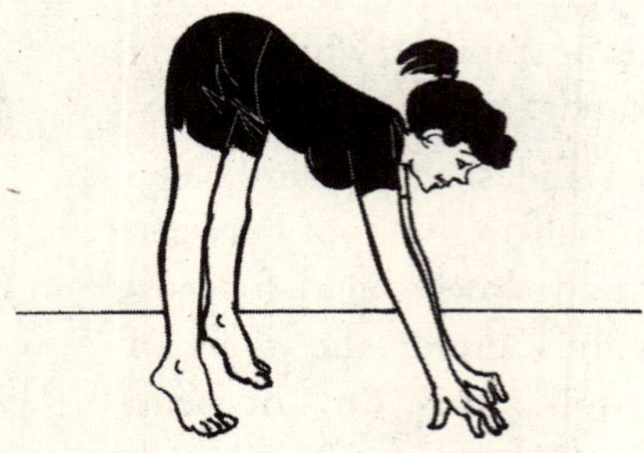

Meaning: 'Shaturmurga' is the name of a bird (Ostrich) which can run very fast and can survive without water for many days.

Method: Stand straight with a joyful attitude. Keep some distance between your feet. Bend forward and touch the ground with the tips of your fingers. Put pressure on your fingers and raise up your body. Keep fingers apart and keep your heels raised. Keep standing on your fingers and toes. In this final posture, the entire weight of the body should be on the toes and fingers. The elbows and knees should not bend. Look in front. You may try to walk a little in this position. Breathe normally in the final position.

Breathing: Exhale while bending forward. Inhale while coming back to the original position.

Benefits:

- Your leg from the toes to the thighs becomes strong and toned by doing this asana.
- Those suffering from gastric problems can do this asana and get rid of gas.
- The fingers, elbows and arms become beautiful, strong and firm by doing this asana.
- It is beneficial in curing the diseases of the eye.
- It reduces obesity.

Note: Some yoga teachers call this asana **Gajasana** (Elephant pose).

Precaution: Those suffering from sciatica and high blood pressure should do this asana carefully and with wisdom.

Sheersha Padangushthasana (Humble warrior pose)

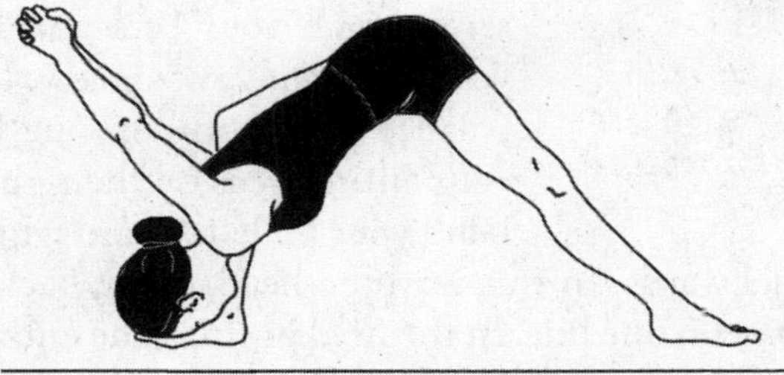

Meaning: 'Sheersha' means head. 'Padangushtha' means the big toe of the foot.

Method: To begin with, stand in Tadasana. Move your left foot about 2-3 feet ahead of the right foot. Take your arms to your back and interlock your fingers. Bend towards your left and try to touch your head to the big toe of the left foot. In this position, the right leg will remain straight and the left leg will be slightly bent. Come back to the original position. Repeat by changing the position of the legs.

Breathing: Exhale while bending down. Inhale while coming back to the original position.

Time: Do for 3-5 rounds

Benefits:

- The spine and the muscles of the legs get strengthened and their ordinary disorders are cured
- It is beneficial in cases of disorders of the wind and constipation
- It cures mental disorders

Precautions:

- If backward-bending asanas are done before and after doing this asana, the difficulty in doing this asana is reduced and other associated disorders do not occur.
- Hold your breath in the final position.
- People suffering from slip disc and sciatica should not do this asana.

Ek Padasan/Veera Bhadrasana

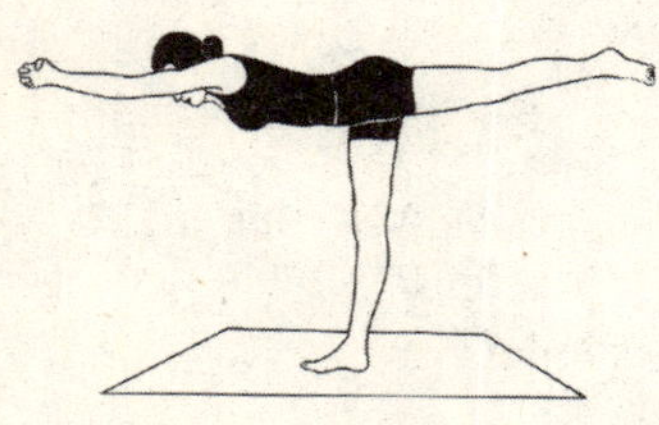

Variation 1: Stand straight. Take your hands above your head. Let your arms touch your ears and interlock your fingers. Now, since you have to balance your body on one leg, keep your entire focus on the right leg and bend your body forward while lifting the left leg backwards. In this way, the head, chest, back and the left leg will come in one line. In the final posture, the entire weight of the body will be on the right foot. Remain in this position for as long as you comfortably can. Then, come back to the original position. Change the leg and repeat the procedure.

Breathing/time: Exhale while bending forward. Breathe normally in the final position. Inhale while coming back to the original position. Hold as per your convenience and do the process 2-3 times with each leg.

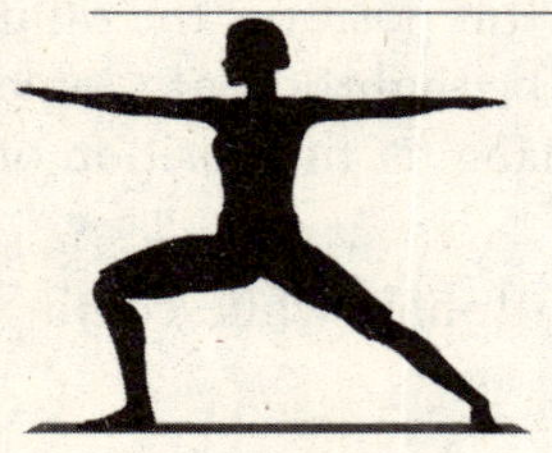

Variation 2: Stand still and touching your ears, take your hands up, and join your palms. Now keep one of your legs by 3 feet apart and bend to form a right angle. Breathe out and keep your chest, hand and face straight outside. Lift your head up and try to look at your toes, hold the position for atleast 20 seconds and return to normal position while breathing out. Now repeat this exercise with another leg.

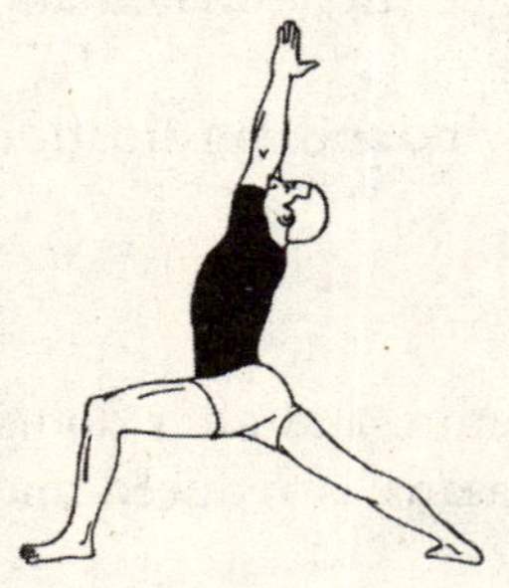

Variation 3: For the 3rd method of this asana, your hands are kept parallel to the shoulders.

Benefits:

• It strengthens the muscles of the legs • It redefines the concept of balance in the body as well as in life • It regularises the blood circulation • It calms down the fluctuations of the mind.

Precaution: People with high blood pressure should not do this asana.

Padangusthasana (Single toe balance pose)

Variation 1

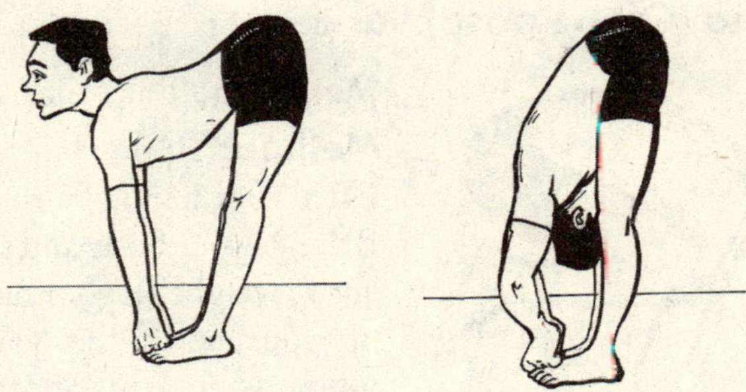

Meaning: 'Pada' means leg. 'Angushtha' means thumb.

Method: Stand in Tadasana. Keep a distance of about a foot between your feet. Exhale while bending forward. Hold the big toes of your feet with your hands in such a way that your palms should face each other. Keep your head in front. Then, apply pressure on your toes and keep your head on your knees. Breathe normally and hold this position for 5-10 seconds. Exhale. Raise your head up. Leave your toes and come back to Tadasans.

Note: Pada Hastasana, Padangushthasana and Uttanasana are similar to each other.

Focus: On the Vishuddhi chakra

Benefits:

- Those who suffer from trembling feet must do this asana. The practitioner who does this asana regularly will never have numbness or trembling in his/her legs. It expels the gas from the body
- Buttocks, waist, spine, stomach and chest – all become attractive which adds beauty to the personality
- It rectifies the digestive system and reduces obesity.

Precaution: Those suffering from high blood pressure, giddiness and sciatica should do this asana slowly and bring it into practice gradually.

Note: The second variation of **Padangushthasana** is given later under 'Exercises of Advanced Order and Balance'.

Asanas of the Medium Category

Bakasana (Crane pose) Variation 1

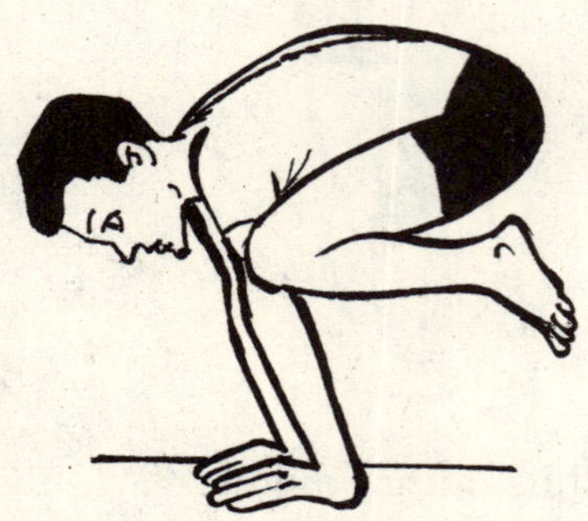

Meaning: 'Baka' means heron.

Method: Sit on your haunches. Place your hands on the ground. Balance your body and shift your entire weight on your hands. Lift up your body. Let your knees touch your arms close to the armpits. Slowly bring your heels close to your buttocks. Lower your head a little. The head and the heels should be almost in one line.

Breathing/time: Keep your breathing normal. Hold the position for 5-10 seconds.

Focus: On Agya chakra

Benefits:

- It increases concentration.
- It rectifies the digestive system and expels the accumulated gas in the abdominal region.
- Since pressure is exerted on the navel, it affects all the 72,000 nadis of the body.
- The muscles of the hands become strong.

Precautions: Those suffering from very high blood pressure and problems of the brain should not do this asana.

Note: Some yoga teachers call this asana **Baka Dhyanasana.**

Comment: There are two or three more methods of doing Bakasana, but all the benefits of those methods can be achieved by this method.

Kagasana (Crow pose)

Meaning: 'Kaaga' is a bird commonly known as a crow.

Method: To begin with, stand in attention position. Sit on your haunches in such a way that there should be no distance between your legs at all. Place your palms on your knees and let your elbows rest between your thighs, chest and stomach. Your hips, spine and neck should be straight.

Breathing: Keep your breathing normal.

Time: Sit in this position for 2-3 minutes.

Benefits:

- The faculties of the abdomen gain benefit from it.
- Disorders of the wind are cured.
- The thighs become beautiful and well-shaped.
- It provides stability in the yogic process to be done during Shatkarma.

Matsyasana (Fish pose)

Meaning: 'Matsya' means fish. The specialty of this asana is that by being in this posture, one can float in water for hours at a stretch. That is why it is called matsyasana.

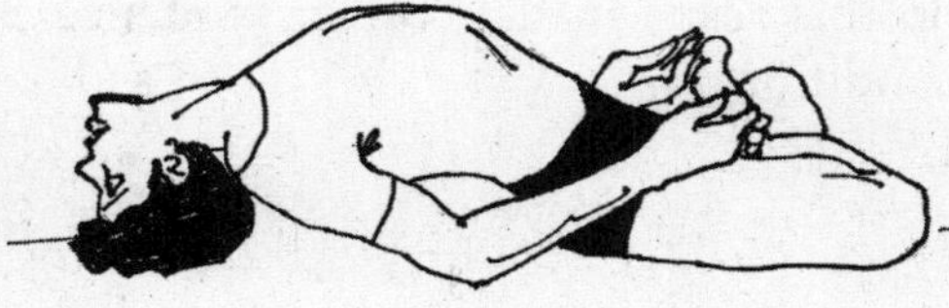

Method: Lie down on the ground in Shavasana. Now place the left foot on the right thigh and the right foot on the left thigh. This is called Vishrama Padmasana. Then, slowly raise your back up, so that the weight of the body is borne by the head and the buttocks. Hold the big toes of your feet with your hands. You can remain in this position for a very long time. But to begin with, do it for only 8-10 seconds. Even though this asana is very simple, it is extremely beneficial.

Focus: On Anahata chakra and the breathing

Breathing/time: In the final posture, practice deep breathing. Do this asana for 3-5 minutes.

Benefits:

- This asana cures piles (with bleeding and inflammation).
- The heart gets strengthened and lungs become strong.
- It works like a medicine for diseases related to respiration.
- It cures constipation and increases hunger.
- It eliminates laziness.
- It strengthens the muscles of the spine, hips/waist, back and thighs.
- Since pressure is exerted on the neck, the thyroids benefit from it. It cures the thyroid glands.
- It gives great relief in cervical spondylitis.

Comment: If this asana is done after doing Sheershasana and Sarvangasana, the disorders that might occur are cured and the benefits from the previous asanas are enhanced.

Note: It can be done in another way. First, sit in Padmasana and then lie down to complete the posture. Some yoga teachers teach this asana by stretching the legs in front.

Precaution: People suffering from problems of the spine, back ache, heart patients, pregnant women and hernia patients should do this asana in the correct sequence considering their physical condition.

Simhasana (Lion pose I) Variation 1

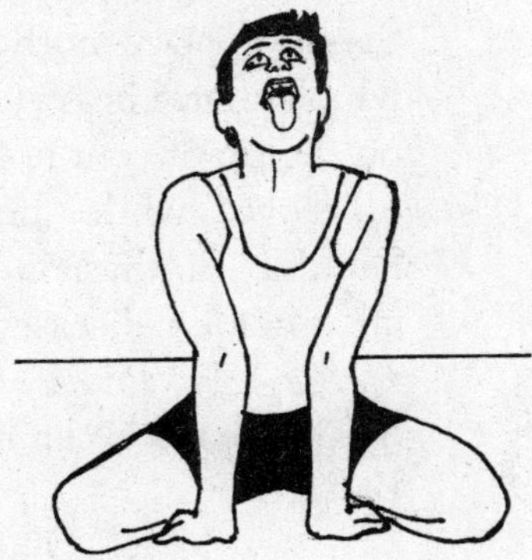

Form: Like a lion

Method: According to Gherunda Samhita – place both your feet under the Seevni nadi (below the Mooladhara chakra) from the opposite sides. Do Jalandhara bandha and fix your gaze either on the tip of your nose or in between your brows. Protrude your tongue out as much as you can and make growling sound from your throat.

Try to exhale from your nose and mouth simultaneously. Bring about a lot of tension on your face, in a way that the face appears to be very fearsome and horrible. Hold this position for 8-10 seconds. Then, change the sequence of the legs and repeat the procedure 3-4 times (If you had placed the right leg over the left leg, this time place the left leg over the right leg.), but maintain the same time for both the rounds.

Focus: On Vishuddhi chakra

Benefits:

- Throat becomes sweeter.
- Stammering stops.
- One becomes sharp-sighted.
- This asana gives all the benefits of Vajrasana.
- Chest becomes strong and stomach soft.

Simhasana (Lion pose II) Variation 2

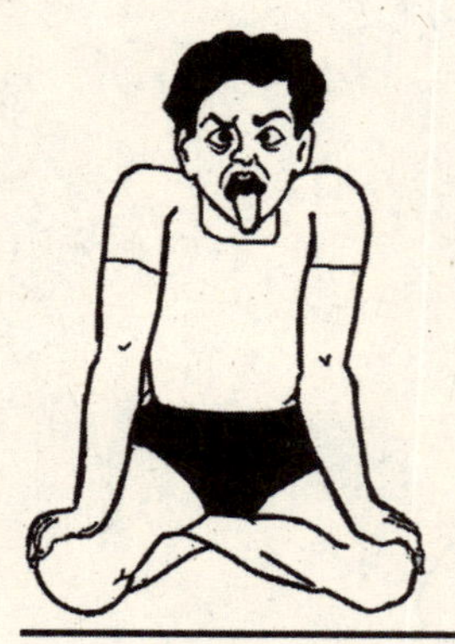

Method: According to Gheranda Samhita place both your heels below Mooladhara chakra (anus). Concentrate on the tip of your nose or between your eyebrows while holding Jalandhara bandha. Simhasana helps get rid of all kinds of diseases. It is written in *Hatha Yoga Pradeepika* that by doing Simhasana, one can master all the three Bandhas.

It is written in Trishikhabramhanopanishad that:

सीवनी गुल्फदेशेभ्यो निपीड्य व्युत्क्रमेण तु।
प्रासार्य जानुनोहस्तावासनं सिंहरूपकम।।

Meaning: Press the Seevni with both the heels from the opposite sides and spread both your knees while placing your hands on them. This posture is called Lion-like asana or Simhasana.

Variation: This can also be done with palms kept flat on the ground, turned inwards and placed under the knees.

Time: Do it everyday for 15-20 seconds and then gradually increase the time.

Benefits:

- Stuttering and stammering are cured by this asana and our voice becomes melodious.
- One becomes fearless.
- The Mooladhara and Agya chakra are awakened by this asana.
- Eye sight is enhanced.

Comment: This asana is also done by slightly changing the position of the hands and legs.

Gomukhasana (Cow face pose)

Form: Like the face of a cow (thin at one end and broad at the other end)

Meaning: In this asana, when we place one knee upon the other, the form obtained resembles the face of a cow and the feet protruding out from both the sides resemble the ears of the cow. Therefore, this asana is called gomukhasana.

Variation 1. (In this method, the heels don't touch each other): Sit down with your legs spread out in front. Bend your right leg from the knee and bring the foot near the left buttock. Similarly, bend the left leg from the knee and bring the foot near the right buttock. Now, take the left hand behind your head and the right hand from the sides of your back. Interlock the fingers of both your hands at the back. This is the final position. Then, change the sequence of the hands and legs and repeat the procedure.

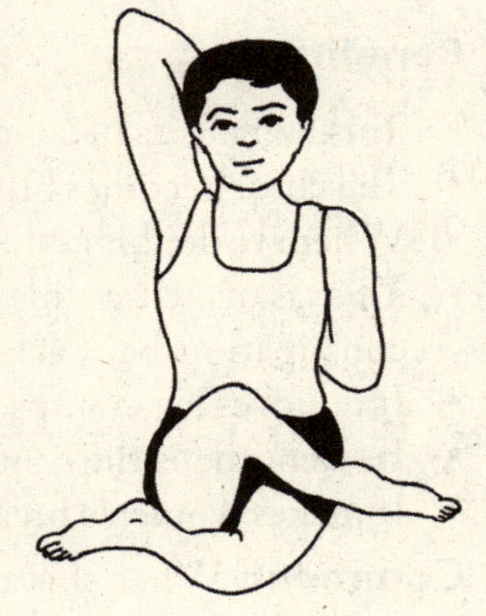

Breathing/time: Breathe normally in the final position. Hold the position for half to one minute.

Variation 2. Sit down in Sukhasana. Place your left foot under the right buttock in such a way that the heel are under the anus. Bend the right leg and place it on the left thigh in such a way that the feet touch the ground. With regular practice, you will be able to bring both the heels close to each other.

Then, take your left hand back from the side of your waist and raise the right hand and take it back from the side of your right ear. Interlock your fingers at the back. Inhale and exhale in this position. Come back to the original

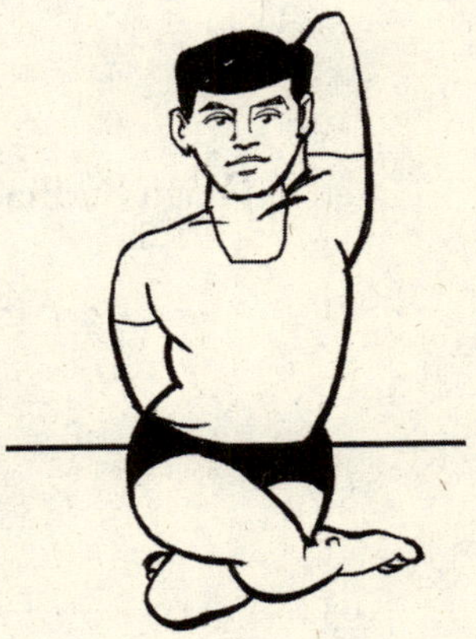

position. Change the position of the legs and hands and repeat the procedure. This is one complete round.

Focus: On Mooladhara chakra

Notes:

1. In the first variation, when the right leg is on the left thigh, the left hand should go behind the head from the top.
2. In the second variation, when the left leg is under the right leg, the right hand should go behind the head from the top.

Benefits:

- This asana is as beneficial as Siddhasana and Padmasana.
- The chest becomes broad and strong by this asana.
- When we do this asana, Moolbandha is automatically executed.
- This asana cures many diseases such as diabetes, arthritis, constipation, back ache and night fall.
- It removes leg cramps.
- It strengthens the shoulders.
- It makes women's breasts firm and well-shaped.

Comment: When this asana is done by keeping the hands on the knees, this asana is called **Supta Gomukhasana.** It is also called **Dhyana Veerasana** in some places.

'Yoga Sadhana' is a simple and easy way of realising the self.

–RJT

Utkatasana (Chair pose)

Method: This asana is done in two ways.

Variation 1. According to Gherunda Samhita: Stand in Tadasana and slowly sit down on your haunches. Place your heels on your buttocks in such a way that they touch your anus. Breathe normally. Place your elbows on your knees.

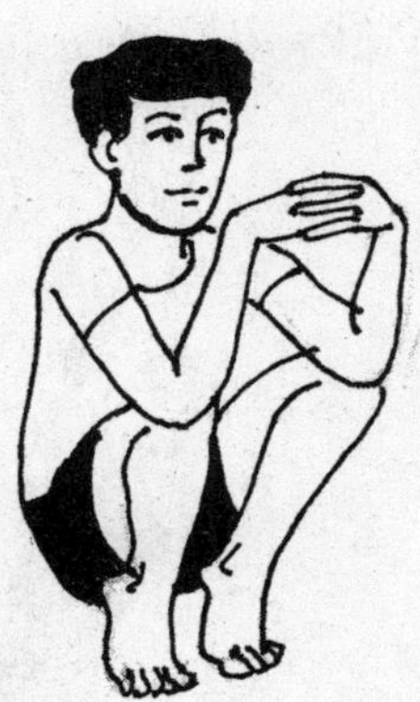

Variation 2. Stand in Tadasana posture. Take both the hands above your head and join your palms in the prayer posture. Then, start lowering your buttocks as if you're trying to sit on a chair. Do not bend your chest forward (imagine that you are sitting on a chair). Hold this position for as long as you can. Then, come back to the original position.

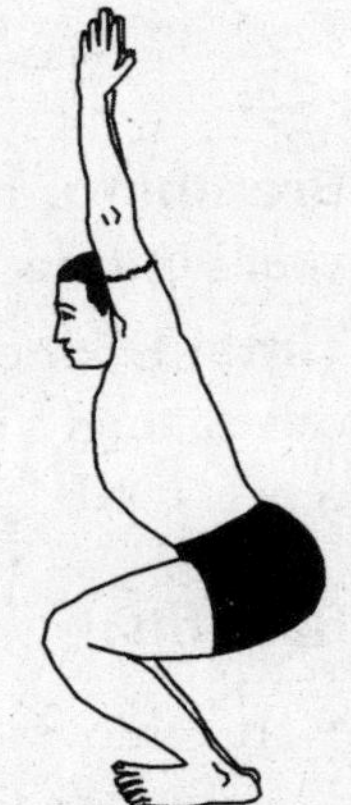

Focus: On Mooladhara and Agya chakra (as per comfort).

Breathing: Breathe out while sitting and breathe in while returning to the normal position.

Time: As per your convenience

Benefits:

- One must do this asana to regularise the flow of Prana in Sushumna. Hence, those who are practising the awakening of kundalini must do this asana.
- It is ideal for increasing your concentration.
- The calves and thighs become strong.
- The brain becomes fresh.
- It is helpful in reducing obesity.
- The spine gets strengthened.

Gatimaya Utkatasana (Dynamic chair pose)

Method: Stand in attention. Keep your hands in front of your chest in the prayer posture. Inhale and raise your hands above your head. Let your arms touch your ears. Exhale and try to sit down. Initially, try to sit as if you are sitting on a chair. Then, with practice, try to bring your buttocks down to the ground. With practice, you can increase the speed of performing this asana (you can also do it by keeping your hands in front, parallel to the ground and palms facing down).

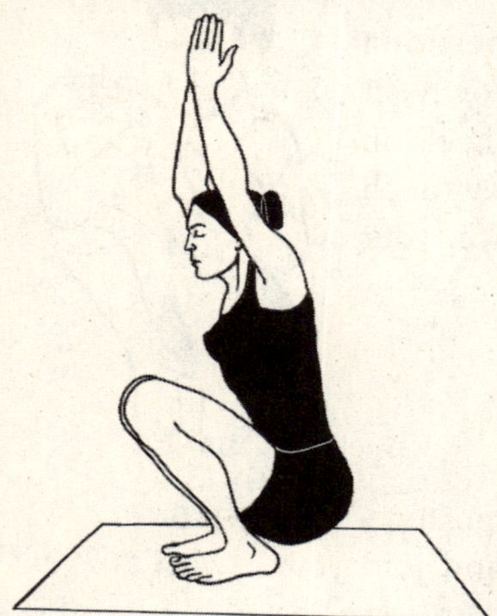

Breathing: Inhale while standing up and exhale while lowering your buttocks to the ground.

Time: Do the asana very slowly in the beginning, and later as the calves, thighs and knees become flexible, increase your speed and repeat it 10-15 times.

Benefits:

- It removes all disorders of the calves, thighs, knees and the entire leg, like leg pain, cramps, numbness, etc.
- It removes the ordinary pain in your knees.
- It gives relief from problems like back ache, slip disc, sciatica, lower back pain etc.
- It makes the digestive system more functional.
- It strengthens your lungs.

Precautions:

- Do not try to sit down on the ground at the first instance.
- Those who have undergone operation in the knees or those suffering from lower back ache should first do specific asanas related to these problems.

Kukkutasana (Cockerel pose)

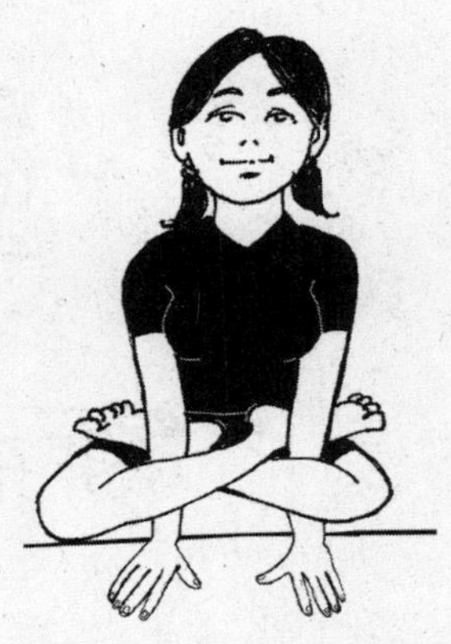

Form: Like a cock. Hence, the name suggests an asana that resembles a cock.

Method: Sit in Padmasana. Pass your hands gently from in between your calves and thighs. Place your palms on the ground in such a way that the fingers point in front. Slowly shift your weight on your palms and lift your body up as much as you comfortably can. Then, come back to the original position. Once you have practised enough, change the sequence of the legs and do the asana.

Focus: Keep your focus on the heart chakra (Anahat chakra), and for spiritual purposes on the Mooladhar chakra.

Breathing: Breathe normally in the final position. Inhale while lifting your body up and exhale while lowering it down.

Time: Repeat this kriya 3-4 times.

Benefits:

- The fingers, palms, elbows and shoulders become strong.
- The muscles of the abdomen become strong.
- One gets all the benefits which one gets by doing Lolasan.
- The body becomes firm and strong.
- Those who play volley ball, basket ball, judo-karate, etc. must do this asana.

Comment: It is easier to do this asana if we apply some oil or cream on the calves, thighs and hands.

Vrishabhasana (Bull pose)

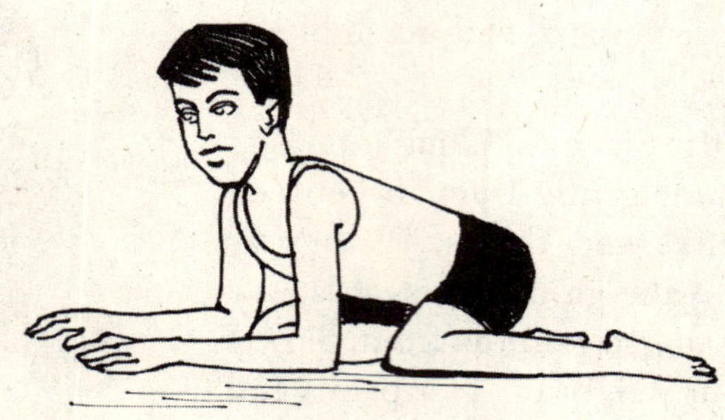

Meaning: 'Vrishabha' means bull. It is the vehicle of Lord Shiva and is the sign of identity carved on the stone slab under the statue of the first Teerthankara Bhagwana Adinatha.

Form: While doing this asana, the posture resembles a relaxing bull.

Method: Sit on a mat in Vajrasana, or sit on your haunches. Shift your position as shown in the illustration. If you sit on your left thigh, place the heel of the left leg close to the Seevni nadi and rest the right leg on the left as shown in the illustration. Then, place both your hands in front just as a bull rests on its fore limbs.

Breathing/time: Breathe normally and repeat the procedure by changing the sequence of your legs. You can practice this asana daily for about 5 minutes.

Focus: For spiritual benefits, meditate on Lord Shiva/Bhagwan Adinatha.

Benefits:

- Shoulders become strong and firm like a bull.
- The thighs, legs, hands, arms, shoulders, knees – all become strong and toned.
- Harmful gases are expelled from your stomach and one starts feeling light.
- One gets many physical benefits automatically.

Trikonasana (Triangle pose 1)

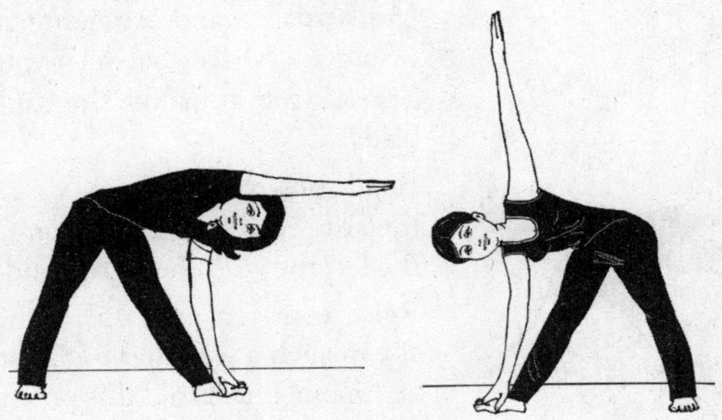

Meaning: 'Tri' means three and 'Kona' means angle Trikona means 'with three angles' or 'three sides'.

Method: Stand joyfully in attention position. Keep your feet about 2-3 feet apart. Raise your arms up to shoulder level, parallel to the ground like the wings of a bird. Slowly bend your body from the waist to the right. Try to hold the right leg with your right hand, or touch the toes with your fingers. Your knees should not bend. In the final posture, the position of the left hand can be done in two ways. First, the left hand can be in one line with the right hand and in the second, the left hand can be placed on the left ear to form a triangle. Repeat the procedure on the left side too.

Breathing: Exhale while bending and inhale while coming back up.

Benefits:

- Cures constipation.
- It repairs the muscles of the legs.
- It makes the spine flexible.
- It cures back ache and diseases of the neck.
- It cures the disorders related to the abdomen.

Comment: This asana can be done in 3-4 ways by making little changes in the procedures.

Trikonasana (Triangle pose 2)

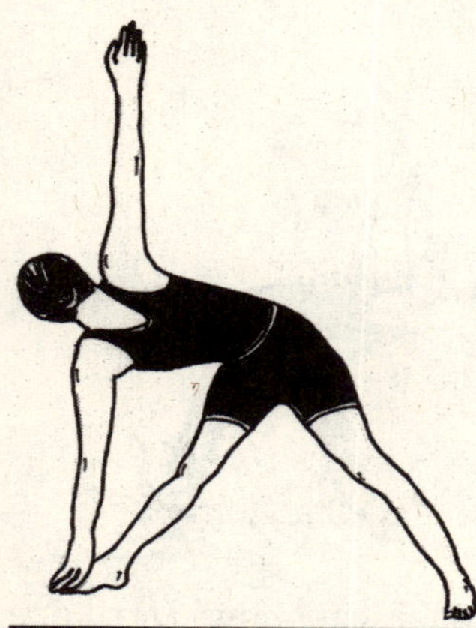

Method: Stand straight with a distance of 3 feet between your legs. Spread your arms like the wings of a bird.

Bend down and twist your torso towards your left. Exhale and touch the left toe with the right hand.

Raise your left arm up towards the sky in such a way that both the arms are in one line. Hold this position for about 5 seconds. Then, come back to the original position and repeat the procedure with the left hand. Gradually increase the time of holding the position.

Note: Some yoga teachers call this asana **Parshva Trikonasana/ Konasana** and **Parivrita Trikonasana.**

Comment: While taking your hand up, turn your head up and fix your gaze at the sky.

Focus: Try to feel the stretch and strain on the muscles of the back, abdomen and the calves. Focus on the Manipuraka chakra.

Gatimaya Trikonasana

Increase the speed of doing this asana.

Benefits:

- The abdomen area benefits by doing this asana everyday in Gatimaya.
- It strengthens the digestive system.
- It reduces obesity.
- The stress from the calves is removed and the calves become strong by doing this asana.
- It cures the disorders of the wind.
- This is a very effective kriya to enhance the strength of the waist.

Ashtanga Namaskarasana (Eight-limbed salutation)

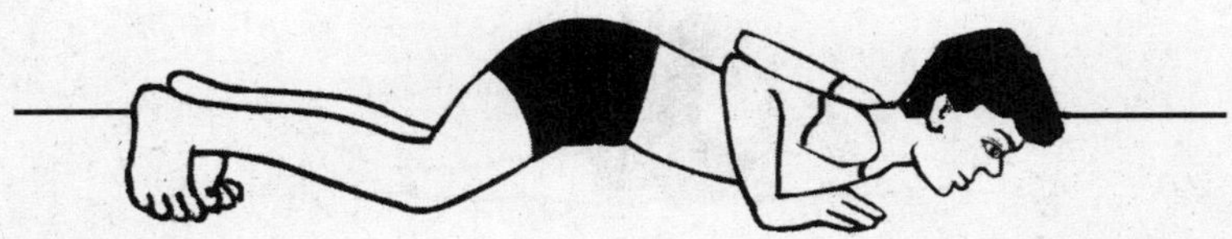

Meaning: 'Ashtanga' means with eight limbs. 'Namaskara' means to pay respect. In other words, to bow down in respect using all the eight limbs (both the legs, both the hands, both the knees, chest and chin). This asana incorporates all these aspects, hence, it is called ashtanga namaskarasana.

Method: Lie down on your stomach with your head towards North or East. The toes of both the legs, both the knees, the palms of both the hands, chest and chin should touch the ground. Keep your abdomen slightly raised above the ground. This asana resembles doing Sashtanga namaskara to God.

Breathing/time: Do normal breathing. Hold the posture as per your convenience.

Focus:

- On your god or your guru.
- Concentrate on the energy generated from the Mooladhara Chakra, which is flowing towards the Sahasrara Chakra.
- Imagine that all the diseases are being destroyed.

Benefits:

- This asana is very beneficial in the ailments of the spine.
- This asana gives total rest to the body and generates new awareness.
- It gives mental peace.

Note: The directions are mentioned due to their spiritual significance. Some yoga masters also call it **Pranipatasana.**

Hanumanasana

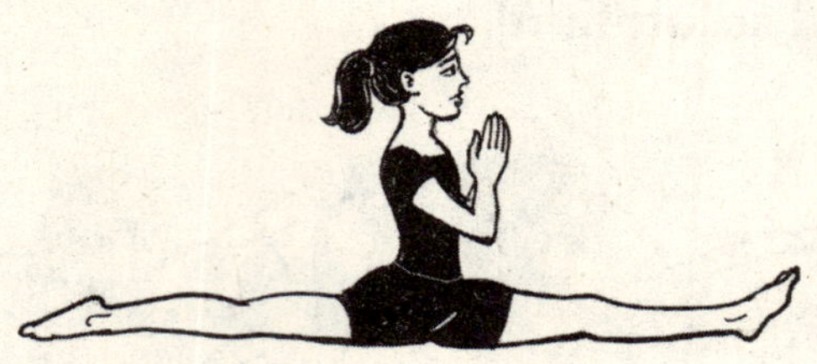

Method: Sit with both the knees on the ground, or with one knee on the ground. Place your palms on the sides. Very slowly, spread your legs in the opposite directions, i.e. in the front and back. Do not try to hurry, because there is a lot of strain in the muscles near the thighs, calves and the anus. It takes a new practitioner considerable time to execute this asana completely. Spread the legs in opposite direction in such a way that the buttocks, thighs and calves touch the ground and the legs form a straight line. Then, take your hands off the ground and bring them in front of your chest in the prayer posture. You can also do it in a different way by taking your hands above your head and joining them in the prayer posture.

Focus: Meditate on Lord Hanumana, think of his character and try to imbibe his qualities.

Breathing: Breathe normally in the final posture

Time: 10-30 seconds

Benefits:

- It calms down lust.
- It removes the diseases of the reproductive organs.
- It increases the blood circulation in the calves, thighs and the pelvic region and benefits to the nervous system.
- It cures arthritis.

Note: Since the most prevalent form of statue of Lord Hanumana is that of holding the mace in one hand and a mountain on the other, many yoga gurus teach Hanumanasan in that posture. Hanumanasana is done in many ways.

Precaution: After doing the asana, do not get up immediately. Bring your legs in front, and sit and relax for some time.

Ardha Chandrasana (Half moon pose) Variation 1

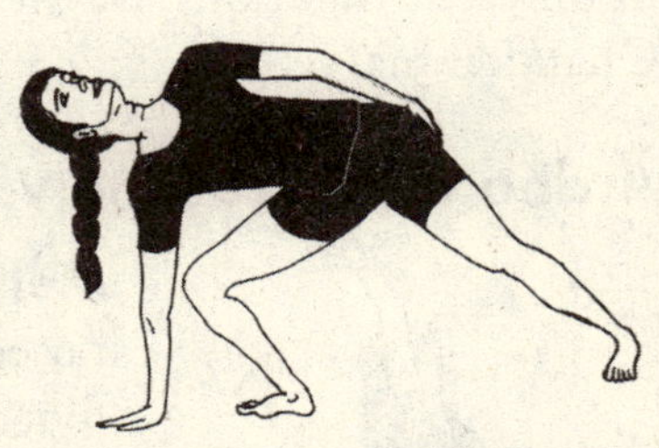

Method: Stand straight in a joyful attitude. Keep a distance of about two to three feet in between your legs. Bring your arms up to shoulder level, parallel to the ground. Since you have to do the asana as shown in the illustration, bend your right knee and simultaneously bend your body to your right. Gradually shift the weight of the body to the right side and raise your left leg up. Your left leg should be raised so much that the right palm should rest on the ground, but the weight of the body should be on the right leg and buttocks. Keep your left hand in line with the left hip. Hold this position for 10-20 seconds. Gradually come back to the original position. Change the sequence of the legs and repeat the procedure.

Breathing: Breathe normally in the final position.

Benefits:

- It strengthens the lower spine and the back.
- Those who have trembling feet must definitely do this asana.
- It cures cramps and knee pain.
- It expels gases from your body and makes the body light.

Ardha Chandrasana Variation 2

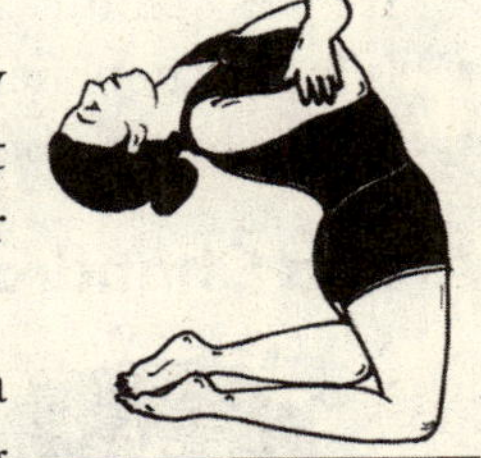

Method: Sit in Vajrasana. Raise your body up and bend it backwards from your waist (see illustration). Cross your arms across your chest.

Breathing/time: Do Antahkumbhaka (Inside hold/Retention full) while bending backwards. Exhale while coming back to the original position.

Benefits:

- It cures constipation and strengthens the digestive system.
- The diseases of the back, hips and spine are cured.

Comment: Since Ardha Chandrasana is done in different ways in different traditions, we are showing these variations of Ardha Chandrasana.

Ardha Chandrasana Variation 3

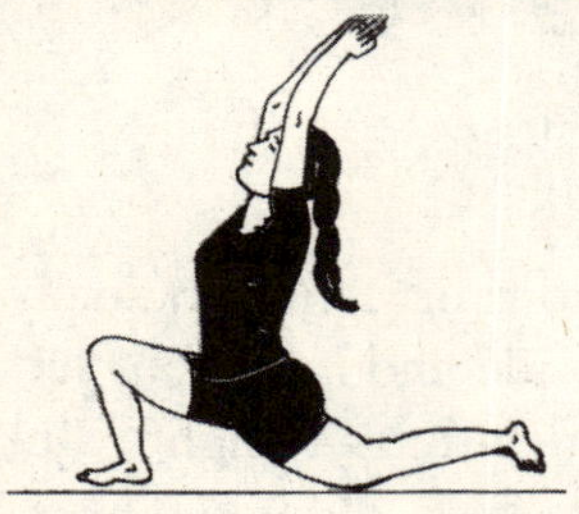

Method: Kneel down with your body raised. Bring your left leg about one foot forward and place it firmly on the ground. Take your right leg back and slowly bend your back and neck backwards as much you comfortably can. You can keep your hands on the sides or raise them above your head in the prayer posture. Bend them back to resemble a half moon and complete the formation of this asana. Come back to the original position. Change the sequence of the legs and repeat the procedure.

Focus: On Swadhisthana chakra

Breathing/time: Inhale while bending back and exhale while coming back to the original position. This is one round. Do five such rounds.

Benefits:

- It regularises the blood circulation in the body.
- It makes the spine strong and flexible.
- It gives stability to leg muscles.
- It is very beneficial for diseases in women.
- It gives ample benefit to the neck and lungs.

Ardha Chandrasana Variation 4

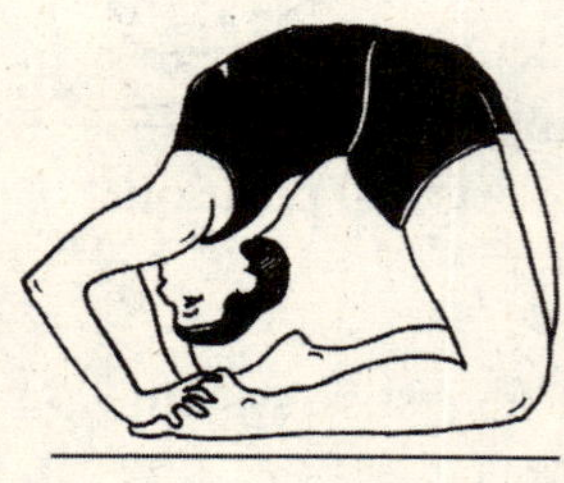

Method: Sit in Vajrasana. Raise both the hands and raise your body on your knees. Gradually, bend your body back from the waist to such an extent that the palms should be able to hold the soles (see illustration). Stay in this position for some time. Come back to the original position.

Breathing: When you are forming the posture, do Antahkumbhaka and exhale while coming back to the original position.

Benefits:

- It makes the spine flexible and supple. It gives relief to the patients of arthritis.
- Gradually, the hips, back, spine, abdomen, neck and head become disease free.
- Women can gain many benefits from this asana.
- One automatically gets all the benefits of Chakrasana from this asana.

Precaution: People with a rigid spine and those suffering from diseases of the stomach should not do this asana.

Lolasana (Pendant pose)

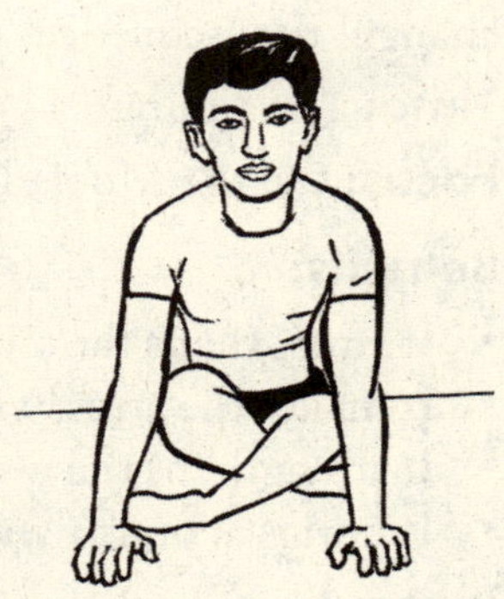

Meaning: 'Lol' means trembling, moving or restless.

Method: Sit with your legs spread in front. Place your hands by your sides. Raising your body a little, bend your right knee towards the back and keep the sole under the left buttock. Sit down your soles. Similarly, bend the left knee, raise your body and place your sole under the right buttock. Sit on your crossed heels. Inhale and by applying pressure on your palms, lift up your body. While maintaining balance, slowly try to swing your body to and fro. Hold your breath while swinging the body and exhale after coming back to the original position. Try to maintain the balance for as long as you comfortably can.

Benefits:

- It tones and strengthens your arm.
- The parts of the abdomen benefits from it.
- It makes the muscles of the back and legs strong and flexible.

Note: This asana is like **Tulasana** or **Jhoolasana.** The only difference is that in Tulasana, the legs are kept one upon the other like Padmasana, whereas in Lolasana, they are placed under the buttocks.

Tulasana/Jhoolasana/Utthita Padmasana (Balance posture) Variation 1

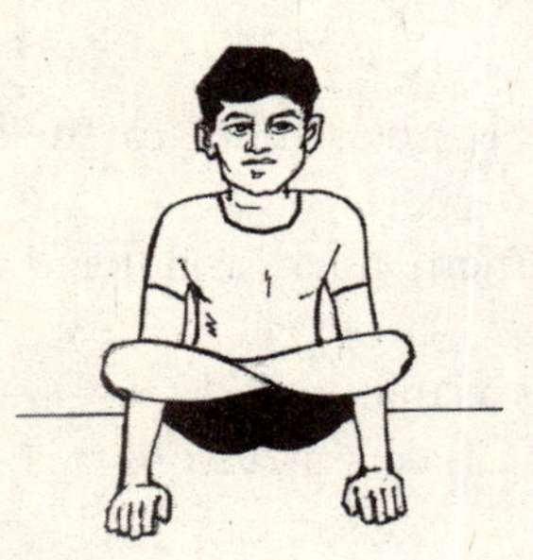

Meaning: 'Tula' means the two sides of a balance, and we can oscillate in this asana like a swing, that is why this asana is called Jhoolasana.

Method: Sit in Padmasana. Place your hands on your sides. Inhale, and by pushing both the hands firmly against the ground, lift up your body. Hold this position for some time. If you want, you can slowly oscillate your body to and fro like a swing. Exhale and come back to the original position. Then, change the sequence of the legs and repeat the procedure.

Time: 1 to 3 minutes

Focus: On the Mooladhara chakra

Benefits:

- It strengthens the chest.
- It makes the arms, wrists and shoulders strong.
- It strengthens the walls of the stomach.
- It brings about balance in life.

Precaution: In this asana, a lot of pressure is exerted on the joint of the wrists. So, those with weak wrist joints should do this asana very carefully and cautiously.

Comment: Some yoga teachers call it Lolasana. The second variation of Utthita Padmasana is given later under 'Exercises of Advanced Order and Balance'.

Practising yoga makes a man calm and active.

–RJT

Meru Akarshanasana/Supta Eka Hastpada Urdhvasana (Spine bending pose)

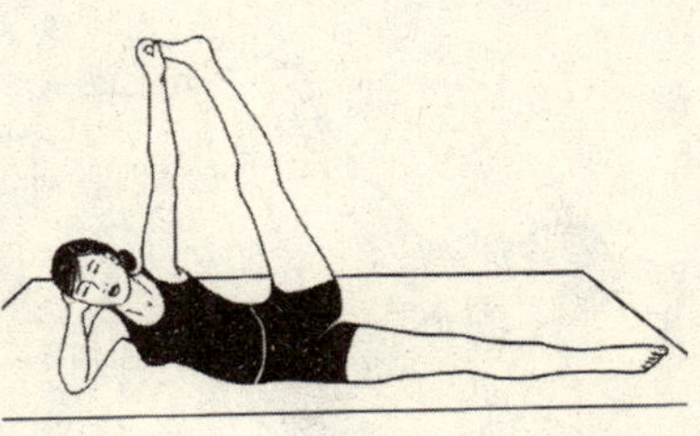

Method: Lie down on your mat. Turn to your right. Taking the support of your right hand, raise your head and let it rest on your right palm. Keep your left hand on the left leg. Then, slowly raise your left leg and try to hold the big toe with your left hand. If you find it difficult, hold on to the calves or the ankles and keep the left leg stretched up. Come back to the original position. Repeat the same procedure with the other leg.

Breathing/time: Inhale while raising the hands and legs. Keep the breathing normal in the final position. Exhale while bringing the hands and legs back to the original position. Repeat 5 times with each leg.

Precaution: Those suffering from slip disc, cervical problems and sciatica should not do this asana.

Benefits:

- This asana stretch whole leg. Hence, the blood circulation in the leg is regularised.
- It brings about flexibility in the joint between the legs and the waist.
- It reduces excess fat around the abdomen and the thighs and makes them well-shaped.

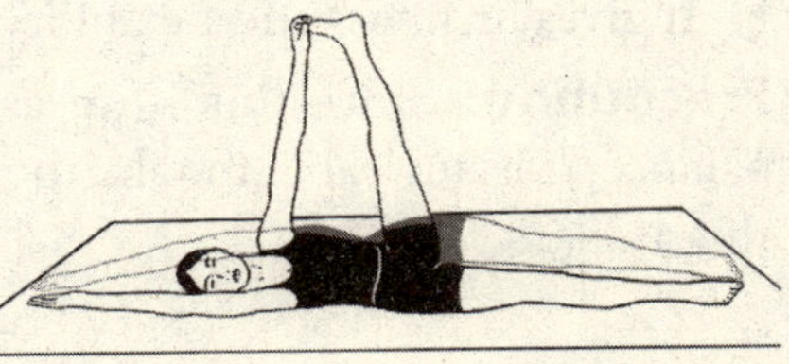

Variation: The same asana can be done in another way. Instead of keeping your hand under the head, both the hands are stretched above the head in the prayer posture. When you raise the left leg, simultaneously raise your left hand and try to hold the big toe. This position is also called **Eka Hasta Pada Angushtha Sparshasana**.

Breathing time/benefits/precautions: Same as mentioned earlier.

Vashishthasana (Side plank pose)

Meaning: Vashishtha is the name of a famous sage, who was the priest of the Suryavanshi kings and is the writer of the seventh Mandala of the Rigveda.

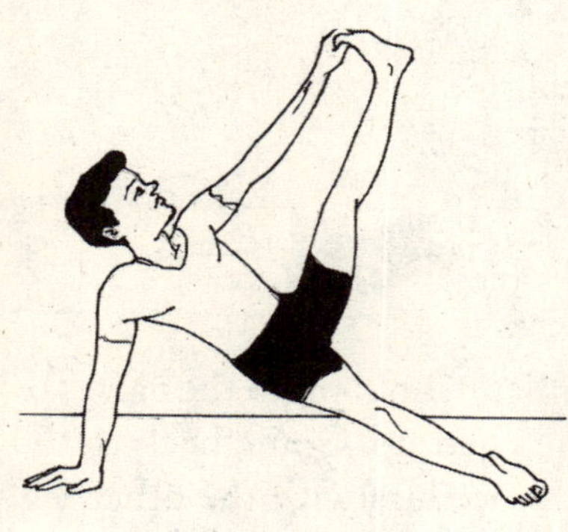

Method: Lie down and turn to your left. Bend your left hand from the elbow and place it close to the shoulder, palms facing down. Shift your entire weight on your left palm and left leg and raise your body up, as shown in the illustration. The whole body should be stretched in one line. When you succeed in coming to this position comfortably, lift up your right leg and hold the big toe with your right hand. Do not bend your knees. Those new to this asana can lean against the wall to do it. Change the sequence of the legs and repeat the procedure.

Breathing: Let the breathing be normal in the final position.

Time: As per your comfort level.

Benefits:

- The arms become strong and firm.
- This asana repairs the regions of the hips and the anus.
- It cures the trembling of hands and legs.
- It gives firmness and flexibility to the entire body.

Precaution: Since this is an asana of the advanced order and balance, it is advisable to take the support of the wall while doing this asana.

Garbhasana/Garbhpindasana (Womb pose)/ Uttana Koormasana (Foetus pose)

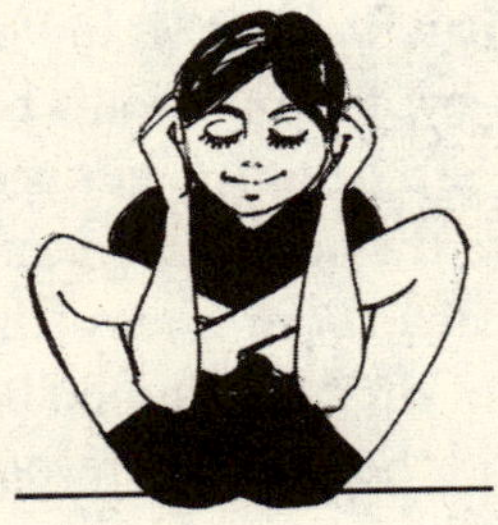
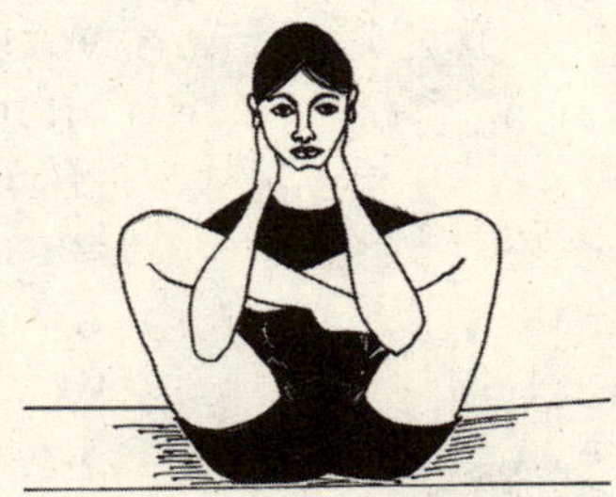

Meaning: 'Garbha-pinda' means a fully developed foetus in the mother's womb.

Method: Sit in Padmasana. Pass both the hands in between your calves and thighs so that they can be bent from the elbows. Then, try to sit on your buttocks and raise your knees. Bend your arms from the elbows and try to hold your ears or interlock your fingers behind the neck. The entire weight of the body should be on the anal joint. Exhale while holding your ears and breathe normally in the final position. Hold the position for 10-15 seconds. Change the sequence of the legs and repeat the procedure.

Focus: On Swadhishthana chakra.

Benefits:

- This asana contracts the abdomen thoroughly as a result of which, the blood circulation is regularised and the abdominal region becomes well toned.
- This asana is beneficial for those who have a weak brain or those suffering from mental ailments.
- It enhances the power of digestion.
- It regularises adrenal glands.
- It maintains the balance between the air, bile and phlegm in the body.
- It makes the entire body beautiful, well-shaped and attractive.
- It destroys the excessive air accumulated in the joints of the hips and the knees. Hence, diseases like arthritis are kept at bay.

Muktasana (Free pose)

Meaning: 'Mukta' means free or carefree.

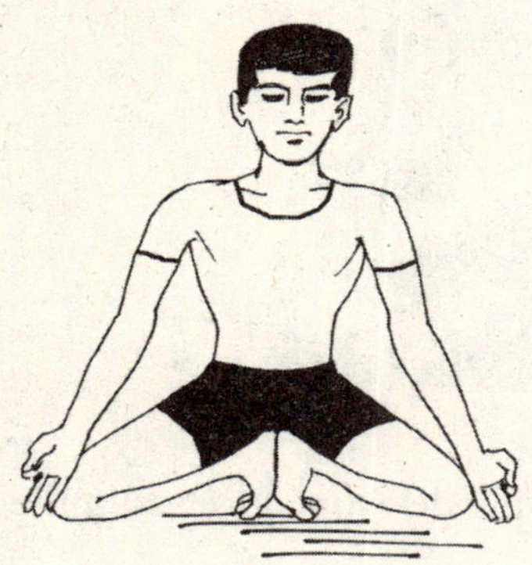

Variation 1. First, sit in Vajrasana. Sit up by joining your toes and place your heels in between your anus and the genitals, on the Seevni nadi. Spread your knees. The entire weight of the body should be on the heels and the toes. Keep your hands on the knees in Gyana Mudra. Sit in this position as long as you comfortably can.

Benefits:

- This asana is beneficial in awakening the kundalini.
- This asana gives strength to the legs and toes. The untimely trembling of the legs can be checked by doing this asana.
- This asana cures the disorders of the reproductive organs in both men and women, and keep their functioning in order.

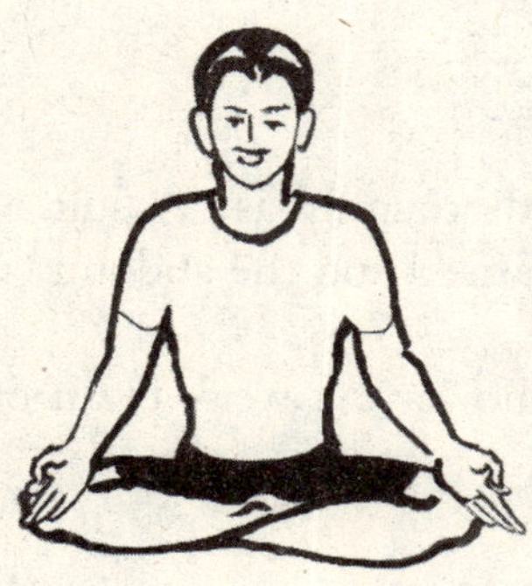

Variation 2. According to Gharanda Samhita – sit with your left heel close to the anus and place your right heel upon it. Keep your spine, neck and head straight. This asana, which grants all the siddhis, is called muktasana.

Focus: Concentrate on the energy being generated in Mooladhara.

Comments: The benefits of the second variation of Mauktasana are the same as Guptasana.

Note: Both these methods are according to different yogacharyas.

Khagasana (Hare pose)

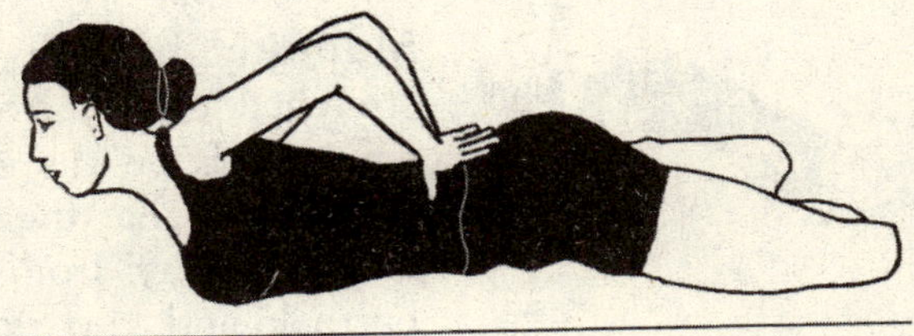

Meaning: 'Khaga' means the one who moves in the sky, and Khagasana is one of the names of Lord Vishnu. While doing this asana, the body resembles a bird flying high in the sky. That is why this asana is called khagasana.

Method: First of all, sit in Padmasana. Then, retaining the posture, lie down on your stomach. Place your fingers on your waist in such a way that the thumbs face the stomach and the fingers face the back. Raise your head and look straight.

Breathing: Do Antahkumbhaka while raising your head. Hold the position as per your convenience and exhale while coming back to the original position.

Benefits:

- It establishes a perfect balance between the wind, bile and phlegm in the body.
- The disorders of the urinary bladder are cured.
- The digestive system becomes more active.
- The pain in hips and back are cured.
- It reduces obesity.

Setu Asana (Bridge pose-1)/Rapatasana/ Vipareeta Dandasana/Purvottanasana*

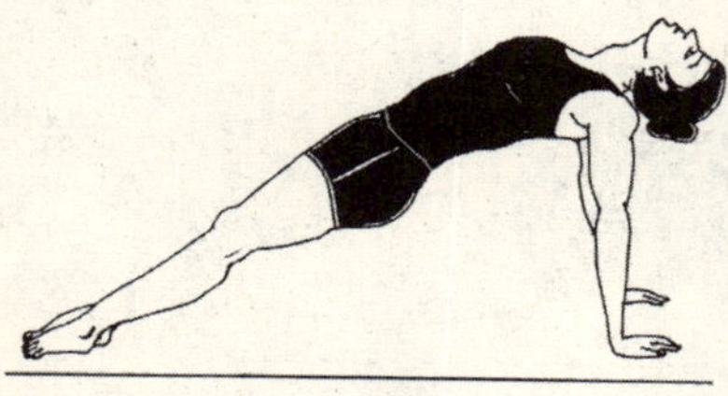

Method: Sit with your legs stretched out in front. Keep your hands on the ground in such a way that the left hand is little away from the left buttock and the right hand is a little away from the right buttock. Let your fingers point back. Bend your torso slightly to the back too.

Then, by applying pressure on your hands, lift up and stretch your entire body. Try to keep your soles flat on the ground. Bend your head towards your back. This position resembles a wooden plank which is used to make a two wheeler go up the steps. Remain in this position for as long as you comfortably can, then, come back to the original position. This is one round. Repeat 10-12 such rounds. Inhale in the sitting position. Hold your breath while raising the body up and exhale while coming back to the original position.

Focus: On Manipuraka chakra

Precautions: Those suffering from high blood pressure and heart patients should do this asana very slowly and cautiously.

Benefits:

- The wrists and joints become strong. It gives strength to the entire body.
- It benefits the waist and the spine.
- It reduces excess fat in the abdominal region.

Comments: While raising the body up, the hands and legs should be stretched fully. Some yoga teachers call this asana Konasana.

---

* Yogacharyas have taught **Purvottanasana** in many different ways:

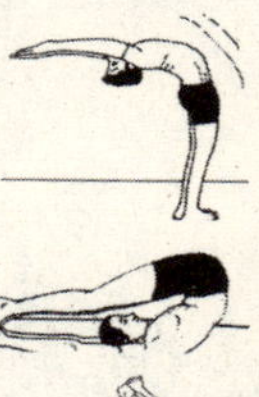

- Stand straight. Raise your hands up and bend your body back from the waist.
- Do **Halasana** and hold your big toes with your hands.

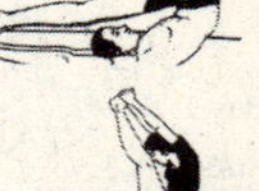

- Stretch your legs in front. Shift your body weight on your buttocks and lift up your legs. Then, the big toes with your hands.

Khanjanasana (Bird pose)

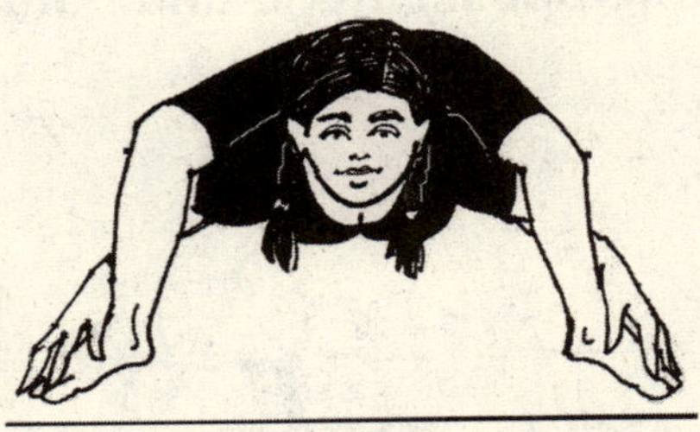

Meaning: 'Khanjana' is the name of a bird. It is said that this bird is very rare and seldom seen; seeing it is considered auspicious.

Method: Stand straight. Place your legs about two feet apart. Bend your knees and try to sit, but do not sit completely. Take your hands back and bring them in front from in between your thighs. Touch your toes with your fingers or hold them. Lift up your buttocks and broaden your chest. Raise your face up.

Breathing: Exhale while being in the process of doing the asana. Breathe normally in the final posture. Inhale while coming back to the original position.

Time: As per convenience

Benefits:

- It cures constipation.
- It keeps the digestive system in order.
- It makes the spine flexible.
- It strengthens the joints of the thighs, knees and the neck.

Precautions: Those suffering from high blood pressure, heart patients and those with chronic problems of the spine should be very cautious towards their body movements.

Practice is not dependent on resources.

Vipareeta Sheersha Dvihasta Baddhasana/ Kalyanasana (Opposite head and hand tied asana)

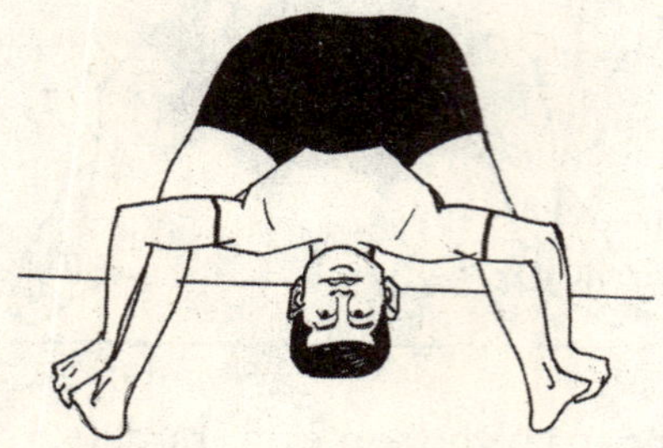

Meaning: 'Vipareeta' means opposite; 'Sheersha' means head. 'Dvihasta' means both the hands; 'Baddha' means held by hand or tied.

Method 1: Stand straight joyfully. Spread your legs. Bend forward and bring your head and hands down. Let them pass in between your legs. Lift your waist. Hold your ankles with your hands. Let the breathing be normal. Hold the position for some time and then come back to the original position. Repeat the procedure.

Method 2. Instead of holding your ankles, take your hands to your back and interlock them.

Breathing: Exhale while bending down. Inhale while coming back to the original position.

Benefits:

- The body becomes healthy, beautiful and energetic.
- The spine benefits from it.
- It is beneficial for those suffering from abdominal disorders.
- It cures indigestion and enhances the digestion power.
- Chances of any diseases related to blood are eliminated.
- Problems of the head like hair fall, premature graying and head ache are cured completed.
- It cures diseases of the eye and disorders of wind.

Precautions: Those suffering from sciatica, high blood pressure and heart patients should not do this asana.

Asanas Done by Bending the Back

Bhujangasana (Cobra pose)

Meaning: 'Bhujanga' means snake. In this asana, the body resembles a snake with its hood spread up.

Method: Lie down on your stomach. Keep your leg stretched and your soles turned up. Now, since we have to raise our body by taking support of our hands, keep your hands on the ground by your sides, next to the shoulders, palms facing down. Apply pressure on your palms and raise your body up from the waist, bending it in the form of a bow. Push your palms firmly against the ground so that the body can stretch properly. Keep looking in front. Do this procedure 5-6 times.

Breathing/time: Inhale while raising your body up. Hold the posture for 10-15 seconds and breathe normally. Exhale while coming back to the original position.

Benefits:

- Since this asana stretches the abdomen and the spine, it makes the body flexible and cures constipation.
- Those suffering from slip disc must do this asana.
- It benefits the spine and all the parts related to the spine.
- It is very beneficial in cases of women's diseases.
- It reduces fat around the abdomen. The body becomes slim and well-shaped.

Precautions: Pregnant women should not do this exercise and those suffering from hernia, peptic ulcers and heart problems should do this asana very carefully.

Comments: Some people call this **Sarpasana.**

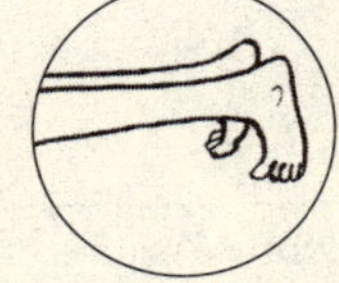

Note: Some practitioners bend their toes while doing Bhujangasana, while some keep them stretched at the back. Both the methods of doing this asana are correct. But the muscles gain more benefit when the toes are stretched. Hence, the practitioner benefits more from the asana. So, it is advisable to do the asana by stretching the toes at the back.

Uttana Prishthasana (Lizard pose)

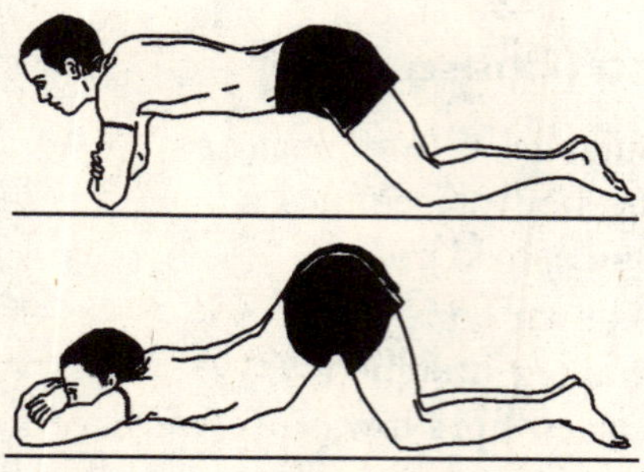

Method: Lie down on your stomach. Interlock your arms. It should appear as if both the hands are holding the other arm. In the first position, lift up your head, chest and the buttocks. Next, bring your chin and chest down and let it touch the ground behind the interlocked hands. Your buttocks should be raised. Come back to the original position.

Breathing/time: Inhale while raising your buttocks and exhale while coming back to the original position. Repeat this asana for 3-5 minutes as per your capability.

Focus : On Svadhishthana and Manipuraka chakras.

Benefits:

- It makes the back and the spine flexible.
- It reduces excess fat around the abdominal region.
- It is beneficial for women.
- It cures the disorders of gas.

Precaution: If your spine is very rigid or if you have any chronic disorder in the spine, then do not do this asana with a jerk.

Note: Asanas done by laying on the stomach such as Bhujangasana, Uttana Prishthasana, Khagasana, Triyaka Bhujangasana, Dhanurasana and Ashtanga Namaskarasana, also come in the same category. They have been included in this book.

Dhanurasana (Bow pose)

Form: Like a bow

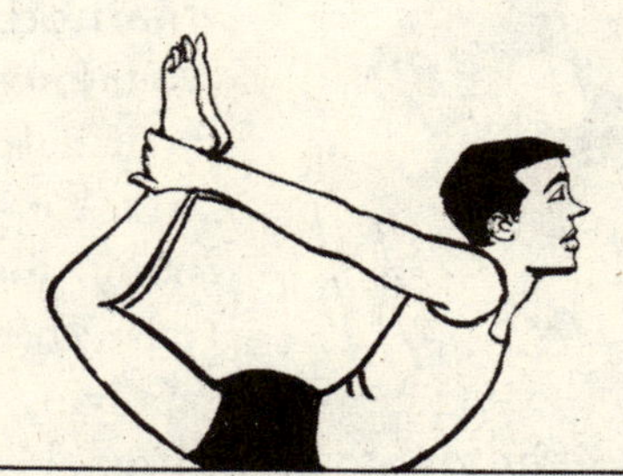

Method: Lie down on your stomach. Bend your legs from the knees and hold them with your hands at the back. Lift your chest and head. Keep your hands straight and try to stretch as much as possible using the muscles of the legs, pulling against them. You can also rock to and fro in this position and do light exercise.

Breathing: Inhale while holding the legs. Hold your breath. Exhale while coming back to the original position.

Time: 15 seconds to half a minute; repeat this asana 4-5 times.

Focus: On Mooladhara and Vishuddhi chakra

Benefits:

- It gives relief from chronic constipation and brings happiness.
- It strengthens the digestive system and improves digestion.
- It is a destroyer of obesity.
- It makes the spine flexible and brings swiftness in the body.
- If this asana is done under the guidance of a guru along with related asanas, it is beneficial in Tuberculosis.
- It makes the reproductive organs of women function well and also cures many other diseases.

Precautions:

- Those suffering from diseases of the intestine, kidney, ulcers and hernia along with the patients of high blood pressure and heart problems should not do this asana.
- Do this asana on empty stomach, because the entire pressure is exerted on the stomach.

Note: Some yoga gurus teach Dhanurasana as seen in the illustration, however, this is actually called **Halasana.**

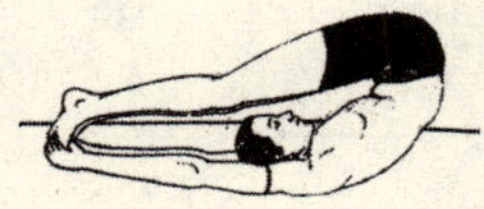

Chakrasana (Wheel pose)

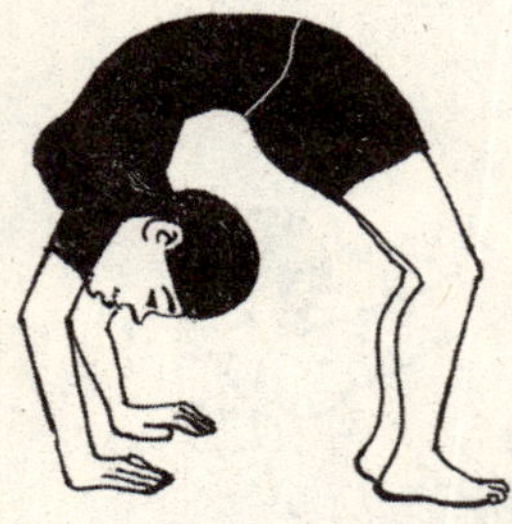

Method: Lie down on your back. Bend your knees and bring your heels close to your buttocks. Place your hands next to your ears in such a way that the fingers point towards the legs. Then, slowly raise the middle part of your body by applying pressure on the hands and shift the weight towards your head. Hold this position for some time. Exhale while coming back to the original position. First, let your head rest on the ground, and then bring the rest of the body down.

Note: Practice this asana as per your capacity. After practising enough, try to slowly bring your hands closer to the heels in the final position.

Focus: On the navel, heart and forehead.

Benefits:

- It is very beneficial for the abdomen, back, stomach and reproductive organs.
- It is very beneficial for the internal diseases in women.
- It makes the body flexible.
- It cures the disease of gas.
- It reduces obesity.
- It strengthens the thighs, spine and arms.

Precautions:

- Do not do this asana if you are pregnant and if you feel weak
- Chakrasana should be practised by holding the breath inside
- Those suffering from ulcers, hernia and diseases of the spine should not do this asana.

Comment: The above mentioned **Chakrasana** is called **Ardha Chakrasana** by some yogacharyas. In some places it is taught in a different way. For example: Stand erect. Raise your hands straight up and bend backwards as much as possible. They call this posture Ardha Chakrasana, whereas, it is **Anu Chakrasana.** Some yoga teachers call this asana **Urdhva Dhanurasana.**

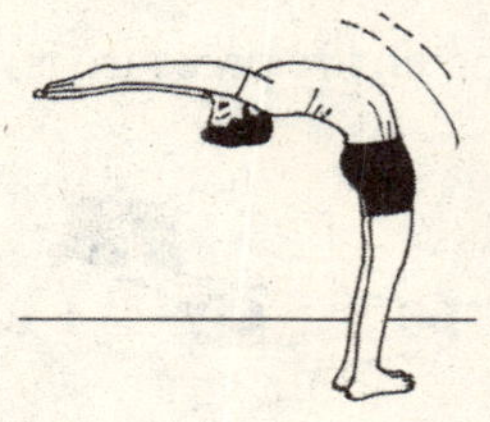

Poorna Chakrasana/Chakra Bandhasana (Round wheel pose)

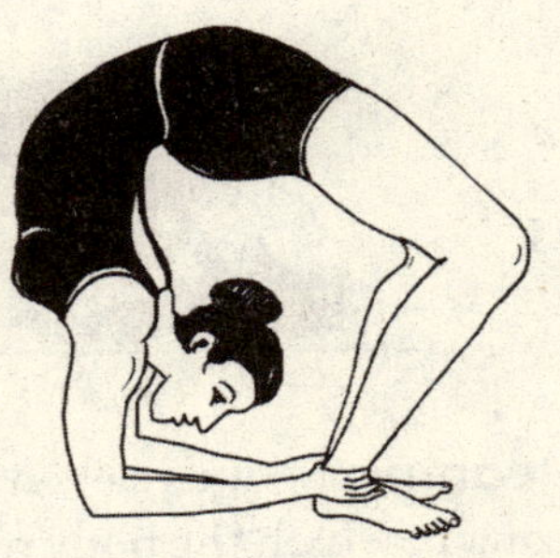

Method: The method of doing Poorna Chakrasana similar to Chakrasana. First, recreate the posture of Chakrasana. Then, to come into Poorna Chakrasana, carefully bring your hands closer and hold the ankles while resting your elbows on the ground to maintain balance.

Breathing/time: See the method of Chakrasana. Do this asana for 10-12 seconds or as per your capacity.

Benefits:

- It gives all the benefits of Chakrasana.
- The spine and the hips become more flexible by doing this asana.

Comments: Poorna Chakrasana can be done in two ways:

1. Lie down on the back and raise the middle part of your body to come into the final posture of Chakrasana. Most of the practitioners adopt this method.
2. In the second method, stand in the attention position. Raise your hands up and slowly bend backwards from your waist. Maintain your balance and let your hands reach the ground. Gradually, hold the ankles and form the posture of Poorna Chakrasana.

Precautions:

- If you are suffering from high blood pressure, if you are a heart patient or if you have a weak wrist, do not do this asana.
- After doing Poorna Chakrasana, you must do Halasana and Sarvangasana.

Setubandhasana (Bridge pose-2)/ Sheersha Padasana

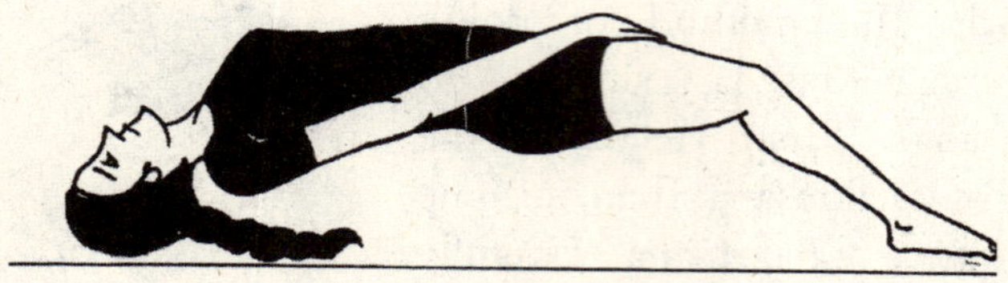

Meaning: 'Setu' mans a bridge, and Setubandhasana means an asana in which the body resembles a raised bridge.

Method: Lie down on your mat in Shavasana, or in other words, lie down on your back. Since we have to raise the middle part of the body by balancing on the head and the feet, first take a deep breath and be cautious about your body. Gradually raise the middle part your body. New practitioners can take the support of their hands. Take your hands either to the back of your head or place them on the ground and take their support to raise your body up. Alternatively, you can lift up your waist and back with your hands. After getting sufficient practice, you can keep your hands in the prayer posture or keep them interlocked across your stomach, or keep them on your thighs. The soles of the feet should be kept firm and flat on the ground. Hold your breath in the final position. Exhale while coming back to the original position.

Benefits:

- The disorders of the neck are cured and the neck becomes strong and toned.
- The endocrine glands of the head, pituitary gland and the thyroid glands receive abundant blood supply and function efficiently.
- The spine becomes flexible and free of all disorders.
- It benefits the digestive system.

Precautions: Do this asana under the vigilance and guidance of an expert yoga teacher. Those suffering from high blood pressure should not do this asana. Keep a thick folded blanket under your head while doing this asana.

Grivasana (Neck posture)

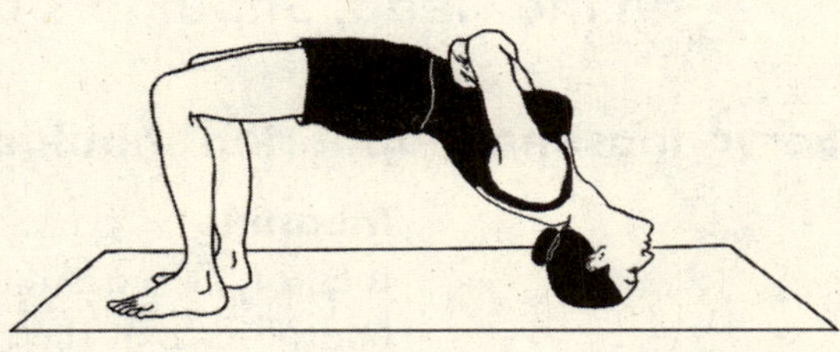

Method: Heavily fold a blanket and spread it on the ground. Lie down on it. Keep your legs a little apart. Bend your knees and bring your heels close to your buttocks. Now to come to the posture shown in the illustration, keep your palms on the ground, near your ears. By applying pressure on the hands and legs, lift up your waist and let the crown of your head rest on the ground. Then, fold your arms together and keep them on your chest. In the final position, balance your body on your feet and head.

Breathing/time: Do Antahkumbhaka while lifting up your waist. Breathe at a slow pace in the final position and exhale slowly while coming back to the final position. Remain in the final position for a maximum period of 5-10 seconds. Do this procedure once or twice.

Benefits:

- It brings flexibility to the spine and neck, and makes them strong, and free of disorders.
- It makes the digestive system effective and functional.
- It is also beneficial for curing diseases in women.

Variation: In Greevasana position, straighten up your legs while keeping the feet flat on the ground. Interlock your arms across your chest or keep them on the thighs. Some yoga gurus call this Sheershpada Bhoomi Sparshasana.

Precautions: Those who have spondylitis, slip disc, cervical problem, high blood pressure, giddiness or heart problem should not do this asana. After doing this asana, one must do Pashchimottanasana, or any other forward-bending asana.

Note: Some yoga teachers call this asana Poorna Setu Asana.

Asanas Done by Balancing/Resting the Body on the Head, Shoulders and Neck

Sarvangasana (Supported shoulder stand)

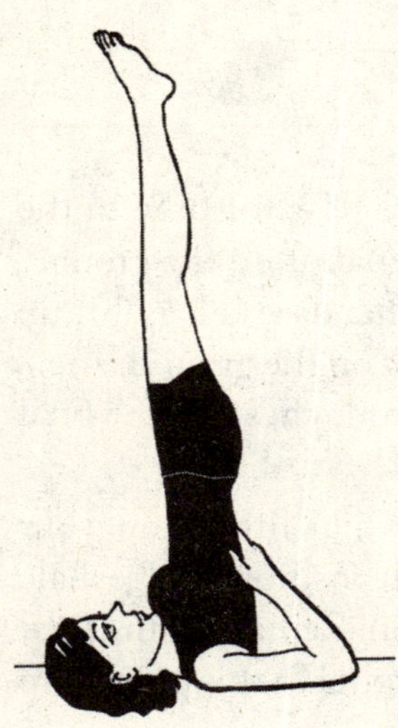

Meaning: 'Sarva' means complete, total or all and 'Anga' means parts of the body. Since all the parts of the body are involved while doing this asana and all the parts of the body benefits from it, this asana is called Sarvangasana. This asana is considered as the second most significant asana after Sheershasana. It is also called the king of asanas.

Method: Lie down on your back. Place your hands by your sides, close to your hips. Keep your knees rigid and without bending them, slowly raise your legs so that your waist and legs are at a right angle. Support your waist with your palms and raise it so that your chin touches your chest. Since you are supporting your body with your palms, this asana is called Salamba Sarvangasana. After enough practice, remove the support of your hands. If this asana is done everyday, it can give extra ordinary benefits.

Breathing/time: Do Antahkumbhaka while doing the asana and while coming back to the original position; breathe normally in the final posture. You can hold the posture for half a minute to five minutes. Increase the time with practice.

Focus: Concentrate on the whole kundalini except the Sahasrara chakra. Concentrate specially on the Vishuddhi chakra.

Benefits:

- If we call it a total body transformation asana (Kaya Kalpasana), it would not be an exaggeration. It affects the diseases related to the thyroid glands, spine, heart and the legs.

- While doing this asana, the endocrine glands receive abundant blood supply, which results in the betterment of their health.
- Those whose are always confused, and those who can't concentrate on their work, must do this asana for at least six months for 3-5 minutes.
- This asana is very beneficial for those who are patients of fits and have weak brain power.
- It cures menstrual problems in women.
- In case of navel displacement, one must do this asana four to six times.
- It stops hair fall and makes the face clear and glowing.
- It gives a positive direction to the sexual power.
- It is very beneficial for disorders related to eye sight, low blood pressure, digestive system, blood impurities and diabetes.

Precautions:

- Those suffering from high blood pressure and diseases related to the heart should do this asana under the guidance of an expert yoga guru.
- Those suffering from cervical spondylitis, slip disc and disorders of the liver should not do this asana.

Note: People who are unable to do Sarvangasana can do Vipareetkarani asana according to their capacity.

Comment: To do Padma Sarvangasana, recreate the Padmasana posture after forming the final posture of Sarvangasana, or do vice-versa. This is called Padma Sarvangasana. For Eka Pada Sarvangasana, after you come into the Sarvangasana position, bend one leg from the waist and bring it down to the touch the floor behind the head.

Vipareetkaranimudrasana/Vilomasana (Half shoulder stand)

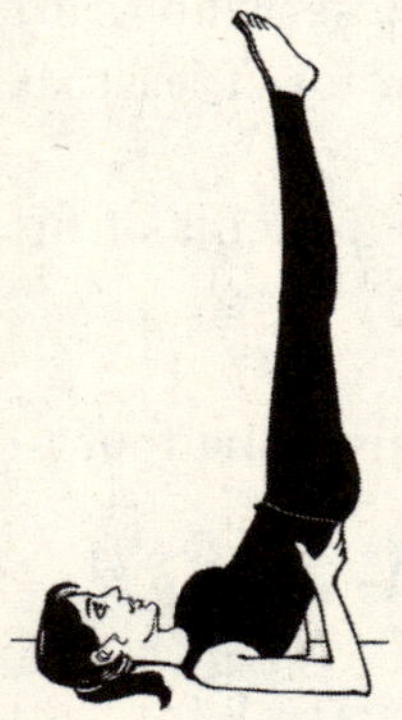

Note: This asana is exactly like Sarvangasana. The only difference is that the chin does not touch the chest. There is a lot of distance in between the two.

Method: This method is similar to Sarvangasana. Lie down in Shavasana. Support your buttocks with both your hands and lift both your legs up slowly. Make an angle of 60 degrees with your legs. Form the posture as shown in the illustration.

Focus: From Mooladhara to the Vishuddhi chakra. This asana is very beneficial for awakening the kundalini.

Breathing: Do Kumbhaka while in the process of doing the asana. Breathe normally in the final position. Hold your breath while coming back to the original position. Exhale after reaching the position.

Time: Gradually increase the time to 5-10 minutes.

Benefits:

- All the diseases related to the throat are cured.
- The voice becomes sweet and melodious.
- The chest becomes strong and all the disorders of the back and stomach are cured by this asana.
- It is beneficial for diseases like elephant feet, numbness in the legs, lack of sensation in the legs, etc.
- It cures all kinds of headaches.
- It enhances the eye sight.
- It stops hair fall and premature graying of hair.
- It is beneficial in cases of hernia.
- It gives quick relief in cases of hypo/hyper thyroid.
- It makes the entire body healthy and beautiful.

Precaution: Patients of high blood pressure, slip disc, spondylitis and heart problems should do this asana with a lot of patience.

Note: There is a mention of this asana in the Mudra chapter too.

Halasana (Plow pose)

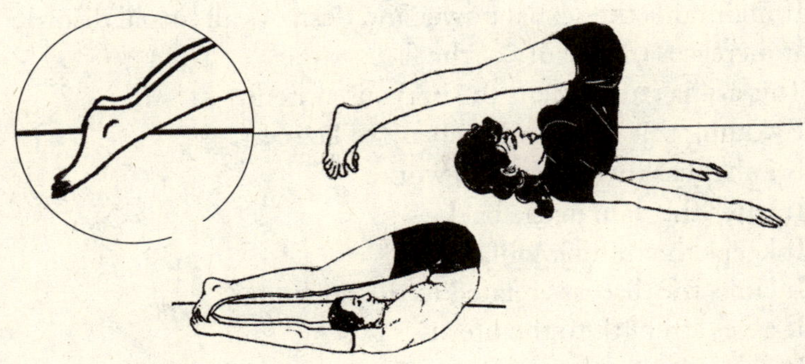

Meaning: 'Hala' means plough (a tool used to plough the fields). This asana is another form of Sarvangasana.

Method: Lie down in Shavasana. Lift up both your legs together and recreate the Sarvangasana position. Take your legs further back (behind the head) and let the toes touch the ground. Remember that in this position, your legs will be straight while touching the ground. In this posture, Jalandhara bandha is automatically formed. The hands can be kept in two positions. In the first position, the hands can be kept under the buttocks or straight on the ground. In the second position, let your hands touch your feet behind your head. Remain in this position for about 10-15 seconds and then gradually, come back to the Shavasana position.

Breathing/time: While coming to the final position, hold your breath inside, and in the final position, inhale and exhale slowly. Do Antahkumbhaka while coming back to the original position. After enough practice, remain in the Halasana posture for 5-7 minutes.

Focus: On Vishuddhi chakra

Benefits:

- This asana grants youthfulness. It does not let the back bone and the waist bend till ripe old age.
- It gives strength to the heart and back.

- It regulates the blood circulation and purifies the blood. It enhances the digestion power and increases hunger.
- It maintains the sexual power and destroys all sexual disorders.
- It increases the beauty of the face.
- This asana strengthens the nervous system.
- By doing this asana, one gets rid of laziness.
- It enhances the capacity to work.
- It cures the pain in the back.
- It keeps the mind joyful.
- It cures the diseases related to the neck.
- It gives strength to the uterus.
- It destroys constipation.
- It is beneficial in thyroid.
- It regulates the kidney. It reduces obesity and activates the small intestine and the large intestine.

Precautions:

- Those who have a rigid body and those who have sustained any kind of injury in the backbone should do this asana under proper vigilance.
- Patients of sciatica, slip disc, hernia and high blood pressure should not do this asana.

Comments: After doing Halasana, you must do Chakrasana, Matsyasana and Supta Vajrasana, or asanas which are done by bending backwards.

Notes:

- When Halasana is done by holding the feet with the hands, some yogacharyas call this posture **Purvottanasana** and in some places it is mentioned as **Dhanurasana**. We have explained Purvottanasana along with Setu Asana and Dhanurasana has been explained in the previous pages.
- Some yoga teaches teach Halasana by changing the position of the feet. See the illustration in the inset.

Vistrita Pada Sarvangasana/Supta Konasana (Reclining angle pose)

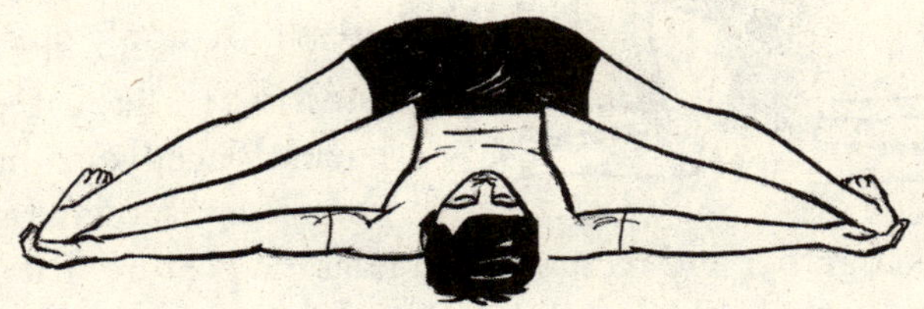

Comment: This is yet another form of Sarvangasana, or it can be considered as a variation of Halasana.

Method: Lie down on your back. Take your hands to your back behind your head. Lift both your legs together and slowly take them behind your head. Do not let your knees bend. Then, spread your legs. Hold the big toe of the right foot with the right hand and the big toe of the left foot with the left hand; or touch the heels. Let the heels point upwards.

Breathing/time: Do Antahkumbhaka while forming the final position. Inhale and exhale normally in the final position. Hold the position for about half a minute. Do it for half a minute or one minute as per your convenience.

Focus : On Svadhishthana or Manipuraka chakra

Benefits:

- It makes the legs firm and strong.
- It makes the spine strong and flexible.
- It keeps the parts of our abdomen in order.
- It also regulates the blood circulation. One gets all the benefits of Halasana from this asana.

Precaution: If you are a patient of slip disc, spondylitis, heart problems, high blood pressure and any chronic disease related to the spine, you should not do this asana.

Note: It is Also known as Vistrita pada halasan by some yoga masters.

Karna Peedasana (Ear-knee pose)

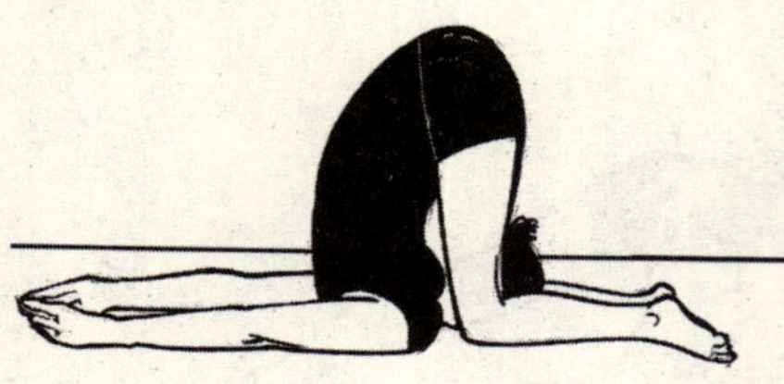

Meaning: 'Karna' means ears and 'Peeda' means to press or to apply pressure.

Method: Lie flat on your back. Place your hands by your sides. Slowly raise both your legs together and recreate the Halasana posture. Then, loosen both your knees and bend them. Bring the left knee close the left ear and the right knee close to the right ear. Press the ears gently with your knees. In this position, the feet will be placed firmly on the ground. Karna Peedasana can be done in two ways. First, with both the hands on the waist as in Sarvangasana. Second, with both the hands on the ground.

Breathing/time: Repeat this asana 5-6 times. Each time hold the position for 10-20 seconds.

Focus: Concentrate on the Agya chakra.

Benefits:

- This asana makes the whole body beautiful, well-shaped and toned.
- It makes the spine flexible. The disorders related to the spine are cured by doing this asana.
- The heart and legs feel relaxed by this asana.
- By doing this exercise, the entire nervous system is strengthened and start working efficiently.
- It regulates the blood circulation in the waist region.

Precautions:

- The spine is under pressure, so do this asana carefully.
- Heart patients and those suffering from high blood pressure should do this asana cautiously.

Comment: In the final position, the thighs are held by holding one wrist with the other.

Eka Pada Sheershasana (One leg head pose)

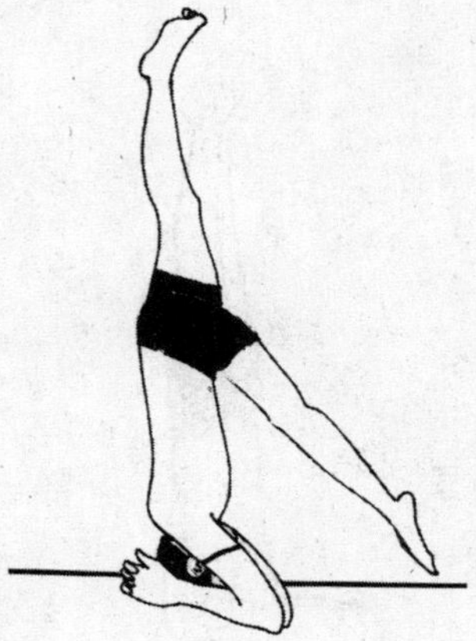

Meaning: This asana is done by bringing one leg down on the floor and raising the other up. That is why it is called Eka Pada Sheershasana.

Method: This method is easier than Sheershasana. The only difference is that in Sheershasana, both the legs are raised up and a lot of care needs to be taken while maintaining balance. However, in this asana, one leg rests on the floor. Therefore, it is also called Eka Pada Alambita Sheershasana.

Note: Rest of the description and benefits are similar to Sheershasana.

Comment: There is yet another way of doing Eka Pada Sheershasana, which is given in the following pages.

Yoga vidya is one of the ancient approaches of
scientific practices in India.

–RJT

Salamba Sheershasana (Supported headstand)

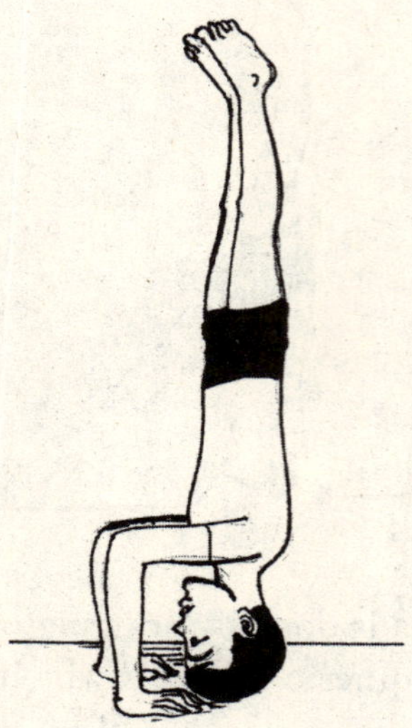

Meaning: 'Salamba' means with support and 'Sheersha' refers to the front of the head. In other words it means to do Sheershasana by taking the support of something.

Method: This method also is like Sheershasana, but the position of the hands is slightly different. In this asana, the palms are pressed against the floor for support. The rest of method, focus and precautions are the same as Sheershasana.

Benefits: It gives all the benefits of Sheershasana.

Comments: In the same position, if the whole body is raised up with the arms stretched straight, it is called **Adhomukha Vrikshasana.** But some practitioners call it only **Vrikshasana.**

Sheershasana (Headstand)

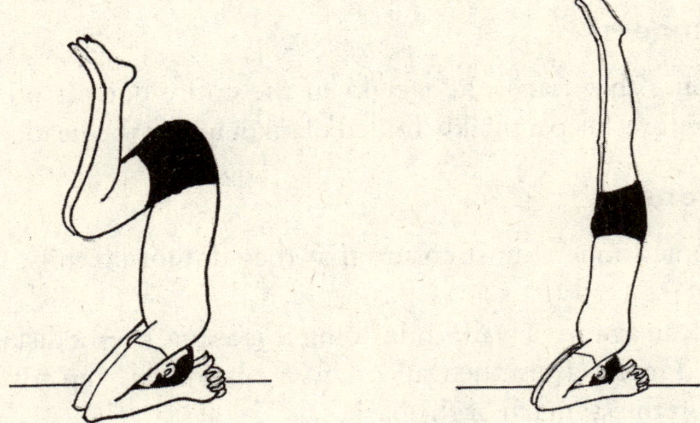

Meaning: 'Sheersha' refers to the front part of the head. In this asana, the practitioner does the asana using the front part of the head, and hence, it is called Sheershasana.

Method: Sit in Vajrasana. Bend your head forward and place the base of the front part of your head on the blanket/mat. Interlock your fingers and place them near your head in such a way that the interlocked fingers encircle your head. Now, shifting your weight on the head and gradually raise your hips (In this position, half of your body weight will be towards the head and half will be towards the legs.). While maintaining total balance of the body, try to lift up both your knees and shift your body weight towards your head. Slowly stretch one leg up towards the sky. Then, maintain balance, stretch the other leg too. This position is called Sheershasana. If you cannot do this all by yourself, take the help of another practitioner or lean against a wall. Hold the position for as long you comfortably can. While coming back to the original position, first bend your legs from the knees, then bring your waist down and finally place your legs on the ground. While being in the final posture, breathing should remain normal. While performing the asana and while coming back to the original position, inhale and do Kumbhaka. This asana is done by balancing the body on the forehead and not on the middle of the head. Therefore do it very carefully.

Focus: Concentrate on normal breathing

For beginners:

While doing this asana, the weight of the entire body is on the head, therefore, keep a thickly folded blanket under the head.

Precautions:

- New practitioners must ensure that they do not do this asana alone.
- If you lean against a wall while doing this asana, keep a distance of 2 to 3 inches from the wall, otherwise it will have an adverse effect on the stomach or the back.
- Do not do this asana in a hurry, or you will pain in the neck or the back.
- While doing this asana, keep your whole body absolutely straight, so that it can gain stability and firmness.
- Both the legs should be kept together, straight towards the sky.
- New practitioners should do this asana for only 2 to 4 minutes.
- After enough practice, lift up both your legs with a jerk and stretch them up towards the sky.
- You must practice Sarvangasana before doing Sheershasana.
- After doing Sheershasana, you must do Tadasana and Shavasana.
- Those suffering from high blood pressure or low blood pressure should avoid doing this asana in the initial stages.
- Those with ailments like heart problems, giddiness, etc. should not do this asana.

Benefits:

- Sheershasana is called the king of asanas. This asana brings about a transformation in the body.
- With daily practice, pure and healthy blood starts flowing through the arteries of the brain. Due to this, slowly, weakness of the brain and other brain-related disorders start vanishing.
- This asana enhances the aura, glow and brightness of the face.

- Since this asana purifies the blood, problems like falling of hair, premature graying and skin diseases are eradicated.
- It grants youthfulness and removes wrinkles from the face.
- It cures disorders of the eyes and makes them beautiful.
- By doing this asana, life gets filled with swiftness and enthusiasm.
- It cures all kinds of disorders of wind.
- This asana is ideal for curing insanity and fits. It brings about a balance in a distracted mind.
- It rectifies the deficiency of Hemoglobin in the blood.
- Patients of paralysis should do this asana regularly under proper guidance.
- Asthma and Tuberculosis can be cured by doing this asana regularly.
- It cures constipation.
- It controls the sexual urge and gives right direction to the sexual power.
- It gives due benefit to the abdominal region and reproductive organs.
- It provides the necessary benefits in all the mental disorders.

Kapalyasana/Kapali Asana (Forehead supported pose)

When this asana is done by shifting the weight on the forehead and not on the front part of the head, it is called Kapali Asana. The rest of the benefits are the same as Sheershasana.

One who does yogabhyas, lethargy stays away
from him/her and one who is lethargic,
yoga stays away from him/her.

–RJT

Padmasana Yukta Sheershasana/Sheershpadmasana/ Urdhva Padmasana (Lotus pose in headstand)

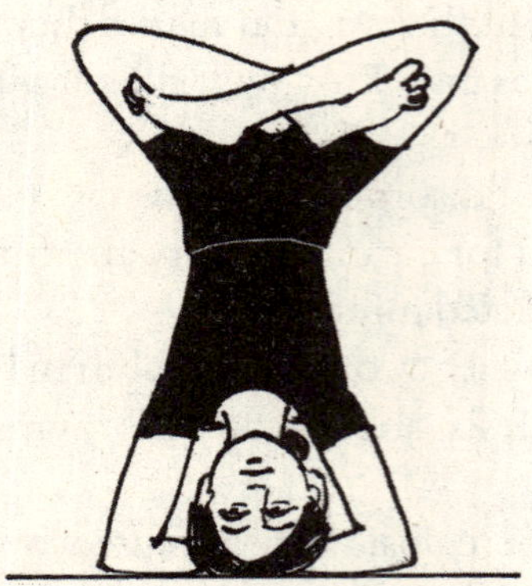

Meaning: 'Padma' means lotus. The aim of this asana is to do Sheershasana in Padmasana posture.

Method: This asana can be done in two ways. In the first method, the practitioner can recreate the Sheershasana posture and then do Padmsana. In the second method, he/she can sit Padmasana. Then, bend his/her head forward and stand up on their knees. Take support of their hands, keep their forehead on the folded blanket and lift their buttocks up in the Padmasana position. This position is called Padmasana Yukta Sheershasana. It is also called Urdhva Padmasana. The rest of the procedure is like Sheershasana.

Benefits: The same as Sheershasana

Note: Do this asana only after you have gained mastery over Sheershasana. The rest of the explanation is similar to Sheershasana.

Pindasana Yukta Urdhva Padmasana in Sheershasana (Womb embryo posture in headstand)

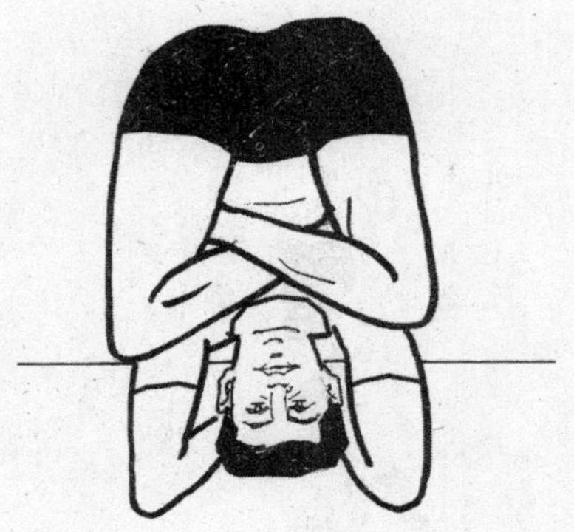

Meaning: 'Pinda' means foetus (child in the womb)

Method: Recreate the Sheershasana posture. Then, do Urdhva Padmasana. In the same posture, bring your knees down in such a way that they touch your armpits or arms. While coming into this final position, relax your buttocks. Inhale twice and exhale slowly to bring your knees closer to the arms. Remain in this position for 20-30 seconds. Inhale and come back to the original position. Repeat the procedure by changing the sequence of the legs in Padmasana.

Benefits:

- It gives all the benefits of Sheershasana.
- The parts of the abdominal region receive abundant blood supply.
- All the benefits of Urdhva Padmasana are received.

Note: This asana should be done only by the practitioner who has mastered Sheershasana. The rest of the explanation is similar to Sheershasana.

Mukta Hasta Sheershasana/Niralamba Sheershasana (Hands free headstand)

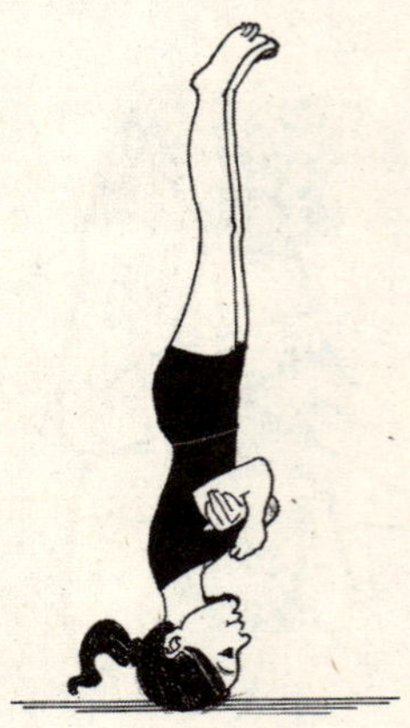

Meaning: 'Mukta' means free. 'Hasta' means hand; 'Sheersha' means head. This asana is called niralamba sheershasana.

Method: This asana can be done only after a lot of practice. You have to slowly give up the support after coming into Sheershasana. Once you have practised enough and are able to master this asana, it will be called mukta hasta sheershasana or niralamba sheershasana.

Notes:

- Rest of the explanation is similar to Sheershasana.
- This is an asana of very advanced order and should be done very carefully under the vigilance of an expert yoga guru.

One must understand all the processes of
yoga in their respective order and thereby,
gain total benefit.

–RJT

Sheersha Chakrasana (Head-wheel pose)

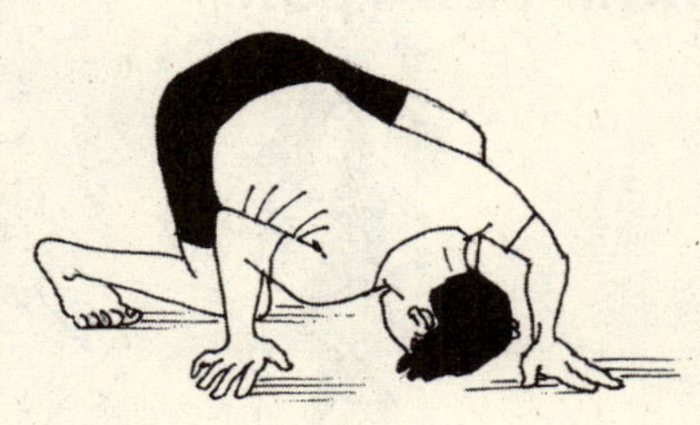

Meaning: 'Sheersha' means head and 'Chakra' means circular.

Method: Since the whole body is balanced on the head in this asana, it is advisable to keep a folded blanket or cloth under the head. Stand straight. Bend your knees and bring your head forward, down on the ground, forming an angle with your legs. In the first position, bring your hands by the sides of your head for support. Then, without moving your head and hands, move on your knees in a circulation motion from left to right, making a full circle and coming back to the starting point (Remember that the head should not move from its place.). Do the same from the right side too. Repeat this procedure a few more times as per your convenience. After enough practice of doing this the asana with the support of your hands, take your hands to your back and hold one wrist with the other, and then do this asana.

Breathing/time: Exhale while bending forward. While moving in circular motion in the final posture, keep your breathing normal and inhale while coming back to the original position. Do this asana 3-5 times.

Benefits:

- It develops memory power.
- The practitioner experiences freshness in his brain by doing this asana.
- The brain, neck, chest, thighs, knees and calves become strong.
- Eye sight is enhanced.
- It regularises blood circulation.
- It enhances the glow on the face.
- It destroys gas.

Moordhasana/Prasarita Pada Uttanasana (Crown-based pose)

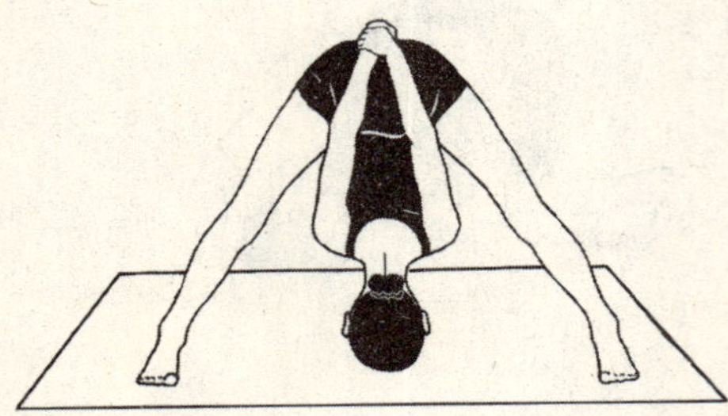

Method: Stand with your legs about 3 feet apart. Bend forward and keep your palms on the ground. Let your weight be balanced in this situation. Bring your head down on the ground in between your hands. Then, lift up your hands and take them behind your back, holding the wrist of one hand with the other. Raise your heels and let the entire weight of the body be balanced on the head and the toes. Remain in this position as per convenience. Bring your hands back on the ground and come back to the original position.

Breathing/time: Exhale while bending forward and breathe normally in the final position. Inhale while coming back to the original position. Hold the position as per your convenience, but gradually increase the time of holding the position. Do 2-3 rounds as per your physical condition.

Benefits:

- It is very beneficial for patients of low blood pressure.
- It gradually cures the disorders related to the brain.
- It increases blood circulation and brings abundant blood supply to the head.
- It removes the wrinkles from the face and enhances the glow.
- It expels the gas.

Precautions:

- If you have any serious wound in the head, or if you have high blood pressure, do not do this asana.
- Those who have giddiness and a weak brain should avoid this asana.

Asanas Done by Bending Forward

Pashchimottanasana (Seated forward bending pose)

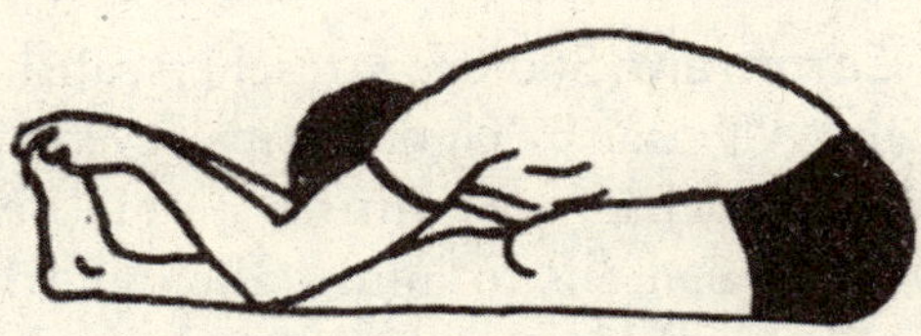

Method: Sit down on the ground and stretch your legs in front. Exhale, and bend forward to touch the big toes of your feet with your fingers. Keep your legs stretched. Do not let your knees bend. Slowly let your head touch the knees. After enough practice, your back will not be bent, but will be flat. Practice gradually. Do not be in a hurry. Inhale while coming back to the original position.

Focus: On Svadhishthana chakra.

Breathing/time: Exhale while bending forward and inhale while coming back to the original position. Repeat this asana at least 5 times and hold the position for 2-5 minutes as per convenience.

Benefits:

- Since the life force starts flowing upwards in the Sushumna by doing this asana, it is very helpful in wakening the kundalini.
- It removes excess fat and makes the body slim.
- It is very beneficial in curing constipation.
- The leg muscles become strong.
- It is very beneficial in diabetes.
- It makes the kidneys and the liver functional.
- It makes the mind stress-free.
- Those practitioners who aspire to become yogis must do this asana. It helps move towards the spiritual path and also helps in practising celibacy.
- This asana is excellent for people of all ages.
- It cures the diseases of the reproductive organs in women.
- This asana increases the height of the body. By practising this asana, arthritis and pain in the calves and thighs can be cured.

- The waist becomes flexible.
- The nerves of the back and waist get toned up.
- The impurities of the marrow are cured.

Precaution: Pregnant women, people with severe back ache and sciatica should not do this asana forcefully.

Comment: Some yoga teachers call this asana 'Bramhacharyasana' and 'Ugrasana'. 'Ugra' means severe, tough, stately, terrible; and 'Bramhacharya' originates from 'Bramha' which means soul; 'Charya' means to infuse. The one who meditates on the soul is called a Bramhachari, because in that state his mind does not divert not be distracted towards anything else, least of all lust. In other traditions Bramhacharyasana and Ugrasana are taught in a different ways.

Special comment: Maharishi Gheranda has named this asana **Ugrasana.**

Gatimaya Pashchimottanasana (Dynamic forward bending pose)

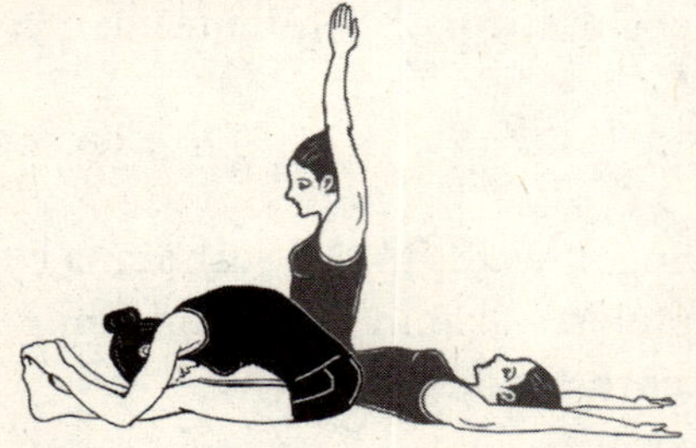

Method: To do this asana in motion, lie on your back. Take your hands behind the head in such a way that the arms touch the ears. Let the palms face up. Raise your torso and in one continuous movement, come to the sitting position then, move on to bend forward to do Pashchimottanasana. Hold the position for some time and then, come back to the original position. This is one round. Do 5-10 such rounds.

Breathing/time: Inhale while coming into the sitting position. Exhale while doing Pashchimottanasana; inhale while coming back to the sitting position and exhale while coming back to the original position.

Note: Benefits and precautions are the same as Pashchimottanasana. Pashchimottanasana is done in many other ways.

Pada-prasara Pashchimottanasana/Prishtha Mushthibaddha Pashchimottanasana (Leg spread back stretch)

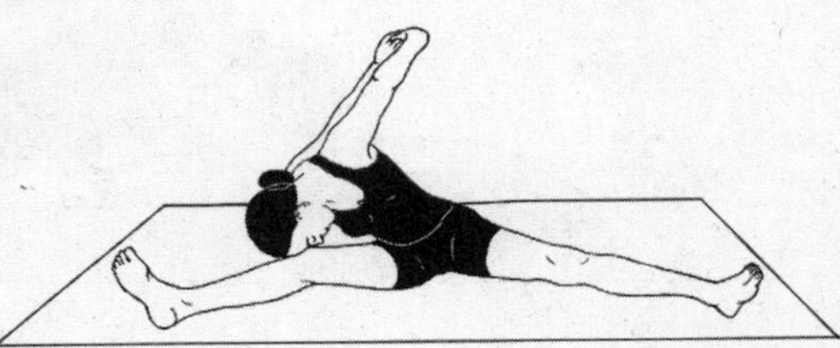

Method: Sit down on your mat with your legs stretched in front. Spread your legs as much as possible. Take both your hands to your back and either interlock the fingers or bind them in a fist. Bend the upper body from the waist to the right and let the head touch the right knee. Keep your hands stretched up behind your back. Remain in this position for as long as you comfortably can. Then, inhale and lift up your head. Come back to the original position. Repeat the same procedure with the left leg.

Breathing/time: Exhale while bending forward. Inhale and exhale normally in the final position. Inhale while lifting up your head. Hold the position as per your convenience or for 5-10 seconds.

Benefits:

- One gets almost all the benefits of Pashchimottanasana.
- It brings about flexibility and suppleness in the joints and in between both the legs; the blood circulation is regularised due to the stretch.
- The disorders of the waist, spine and back are cured.

Precaution: Those with a rigid body should first do other related asanas or do this asana with a lot of care and caution.

Variation: In variation of the above mentioned position, bend forward and place your head in between your legs and try to touch the ground with the forehead.

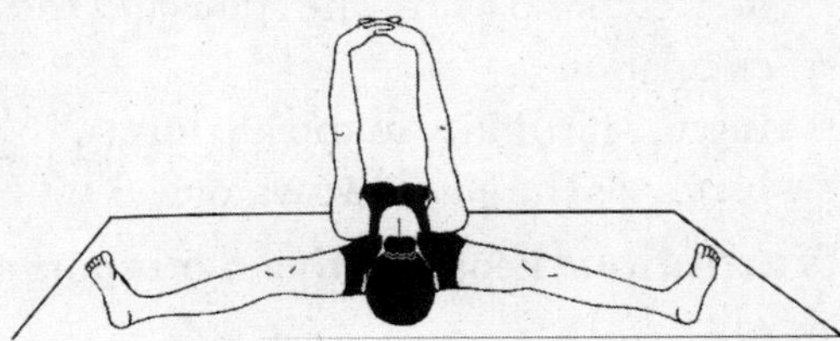

Supta Janusheersha Sparshasana/Shaithalyasana (Head-to-knee sleeping pose)

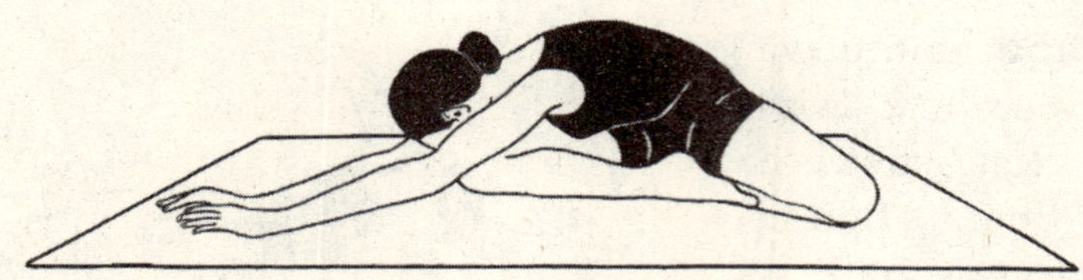

Method: Sit with your legs stretched in front of you. Bend your right leg from the knee and place the right heel close to the right buttock. Bend the left leg from the knee and place the sole and heel against the thigh of the right leg. Then, raise both your hands and bring them down along with your head. Let your hands touch the ground and remain straight. Bend your head forward to touch the knee. Then, lift your head, and again bend it forward, but this time don't touch the knee, rather touch the floor to the left of your knee. Again lift up your head and bend it forward. This time let the head touch the floor to the right of your knee. In this way, the head will touch the knee, followed by the floor to the left and then, that to the right of the knee. Repeat the procedure by changing the sequence of the legs.

Breathing/time: Exhale while bending the head forward. Inhale and exhale normally in the final position and inhale while lifting up your head. Every time when you touch the knee or the floor with your head, hold the position for 5-10 seconds.

Benefits:

- It massages the internal organs of the digestive system.
- It stretches parts of the spine and the back and regulates blood circulation.
- It gives flexibility to the hip joints.
- It pushes the gas downwards.

Precaution: People with a rigid spine should do this asana very slowly.

Utthita Janushirasana (Head-to-knee standing pose)

Method: Stand with your legs about 2 to 3 feet apart. Bend your torso forward and bring your head in between your knees. Take your hands behind the legs and interlock them or hold your calves. In the final position, let your chest touch the thighs and keep your legs straight.

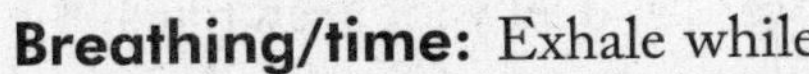

Breathing/time: Exhale while bending forward. Keep your breathing normal in the final position. Inhale while coming back to the original position. Remain in the final position for 10-15 seconds or as per your convenience. Repeat the procedure 4-5 times.

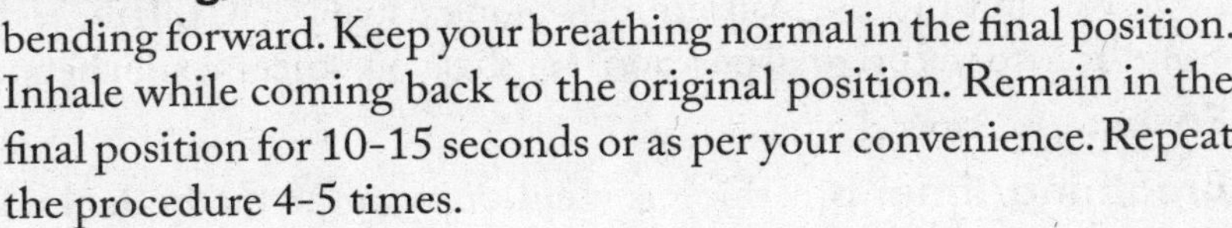

Benefits:

- It expels harmful gases from the body.
- If this asana is done regularly, all the disorders of the head will be cured along with the disorders of the eye.
- It enhances the glow on the face.
- It regularises blood circulation in the waist, spine and the back.
- It keeps hair fall in check.
- It improves parts of the digestive system.

Precautions:

- Those with a rigid spine and suffering from severe back ache should not do this asana.
- After doing this asana, do Dhanurasana, Bhujangasana, etc.

Note: This asana is also called **Uttanasana Sthita Hastbaddha Janushirasana.**

Ugrasana (Ferocious pose)

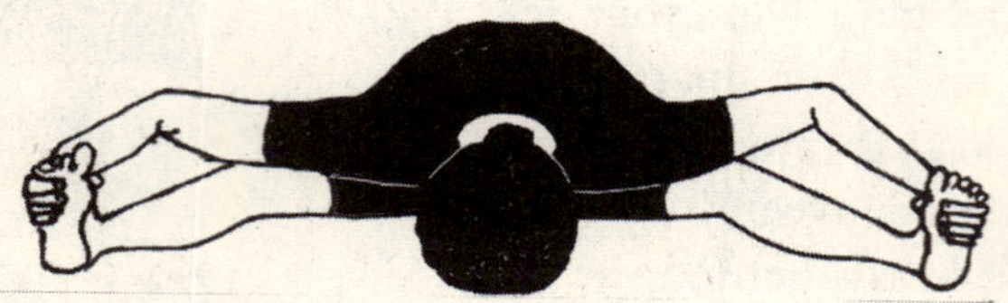

Method: Sit with your legs spread in front. Let there be a distance of two and a half to three feet between your legs. Exhale and hold the big toe of the right leg with your right hand and that of the left leg with your left hand. Bend forward and let your head touch the floor. Remain in this position for as long as you can. Inhale and come back to the original position. Try that your knees do not bend.

Focus: On Agya chakra

Breathing/time: Breathing is mentioned in the method. Hold the position for 3-5 minutes or as per your convenience.

Benefits:

- It benefits the abdominal region.
- It cures the disorders caused due to air.
- It gives all the benefits of Pashchimottanasana.

Note: Yogi Iyengar has called this asana **Pashchimottanasana** and **Bramhacharyaasana**. The practitioners should focus on the benefits and practice with wisdom.

Precaution: People with a rigid spine, severe back ache, sciatica as well as pregnant women should not do this asana.

Janu-sheersha Asana/Janu Shirasana (Head-to-knee forward bending)

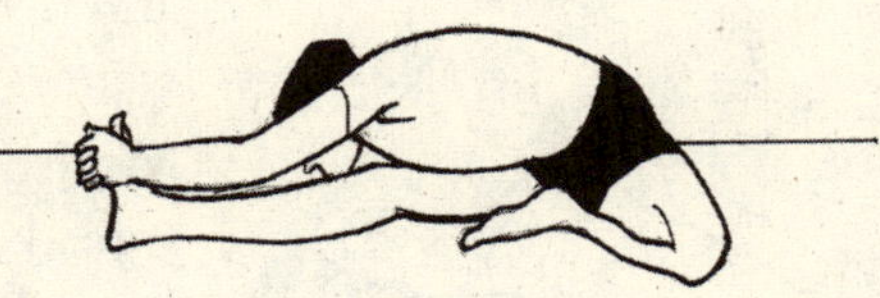

Meaning: 'Janu' means knee and 'Sheersha' means head. The process of keeping one leg straight and touching the knee with the head is called janusheersha asana.

Method: Sit on the floor with both your legs stretched in front. First, bend your left leg from the knee and place the heel near your genitals. Then, try to hold the big toe of your right leg with both your hands. Interlock your fingers and try to slip your hands down to the soles. Bring your head down to touch the knee. Exhale while bending your head. Hold this position for some time and then, come back to the original position. In the final position, take deep breaths and hold the position for half to one minute. Inhale while coming back to the original position. Change the sequence of the legs and repeat the procedure. Do the procedure for the same time duration.

Focus: In order to make the energy flow upwards, concentrate on the Agya Chakra, and for relief from diseases, focus on the Svadhishthana and the Manipuraka Chakra.

Benefits:

- It repairs the kidneys and makes them more functional.
- It makes the energy move in the upward direction, which enhances the glow on the face.
- The practitioners who are suffering from enlarged testicles should do this asana for a longer time period.
- It cures diseases related to spleen and liver.

Note: It is called **Pashchimottanasana.** When this asana is done by placing the left foot on the right thigh and holding the big toe, it is called **Utthita Janu Sheershasana.** Repeat the procedure by changing the sequence of the legs. All the above mentioned benefits are received.

Precaution: Pregnant women and those having sciatica and a rigid spine should not do this asana.

Mahamudrasana (The great gesture)

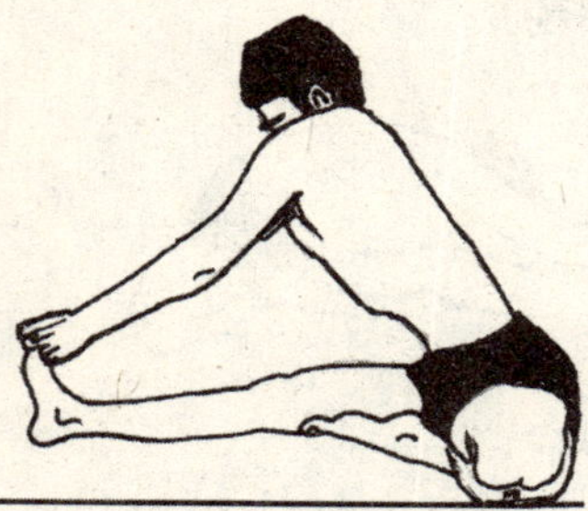

Meaning: 'Maha' means great, big, and excellent; and 'Mudra' means stance or posture.

Method: Sit down with your legs spread out in front. Bend your left leg from the knee and place the feet close to the right thigh in such a way that the heel touch the genitals near the Mooladhara. At this point you will note that your straight right leg and the bent left leg are forming a right angle. Bring your hands forward and hold the big toe of the right leg. Keep the spine straight and stretched then, place the chin on the sternum.

Slowly relax your body and come back to the original position. Repeat the same procedure by bending the right leg.

Breathing/time: Inhale, but contract your stomach in and keep it tight. Try to bring your stomach as close to the back as possible. Then, bring the stomach back to the normal position. Exhale, then inhale and repeat the procedure. Do not do it forcefully. Hold the position for 1 to 3 minutes.

Benefits:

- It benefits the entire abdominal region.
- It repairs the kidneys and strengthens them.
- This asana cures the diseases of the testicles.
- Women who have problems of displacement of the uterus should do this asana. This asana brings the uterus back to its original position.
- It eliminates all disorders caused due to constipation. In *Hatha Yoga Pradeepika*, it is written that this asana destroys great diseases and keeps even death away. What is it that the practitioner of Maha Mudra cannot digest? He can digest even poison.
- The practitioner of this asana will never suffer from leprosy, constipation, piles, spleen and many other rigid diseases.

Precaution: Those suffering from heart diseases, high blood pressure and those with a hot temperament should not do this asana.

Note: Please be very cautious while doing this asana. Only after you have practised it thoroughly should you do this asana in its complete form.

Baddha Konasana (Bound angle pose)

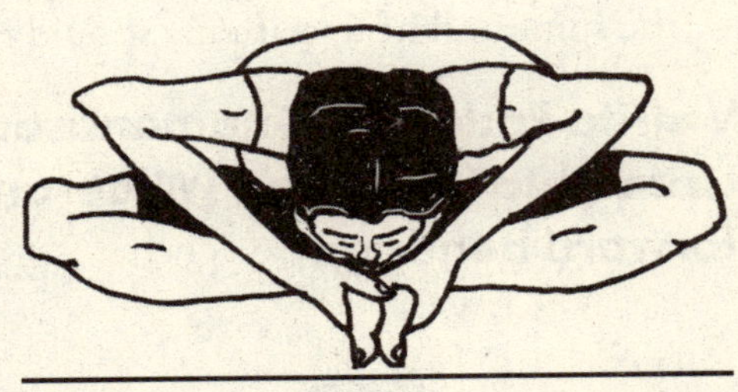

Meaning: 'Baddha' means tied, held or firmly established, joined with something or attached.

Method: Sit with your legs spread in front. Bend both the knees and bring your feet together. Join the heels and pull them towards your genitals and bring them to the Mooladhara Chakra. Let your thighs and knees touch the ground. Your spine should be absolutely straight. Look in front and hold the feet firmly. Then, exhale and bend forward to touch the ground with your nose. Let your chin too touch the ground. Breathe normally. Hold your breath for 10-20 seconds, inhale and come back to the original position.

Breathing/time: Already mentioned in the method.

Benefits:

- It is very beneficial for diseases in men and for women.
- It makes the kidneys, the genitals, and the urinary bladder disease free.
- This asana is a blessing in cases of hernia, pain in the hips and generally, for the testicles.
- It regularises the irregular menstrual bleeding in women and strengthens the uterus.
- Pregnant women should sit in this posture (but not bend forward) regularly. As a result, they will not have too much

pain during delivery and there will be no swelling in the blood vessels.

- This asana increases the blood circulation in the back, stomach and the lower abdomen area.

Precautions:

- It is not possible to do this asana perfectly in the first attempt. So, do it regularly.
- People suffering from high blood pressure, chronic problems of the spine and heart patients should not do this asana.

Vistrita Pada Bhoo-namanasana/Bhumasana/ Upavishta Konasana (Wide-angle seated and forward bending)

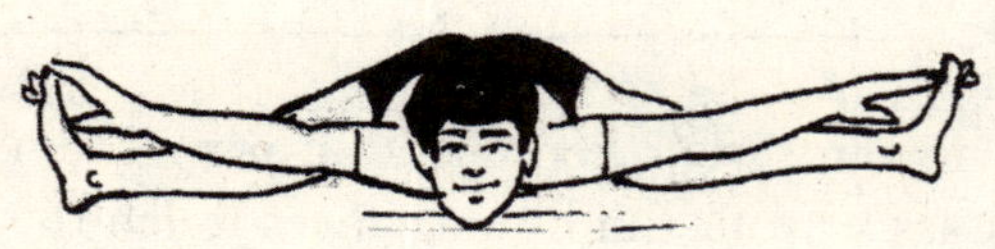

Meaning: 'Bhoo' means earth. 'Namana' means to bow or salute. Bhoonamana means to bow to the mother earth with respect.

Method: Sit on your mat with your legs spread out in front. Gradually, spread your legs further like the wings of a bird (see illustration). Hold the big toe of the right foot with your right hand and that of the left foot with your left hand. The entire leg from the heel to the thighs should touch the ground. Exhale and bend forward from your waist to bring the stomach, chest and the chin to touch the ground. Hold this position for 5-10 seconds and then, come back to the original position.

Benefits:

- It increases the spiritual energy.
- It helps enhance the concentration during meditation.
- It benefits women by making their breast firm.
- The whole body is put to use. Therefore, all the nerves, veins, and bones become healthy.
- It reduces obesity to some extent. It cures the disorders of the urinary tract.

Notes: After sufficient practice, this asana can be done by touching the ground with the forehead. Some yoga teachers call this asana Pakshi asana.

Precautions: Be cautious towards the movements and the breathing. Since this is a difficult asana, do not do it in haste. Do it with patience.

Utthita Padahastasana (Extended hand to big toe pose)

Method: Sit on your mat with your legs stretched in front of you. Hold the big toe of your right leg with the right hand and that of the left leg with the left hand. Inhale, and lift both your legs together and touch the knees with your forehead. Let the whole weight of the body be on your buttocks. Hold this position for as long as you comfortably can, and then, come back to the original position and exhale. Repeat this procedure as per your capacity.

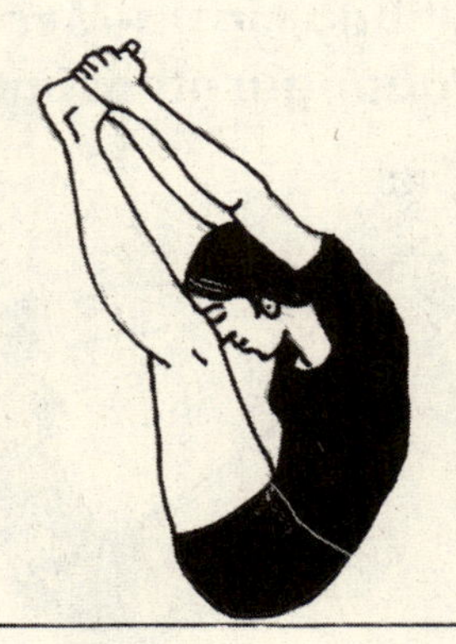

Eka Pada Padmottanasans (One leg forward bending for abdomen)

Method: If you find it difficult to raise both the legs together, you can first do Eka Pada Padmottanasana. In this asana, keep one leg in Padmasana posture by placing the heel near the Mooladhara or the Seevni, and hold the other with both the hands and lift it straight up. Let the forehead touch the knee. Repeat the procedure by changing the sequence of the legs.

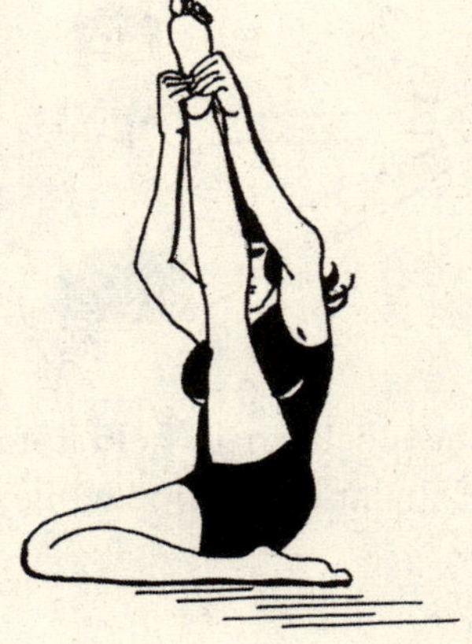

Niralamba Pashchimottanasana/Urdhvmukha Pashchimottanasana (Upward facing intense west stretching pose)

Method: This asana is also a variation of Utthita Pada Hastasana. The only difference is that you have to sit with your knees bent upwards. Hold the soles of your feet with both the hands and lift up both the legs together. Rest of the procedure is as mentioned above. The entire weight of the body will be on the buttocks.

Utthita Hasta-Merudandasana/Ubhaya Padangushthasana (Raised hand spine pose)

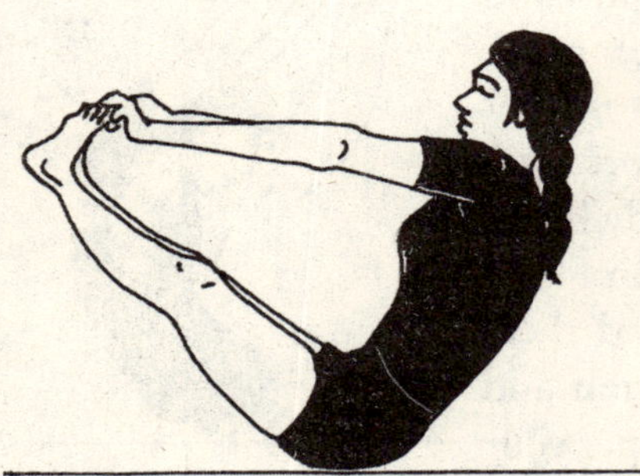

This asana is similar to Utthita Pada Hastasana. The only difference is that the head does not touch the knees. Only the legs are lifted and stretched straight up.

Comment: Some yoga teachers call this asana Poorvottanasana.

Merudandasana (Spinal column pose)

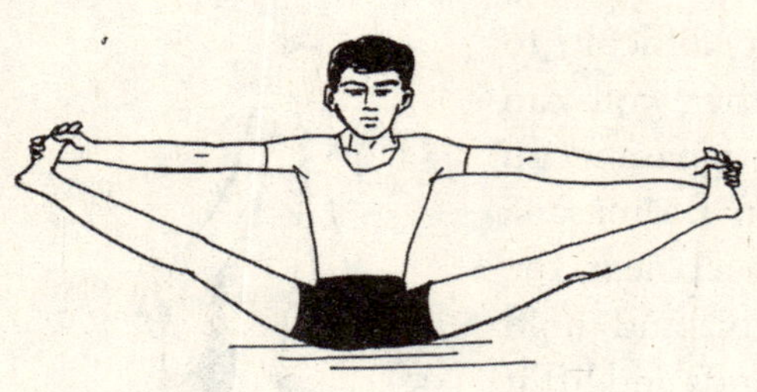

In this asana, instead of touching the knees with the head, the legs are spread to the left and right sides, as much as possible. The toes are held with the respective hands and the position is held for some time by doing Antahkumbhaka. Exhalation is done while coming back to the original position.

Benefits:

- All the above mentioned asanas benefit the abdominal region.
- They reduce the fat around the abdomen. They benefit the reproductive organs.
- The legs become well-shaped and beautiful.
- The balancing power is enhanced.
- The spine becomes flexible, strong and disease free.

Precaution: Those suffering from sciatica, slip disc and diseases related to the spine should not do this asana.

Note: We have presented all the above mentioned asanas here because they are similar to **Utthita Pada Hastasana.**

Anyone in this world can study yoga and gain its experience, and then enjoy its benefits. One needs to give a practical form to yoga in one's life.

–RJT

Asanas Done by Twisting the Spine

Tiryaka Bhujangasana (Twisting cobra pose)

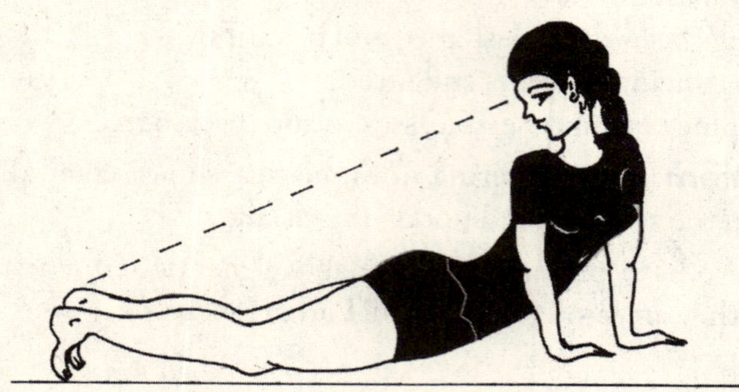

Method: This kriya is used in Shankha-prakshalana. Recreate the Bhujangasana posture. First, turn your head and torso to the right and look at the heel of your left leg. Then, repeat the process on the other side. This is one round. Do 5 such rounds on each side. Be cautious about the breathing.

Breathing:

- Inhale while raising the body up.
- Exhale while turning to the sides.
- Inhale while Returning.
- Exhale while coming back down to the original position.

Time: Do 10 rounds each while doing Shankha-prakshalana.

Focus: On Svadhishthana chakra

Benefits:

- It gives all the benefits of Bhujangasana.
- It gives special benefits when done in Shankha-prakshalana.
- It gives a thorough massage to the digestive system.
- When done slowly, it cures chronic diseases of the spine.

Note: If the legs are kept about half to one foot apart, the torso and the head have to be twisted at a greater angle. Hence, the practitioner gets greater benefits.

Ardha Matsyendra Asana (Half spinal twist)

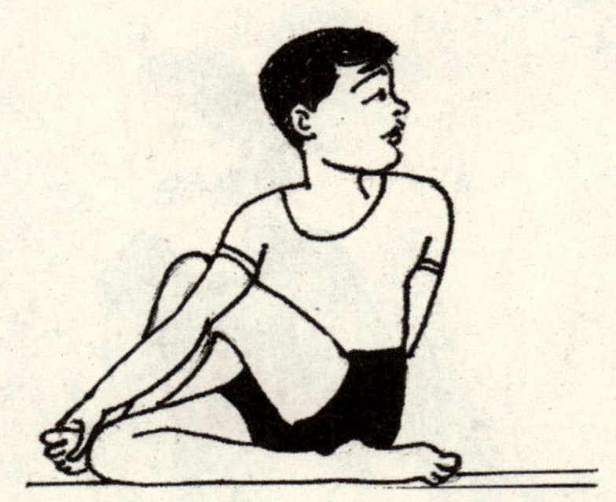

Meaning: This asana was probably taught by Yogi Matsyendranatha to his disciples, that is why it is named after him.

Method: Sit with your legs spread in front. Bend your left leg from the knees and place the heel near the Mooladhara at the Seevni, or place it near the right buttock. Then, bend the right leg from the knee and place it by the outer side of the left knee. Keep your left arm pit over the right knee. Push the knee with your arm to your side and twist your body to the right. Fix your gaze in between your brows. Twist your body as much as possible, but do not forget to hold the big toe of the right foot with your left hand. Repeat the procedure by changing the sequence of the legs.

Breathing/time: Hold the position for 5-10 seconds as per your capacity. Exhale while twisting the body to the sides, then do Bahyakumbhaka. Inhale while coming back to the original position.

Benefits:

- It is a sure shot remedy for constipation.
- It completely strengthens the spine.
- It massages the abdominal region and fixes the digestive system.
- It cures the disorders of 72,000 nadis and thousands of other diseases.
- It is helpful in awakening the kundalini.
- It reduces obesity.
- It is beneficial in cases of hernia and diabetes.

Precautions: Pregnant women, and people suffering from sciatica, ulcers in the stomach, injury in the spine, slip disc, etc. should do this asana with a lot of care and caution.

Poorna Matsyendra Asana (Full spinal twist)

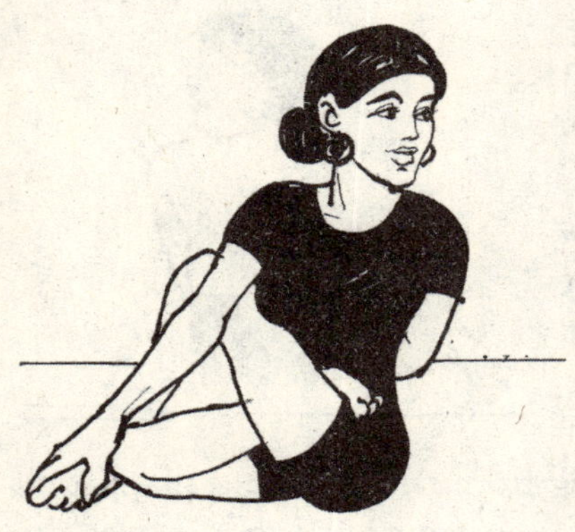

Comment: This asana is dedicated to the Hatha Yogi Matsyendranatha.

Method: In this asana the left leg is kept in the Ardha Padmasana position, which means the left leg is kept under the right buttock, and in Poorna Matsyendra Asana, the left leg is placed on the right thigh. The rest of the procedure is the same and benefits are also almost the same.

Breathing: Exhale while twisting your body to the sides, then do Bahyakumbhaka. Inhale while coming back to the original position.

Time: Twist your body for a maximum period of 2 minutes. If you experience any difficulty, come back to the original position.

Benefits:

- It gives all the benefits of ardha matsyendra asana.
- While performing this asana, the faculties of the abdomen contract on one side and stretched on the other side. So, they get a lot of benefit.
- The pain in the joints of the buttocks is cured very soon.
- Due to the spine twisting backwards, the pain in the back, waist, and the joints of the buttocks is cured.
- It cures the diseases of the reproductive organs and reduces fat around the abdomen.

Precaution: Pregnant women, and people suffering from sciatica, ulcers in the stomach, injury in the spine, slip disc, etc. should not do this asana.

Meru Vakrasana (Simple spinal twist)

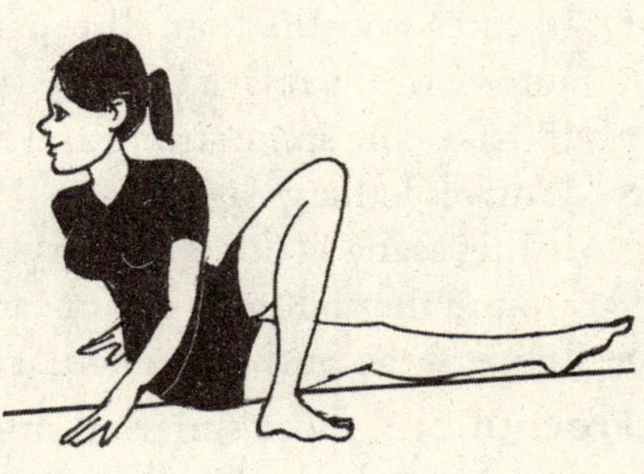

Meaning: 'Vakra' means twisted or something which is not straight.

Method: Sit with your legs spread in front. Bend your right leg and place it on the outside of the left thigh. Turn your upper body from the waist towards your left. Bring your right hand near the left buttock and take the left hand back to the right side. Keep your palms firmly on the ground. Inhale, then do Kumbhaka while twisting the body to the sides. Exhale while coming back to the original position. Repeat the same procedure by changing the sequence of the legs and twisting the body on the other side. This is one round.

Breathing/time: Breathing is mentioned in the method. Repeat the procedure 5 times on either sides.

Focus: On Mooladhara and Svadhishthana chakra

Vakrasan/Mareechyasana (Sage twist pose)

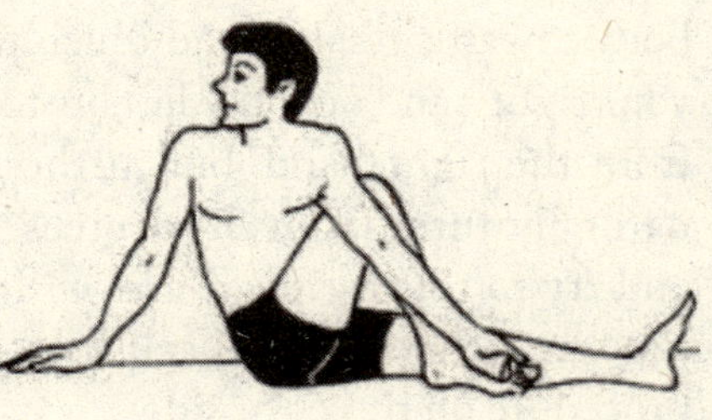

Method: Stretch your legs forward while sitting. Fold your right leg and keep it near your left knee, now turn your body to right side and breathe out. Taking your left hand towards the right knee, hold the thumb of your right foot. Keep your right hand back on the floor. Keep your back straight. Hold it for 10-30 seconds. Now breathe in and return. Repeat the same in the opposite direction.

Benefits:

- It cures constipation. The parts of the digestive system are automatically revived.
- It makes the spine strong and flexible.
- It drives lethargy away.
- If this asana is done regularly, the waist becomes slim and fat around the abdomen disappears.
- It opens the Sushumna nadi if done regularly.

Precaution: Those suffering from chronic diseases of the spine and back should do this asana with a lot of patience and care.

Tiryaka Meru Bhoo-namanasana (Spinal twist prostration pose)

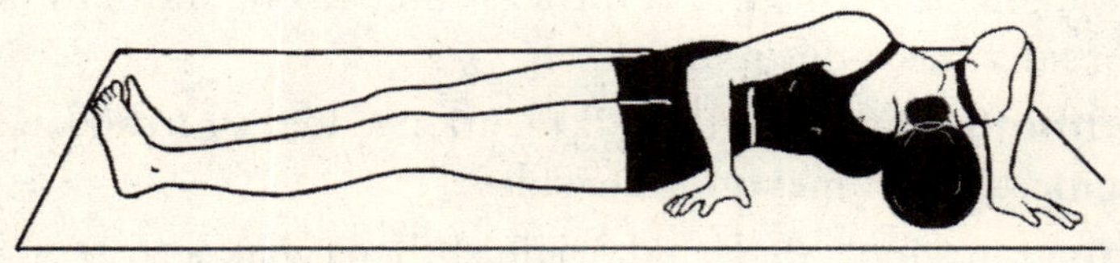

Method: Sit with your legs stretched in front. Keep your feet together (see the illustration). Since you have to twist the upper body towards the left and touch the forehead to the ground, keep your right hand near the left buttock and the left hand a little away from the right hand, but in the same line. The upper body will naturally turn about 90 degrees. Then, bend your head forward and try to touch the ground with it. Hold this position for some time and then, come back to the original position. Repeat the procedure on the right side.

Notes:

- While turning the body to the left, bring the head towards the left hand.
- While bending the head, the spine should be absolutely straight and the buttocks and legs should not be lifted from the ground.
- Repeat on both the sides for the same time duration.

Breathing/time:

- Inhale while twisting the upper body. Exhale while bending the head and inhale while lifting your head up.
- Hold the position for 5-10 seconds and do five rounds on each side.

Benefits:

- It brings flexibility in the spine.
- It stretches the back and the waist and regulates blood circulation.
- It massages parts of the digestive system and makes them active.
- It reduces fat around the waist.

Tiryaka Kati Chakrasana (Swaying and rotating waist)

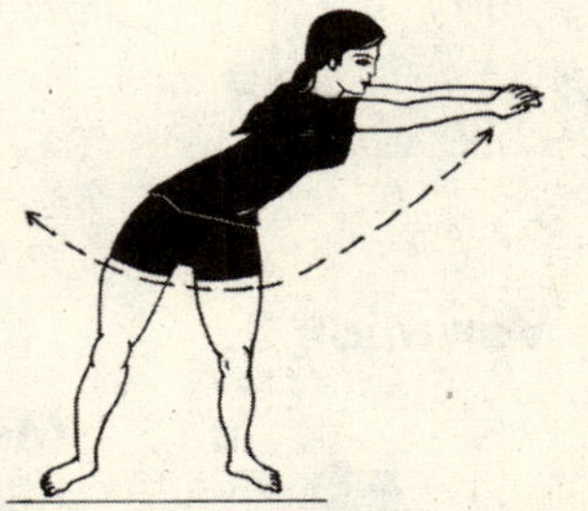

Comment: This asana cleanses and purifies the body. This is specially used in Shankha-prakshalana.

Variation 1.

Method: Stand straight with your legs about one to one and a half feet apart. Interlock your fingers and stretch your arms in front, parallel to the ground. Then, bend your body from the waist, but do not bend the spine. Keep looking in front and slowly turn to your right and keeping the same pace, to the left. Maintaining the pace, come back to the original position.

Notes:

- Turn, to the right and left, as much as possible.
- While doing the asana, inhale and do Kumbhaka.
- Exhale in the original position.
- You can also pursue the following breathing pattern: Inhale while turning to the right and exhale while coming back to the original position. Similarly, inhale while turning to the left and exhale while coming back to the original position. This method is more beneficial in Shankha-prakshalana kriya. Do this kriya at least 4-8 times.

Variation 2.

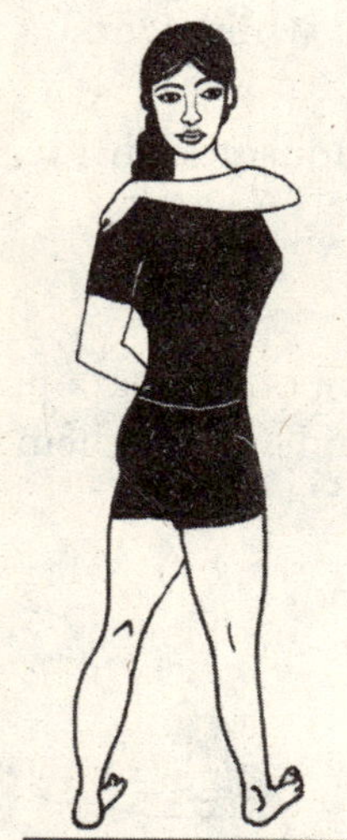

Method: In this method, the position of your hands changes. The left hand is kept on the right shoulder, and the right hand goes to the back. Turn the body to the right as far as possible. Then, come back to the original position. Keep the right hand on the left shoulder and take the left hand to the back. Turn the body to the left as far as possible. Then, come back to the original position. Repeat this kriya 4-8 times.

Variation 3.

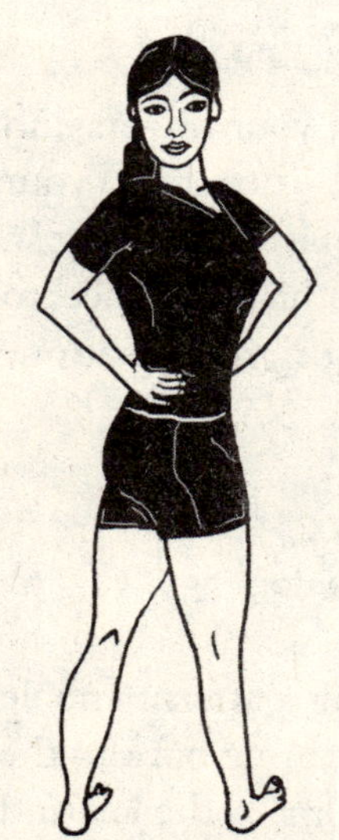

Method: In this method, change the position of the hands and keep them on the waist. The rest of the procedure is the same as above.

Benefits:

- It cures the disorders of the waist, spine, back, lungs, neck, etc. and grants them good health.
- It cures constipation. It enhances the digestive power.
- It reduces fat around the waist.
- In case of gas, drink some water and then, do this kriya.
- It makes the spine flexible.
- It drives away physical/mental stress.

Asanas Done by Lying on the Back

Supta Pavanamuktasana (Leg lock pose)

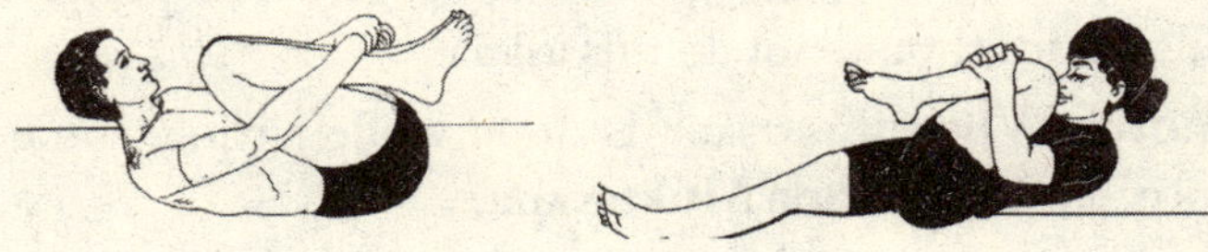

Meaning: 'Pavana' means air/wind. 'Mukta' means to be free. The asana which helps relieve air from the body is called pavana muktasana.

Method: Lie on your back. Keep your legs straight on the ground. Exhale, do Bahyakumbhaka, and bend your right knee. Wrap your arms around the right knee and bring the knee towards your head. Lift up your head to touch your nose to the knees. Try to press your stomach with your thighs. Hold this position for some time. Inhale and come back to the original position. Repeat the same procedure with the left leg. Then, do the same using both the legs together. Pavana Muktasana done with the right leg is called **Dakshina Pavana Muktasana** and the when done with the left leg is called **Vaama Pavana Muktasana.** When it is done with both the legs, it is called **Poorna Supta Pavana Muktasana.**

Breathing/time: Exhale while touching the knee with the nose. Inhale while coming back to the original position. Do this kriya 5-10 times.

Note: When you bend one leg forward to touch the knee with the nose, keep the other leg straight on the ground.

Benefits:

- As the name suggests, it expels the Apana Vayu from the body.
- Chronic arthritis and backache can be cured in due course by doing this asana regularly.
- It is a sure shot remedy for ailments like constipation, lack of appetite, lethargy, enlargement of intestine, disorders of the blood, etc.

- It is beneficial in curing giddiness, mental weakness, headaches, etc.
- It reduces fat and strengthens the spine and the neck.

Precaution: Those suffering from very high blood pressure, slip disc and sciatica should not do this asana.

Comment: When this asana is done while sitting, some yoga teachers call it just **Pavana Muktasana.**

Supta Padangushtha Nasa-sparshasan (Reclined big toe to nose touching pose)

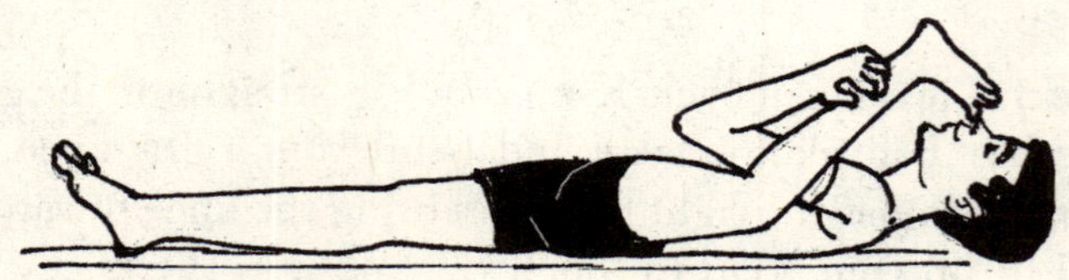

Meaning: 'Supta' means asleep, or lying down, or to lie down. 'Pada' means leg. 'Angushtha' means thumb. 'Nasa' means nose. 'Sparsha' means to touch.

Method: Lie flat on your back. Lift your right leg with both the hands and bring it towards your face. Try to touch the nose with the big toe of your leg. Let the left leg be on the ground. Then, slowly come back to the original position. Repeat the procedure with the left leg. After enough practice, lift both the legs together and try to touch the nose.

Breathing: Do Antahkumbhaka while touching the nose with your knees. Exhale while coming back to the original position.

Time: Repeat this kriya 3-5 times with the left leg, then 3-5 times with the right leg, and then 3-5 times with both the legs.

Benefits:

- It reduces the pain in the waist and back.
- The waist becomes more flexible and slim by doing this asana.
- The buttocks and the thighs become strong and toned by doing this asana.

- It enhances the digestive power.
- It benefits the spine.

Note: When one leg is touching the nose, the other leg should be flat on the ground. After enough practice, do it by keeping your head firmly on the ground.

Precaution: Since this asana is complicated, do not do it in haste. Do it carefully with a lot of wisdom.

Kandharasana (Shoulder pose)/ Setu Asana Type II – (Bridge pose-3)

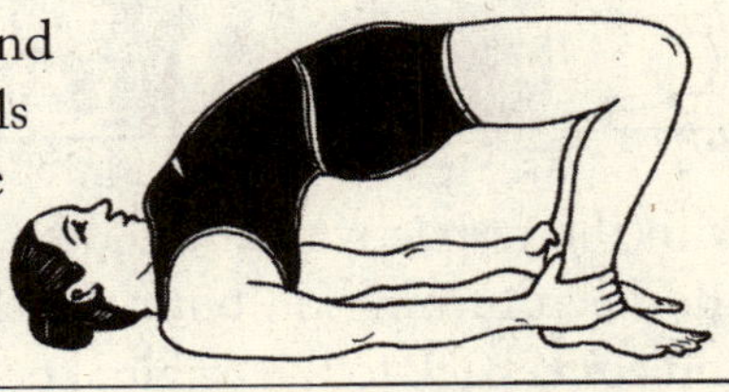

Method: Lie on your back. Bend your knees and bring your heels close to the buttocks. Hold the left ankle with the left hand and the right ankle with the right hand, and try to lift your buttocks up. Push your back up and make a bow-like formation. To come to this position, lift your chest and abdomen too. Hold this position for some time. Then, come back to the original position. Leave your ankles and spread the legs in front.

Breathing: Hold the breath inside while lifting up your buttocks. Exhale while coming back to the original position.

Time: Do this kriya 5-10 times.

Focus: On Vishuddhi and Anahata chakra.

Benefits:

- This asana is very beneficial for women diseases. It cures ailments like irregular menstrual bleeding, miscarriage, etc. and strengthens their reproductive organs.
- It generally removes lethargy in the internal abdomen area.
- Those who work in the office can do this asana and get rid of the pain in the back and spine.
- It rectifies the spine and cures backache.
- It cures asthma and regulates the respiratory system.
- It is beneficial in diseases related to thyroid.

Precaution: If you have any chronic disease in the abdomen, if you have a rigid spine, or if you are suffering from hernia, ulcers and disorders related to the neck, you should do this asana very slowly.

Note: Some yoga teachers call it **Setu Bandhasana.**

Dvi-parshva Asana/Parshva Dhanurasana (Side bow pose)

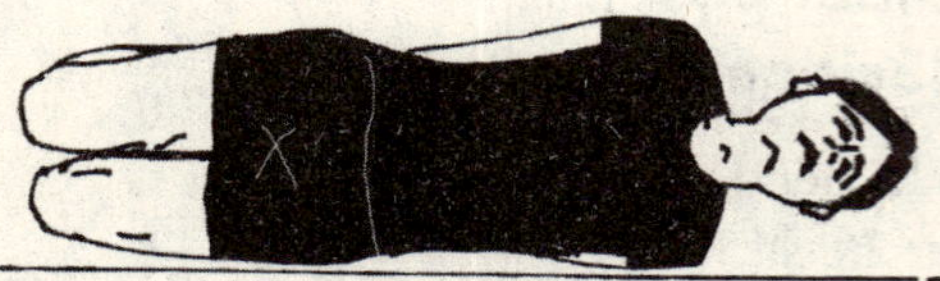

Method: Lie on your back, on the blanket and turn to your side. Exhale, bend your legs to your back and hold your feet with the respective hands. Then, inhale and do Antahkumbhaka, and keep turning on both the sides as much as possible. Exhale and come back to the original position.

Breathing/time: Do Antahkumbhaka while doing this asana. Repeat it 4 times.

Benefits:

- It cures constipation and strengthens the digestive system.
- By doing this asana, fat around the abdomen is reduced.
- The chest becomes strong and broad.
- Those suffering from sciatica must do this asana to gain benefits.

Precaution: Those who have a rigid body or are suffering from heart diseases should use their wisdom while doing this asana.

Note: This mobile movement is specifically done for Shankha-prakshalana kriya.

Comment: In this book, mentioned earlier are some more asanas done by lying on one's back. Please study the following asanas as well:

Chakrasana, Poorna Chakrasana, Chakra Bondhasana, Setu Bandhasana, Sheersha Padasana, Greevasana, Rapatasana, Setu Asana, Veepreeta Dandasana, Poorvottanasana

Exercises of the Advanced Order and Balance

Pada Prasara Kachchhapa Asana/Kurmasana (Master tortoise pose) Variation 2

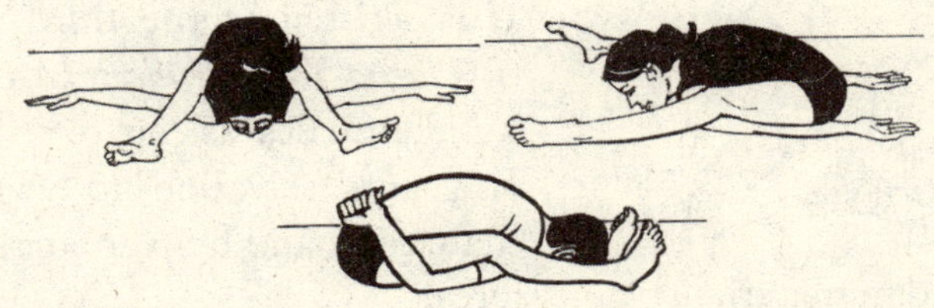

Meaning: 'Koorma' means tortoise.

Method : Sit with your legs stretched in front. Keep a distance of one or half a feet between both the knees. Bend your head forward and let your right arm pass under the right knee and the left arm pass under the left knee. Slowly take your arms to your back and either interlock them, or spread them flat on the floor. To complete the asana, lift your knees and let your soles rest on the ground. Keep the breathing normal. Exhale when you bend forward. In this posture, if you interlock your ankles and interlock your hands behind your back, this asana will be called as **supta koormasana.**

Breathing: Exhale while bending forward. Breathe normally in the final position and inhale while coming back to the original position.

Time: As per your convenience. Do it for a longer duration for spiritual benefits.

Focus: On Svadhishthana and Manipuraka chakras

Benefits:

- This asana provides physical balance.
- It keeps the brain tension free and the mind joyful.
- It is beneficial in cases of backache, pain in the waist and neck.
- It activates parts of the abdomen.
- It cures constipation.
- This asana teaches how to win over materialistic desires.
- It strengthens the kidneys.

Precaution: Those suffering from slip disc and sciatica should not do this asana.

Kandpeedasana/Kandasana (Upward ankle twist pose)

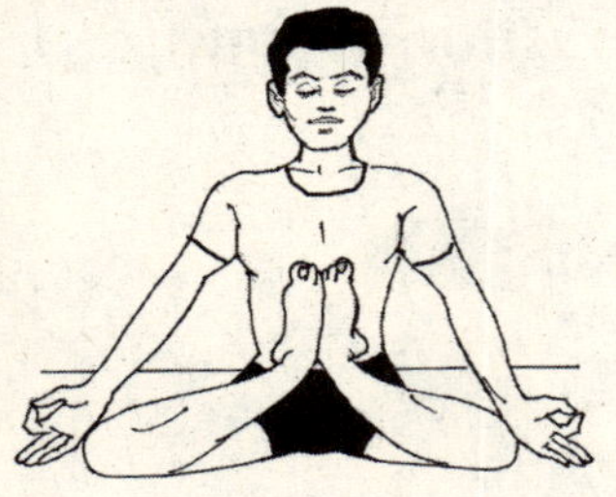

Meaning: 'Kanda' means the main gland, root, or knot.

It is written in the third chapter of *Hatha Yoga Pradeepika* that the kundalini lies asleep on the root. It grants salvation to yogis and mahatmas and help entangle those engrossed in materialistic pleasures.

Method: Sit on your mat joyfully. Spread your legs straight in front. Bend your knees and keep your thighs apart. Bring your heels to face each other and join them (almost similar to Baddha Konasana). Hold the right foot with the right hand and the left foot with the left hand. Then, pull the feet towards your torso using your hands. Upturn your ankles. Hold your feet and pull your knees and thighs. Bring your heels and the outer part of the feet (soles) to touch your navel and chest. Beginners should continue to hold the feet, and after enough practice, keep the hands on the knees.

Breathing/time: Keep your breathing normal in the final position. Do as per your capacity and convenience.

Focus: On Svadhishthana and Manipuraka chakras

Benefits:

- It controls materialistic desires.
- It makes the energy move upwards. Every muscle under the navel area gets enough exercise.
- It makes the joints of the buttocks, knees and ankles flexible, due to which their rigidity is cured.
- It calms the instability of the mind.

Precautions:

- Since this is an asana of the advanced order, do it with a lot of caution.
- Only people with strong and flexible knee joints should do it.

Nabhi Peedasana (Navel pressing pose)

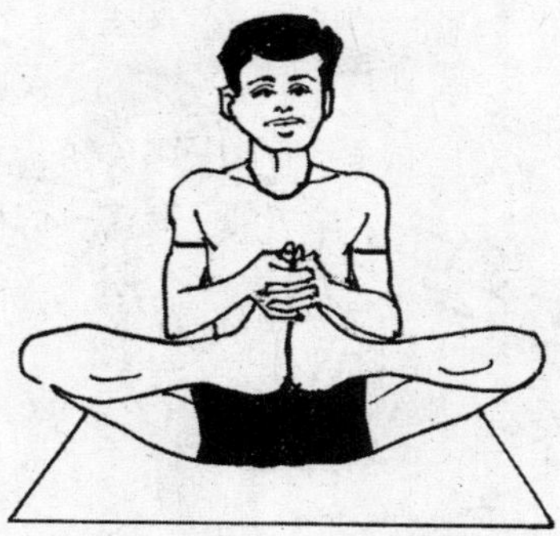

Method: Sit on your mat with your legs spread in front. Bend your knees and join the soles of your feet. Hold the feet together with both the hands. Pull the feet inwards and place them at your navel. Since your knees are lifted while practising this asana, the entire weight of the body will be on the buttocks. Therefore, try to do this asana while maintaining your balance.

Breathing/time: Do Antahkumbhaka while lifting your legs and exhale while coming back to the original position. Repeat this asana 4-5 times.

Benefits:

- It enhances the strength of the digestive system, abdomen and the intestines.
- The movement of the life force is balanced and occasionally affects the Sushumna.
- The nerves carrying the semen are nourished.
- It brings about self-improvement and balance in life.

Precaution: Those suffering from sciatica, slip disc and knee pain should not do this asana.

Akarna Dhanurasana/Dhanurakarshana (Shooting bow pose) Variation 1

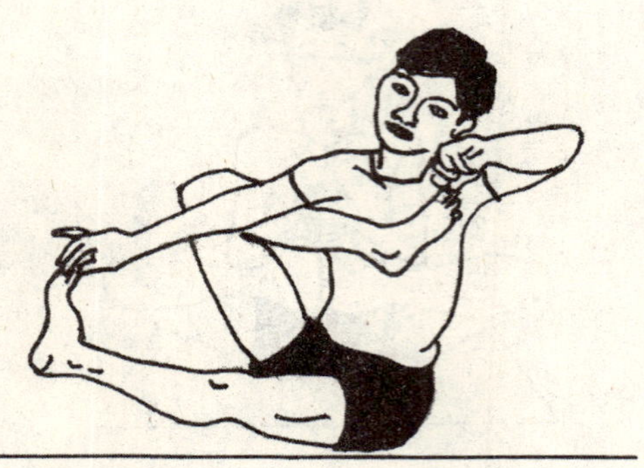

Method: Sit with both your legs spread in front. Keep your right leg on the left thigh in Ardha Padmasana position. Hold the big toe of the left foot with your right hand. Keep the knee firmly on the ground. Hold the big toe of the right foot with your left hand and bring it up to your left ear. Keep the back, neck and head absolutely straight.

Breathing/time: Inhale in Ardha Padmasana position. Do Kumbhaka in the final position and exhale while coming back to the original position. Repeat the same procedure by changing the position of the legs. Do 5 times or as per your convenience.

Benefits:

- All the parts of the limbs like thighs, calves, knees, toes, etc. become stable by doing this asana.
- Trembling of legs is cured.
- The lower abdominal area is strengthened.
- It helps in easing the motions.
- Those suffering from hydrocele can benefit from this asana.
- It benefits the spine and helps one gain self-respect.
- It enhances self-confidence.

Precaution: Those suffering from sciatica and slip disc should not do this asana.

Akarna Dhanurasana (Shooting bow pose)
Variation 2

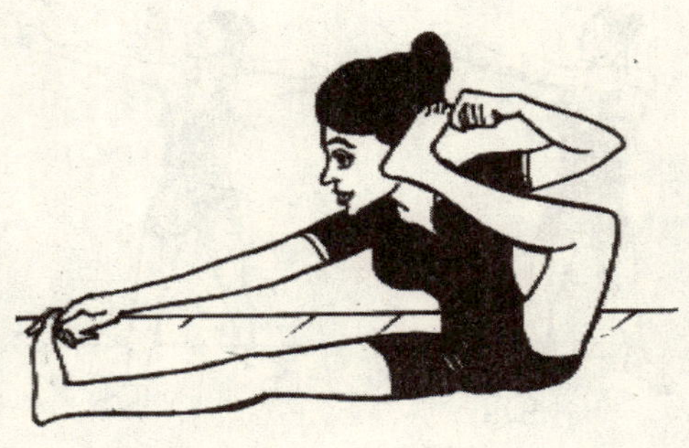

Meaning: 'Karna' means ears. The prefix 'a' means till, and 'Dhanu' means a bow.

Method: Sit with the legs spread in front. Hold the big toe of the right foot with your right hand and bring it up to the right ear. Hold the big toe of the left foot with the left hand. Remain in this position for 5-10 seconds. While doing this asana, when the big toe of the right foot is near the ears, the left leg should be kept straight (Do not let the knee bend.). Repeat the asana by changing the sequence of the legs.

Breathing/time: Do Antahkumbhaka while taking the big toe near the ear, exhale while coming back to the original position. Do it 5 times with each leg.

Benefits:

- The muscles of the legs become flexible.
- The buttocks become well-shaped.
- The disorders of the abdomen are cured.
- It helps in easing motion.
- It promotes the ideal development of the body.

Precautions:

- Keep the spine straight. Those suffering from severe backache should use their wisdom.
- The leg which is not bent should be kept straight.
- Those suffering from sciatica and slip disc should not do this asana.

Comment: Some yogacharyas teach this asana in a different way.

Akarna Dhanurasana/Dhanusha Bana Chalana Kriya (Shooting bow pose) Variation 3

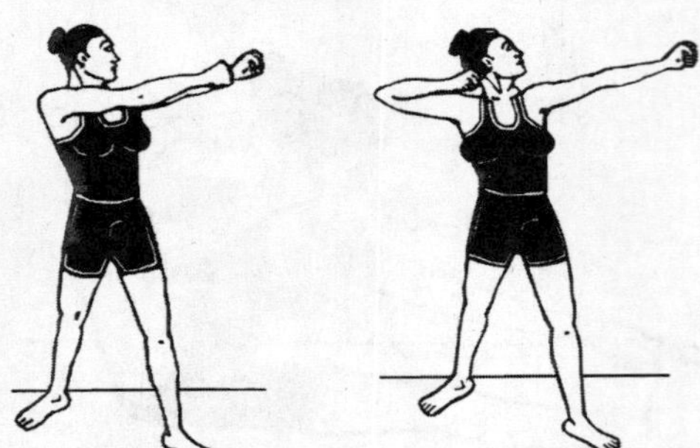

Method: Stand with your legs apart, keeping them exactly in line with your shoulders. Move the left foot slightly ahead by about one step. Stretch your left arm forward and form a fist. Keep your arm a little high (see illustrations). Then, form a fist with the right hand and keep it a little behind the left fist. Imagine that you are holding a bow and arrow. Inhale and slowly pull the left hand back up to your ear as if you are pulling the strings of a bow. Both the arms should be stiff. Take your head slightly back. Then, exhale and imagine that you have shot the arrow. Reduce the stress on your arms and bring your left fist back near the right arm. Do this kriya 5 times and then, change the sequence of the legs and hands before repeating the procedure 5 more times.

Comment: Do not take this kriya lightly because it teaches us two things: First, concentration and the second, focusing on the goal. When we pull the strings of the bow, we look at our goal or target with absolute concentration. In the same way, when we aim at our own development and growth in life, working in that direction with concentration, we will certainly succeed. We must always remember these two values in our life.

Benefits:

- We get the mantra to develop our life.
- The power of concentration increases. We enable new paths to attain our goals.
- The disorders of the shoulders, hands and neck are cured.

Note: The practitioner tries to pull the string of the bow in this method.

Prishthasana (Back bending pose)

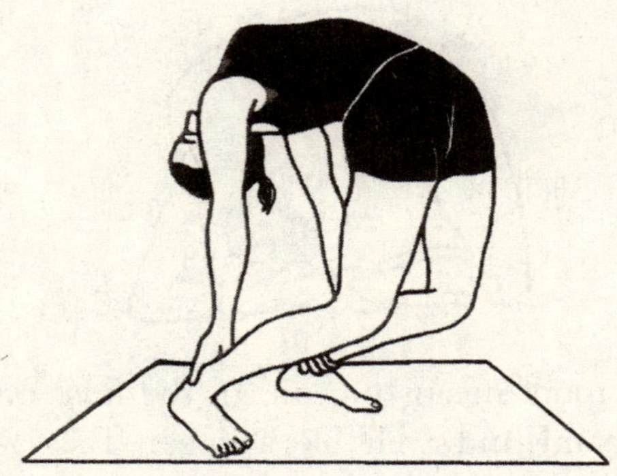

Method: Stand straight. Keep a distance of one foot between your legs. Bend your knees slightly forward and hold the lower part of your calves (ankles) by taking your hands back. When you do this, your waist and chest will bend to form a bow-like shape. Bend your head back (Try to bend your head as much towards the floor as possible.). This is the final position of this asana.

Breathing/time: Exhale while bending backward. Breathe slowly in the final position. Do Antahkumbhaka while coming back to the original position. In the beginning, do as per your capacity, gradually, increase the time.

Benefits:

- This asana is ideal for improving the strength of the neck.
- It makes the parts of the abdominal region more active.
- It cures the disorders of the waist, back and the spine.
- It strengthens the legs.

Precaution:

- Those suffering from ulcers, high blood pressure, or chronic diseases of the back or stomach should not do this asana.
- After doing this asana, you must do forward-bending asanas.

Kapotasana (King pigeon pose) Variation 1

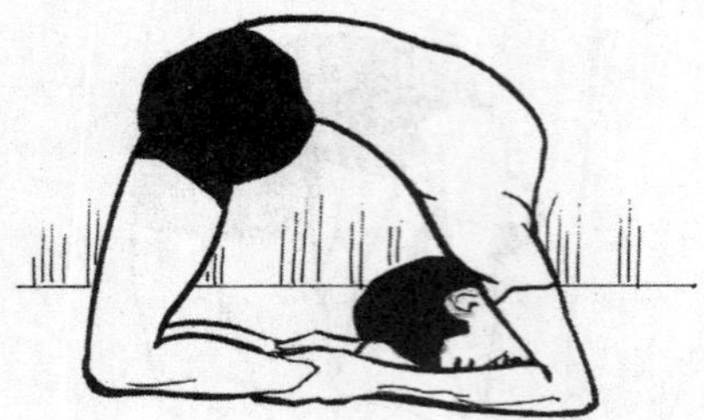

Meaning: 'Kapota' means pigeon. In the final position of this asana, chest expands and swells like a pigeon. That is why it's called 'kapotasana'.

Method: Sit in Vajrasana, and then, lie on your back. Bring your hands behind you and keep them near your ears. As you do this, slowly lift your stomach, chest and head. Allow your thighs to be perpendicular to the floor, and your legs from the heels to the knees to be parallel to the floor. Since to complete this asana, your head should touch your feet, it requires a lot a practice to perform it. Slowly raise your body and rest the back of your head on the soles of your feet. Hold the pose for a few seconds while breathing normally. Exhale and slowly lift your head up. Place your neck, back and head on the ground. Then, slowly straighten up your legs and relax.

Focus: On Svadhisthana chakra or Agya chakra.

Benefits:

- The muscles of the chest, neck and shoulders are stretched which improves the body posture.
- It strengthens the backbone, realigns the spine and relieves backache.
- It stimulates all the organs in the abdominal region, and is considered ideal for women trying to conceive.
- If flexes the hips, thigh and the groin.

Precaution: Avoid this asana you have serious injury in your back or neck, suffer from insomnia, migraine or hypertension.

Note: Some teachers teach this asana with a few variations.

Kopatasana (King pigeon pose) Variation 2

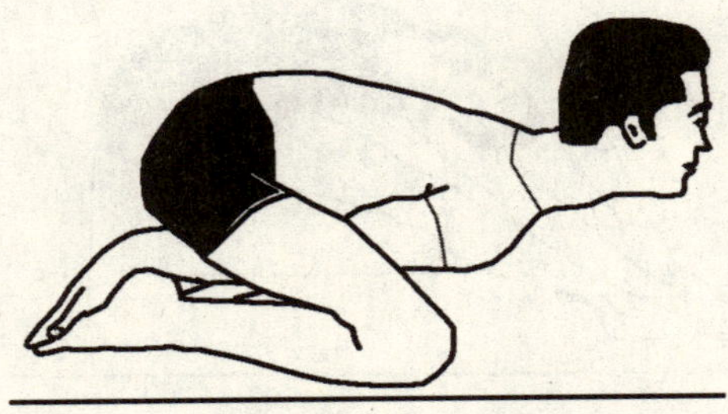

Method: Sit by bending your knees in front. Keep a distance of one and a half feet between the knees. Join the feet at the back. Take your hands to your feet from the space between your thighs and bend forward (Cover your feet with your hands.). Locking your neck, raise your head a little. Exhale and open your chest. Bring your head down again. Repeat 6-8 times.

Focus: On Anahata chakra

Benefits:

- It expands the thorax and strengthens the lungs.
- It tones the muscles of the throat, abdomen and chest.
- It activates the nervous system and also increases oxygen intake.
- Hands and legs become strong by doing this asana.

Knowledge of yoga is a divine gift given
to us by sages, saints and great souls.
Let's keep it safe by spreading it extensively.

–**RJT**

Parighasana (Gate pose)

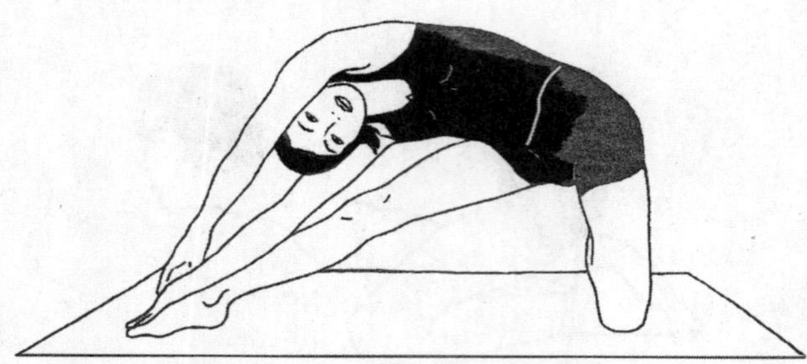

Method: Stand on your knees. Keep them close to each other. Stretch your right leg to the side and establish the foot firmly on the ground. The foot of the right leg should be in line with the left knee. Spread your arms to the sides at shoulder level. Bend the right hand and the upper body from the waist to the right side and bring the arm down on the right foot, palms turned up. The lower part of the elbow should touch the ankle. Bend your head in such a way that your right ear touches the right arm.

Then, bring the left arm down in such a way that it touches your left ear. Place the left palm on your right palm. Your right leg, hands and head will be in line with the left knee. This is the final position of this asana. Remain in this position for about 20-30 seconds and then come back to the original position. Repeat the procedure with the left leg too.

Breathing/time: Exhale while bending the head. Breathe normally in the final position. Inhale while coming back to the original position. Remain in Parighasana for 20-30 seconds on each side. After enough practice, you can hold the position for one to one and a half minutes.

Benefits:

- It cuts out the fat around the waist and makes one slim.
- The internal organs get massaged due to the contraction and expansion of the abdomen.
- It activates the digestive system.

Precaution: Pay special attention to the balancing of the body.

Moolbandhasana (Root lock pose)

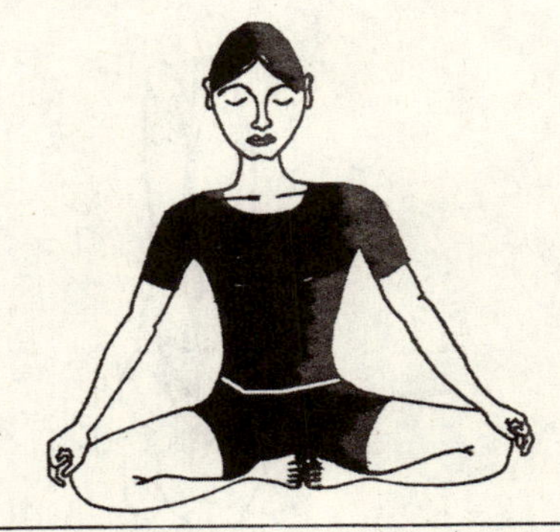

Meaning: 'Moola' means root or source and 'Bandha' means to tie or lock.

Method: Sit on your mat joyfully, with your legs stretched in front. Bend your knees and join your soles. This posture is similar to Baddha Konasana. Then, place both the heels between the genitals and the anus (Seevni nadi or the perinium) and try to sit on your heels. The pressure of this posture will be exerted on the Mooladhara. After enough practice, you can your heels with the big toes of your feet.

Breathing/time: Take deep breaths. Hold the position for half to one minute.

Focus: Try to imagine that the energy is flowing upwards from Mooladhara chakra.

Benefits:

- The practitioner moves towards spirituality; the energy moves upwards by doing this asana.
- It is beneficial for the reproductive organs and the penis.
- The sexual urge is brought under control by this asana. This is an ideal asana for those who observe celibacy.
- It provides mental peace and destroys negative thoughts.

Precautions:

- The maximum impact of this asana is on the knees, therefore, those with have pain in their knees or those who suffer from any kind of severe pain should not do this asana.
- Those who have severe pain in their buttocks and waist should not do this asana either.

Note: Some yoga teachers call this **Gorakshasana.**

Vrishchikasana (Scorpion pose)

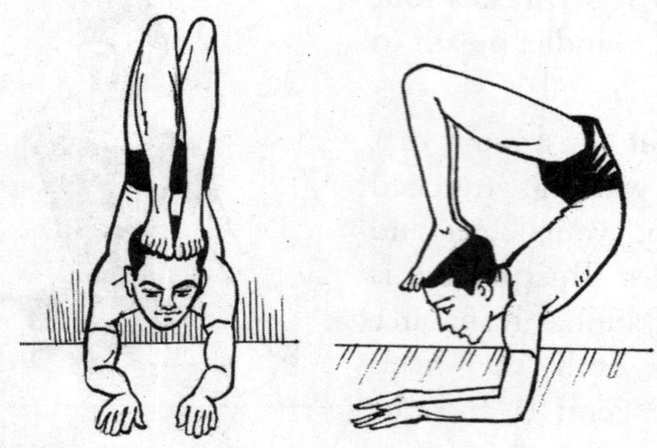

Meaning: 'Vrishchika' means scorpion. When it stings, it turns its tail towards its head. In the final position, our body resembles a scorpion ready to attack, that is why it is called vrishchikasana.

Method: Sit with your knees on the mat. Bend forward and place your hands on the floor in such a manner that the hands (from the elbows to the palms) touch the floor. Lift your neck and head up. Exhale. Lift your lower body and throw it up with a jerk to make a position like Sheershasana, while maintaining your balance. Bring your feet up to your head by bending the waist and the knees. Try to lift your neck and head upward as much as possible. Since this is an asana of the advanced order, do it very carefully. Try to bend your spine so much that the heels touch the crown of your head. Your arms should remain straight from your elbows to the shoulders. Your arms and the forearms on the floor should form a right angle. In the final position of this asana, the neck, shoulders, chest, spine, back and the abdomen are all kept tight. Hence, the breathing becomes fast. Try to breathe normally. Hold this position for as long as you comfortably can do and then come back to the original position.

Breathing: While recreating the Sheershasana-like posture, inhale and hold the breath, and then, breathe normally.

Focus: On Agya chakra

Benefits:

- This asana helps in enhancing the glow, beauty and grace of the face.
- The shoulders and arms become strong.
- The disorders related to the abdomen are cured and the digestive system becomes active through this asana.
- The parts of the back become strong and healthy.
- It is beneficial in case of diseases of the spine and the neck.
- Yogacharyas believe that this asana has psychological effects too. In this asana, the practitioner touches or hits his head with his feet and drives away the negative emotions like hatred, enemity, jealousy, etc. This makes the practitioner kind, humble and full of self-control. Therefore, it will not be an exaggeration to say that this asana fills the practitioner with spiritual energy.

Precautions:

- To reduce the stress on the back, do forward-bending asanas such as Pashchimottanasana after this asana.
- If you are suffering from high blood pressure, disorders related to the spine, or if you are a heart patient, you should not do this asana.
- Always take help while practising, untill you have not mastered this asana.
- Since this asana calls for high level of practice, keep patience till you master it.

Note: Some yoga teachers call this asana **Poorna Virishchikasana.**

All the practices which are instrumental in purification of the soul and lead to salvation can be called yoga.

– Shri Yashovijayakriya Dvatrinshika 10/1

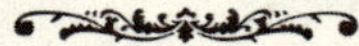

Utthita Vrishchika Asana (Extended scorpion pose)

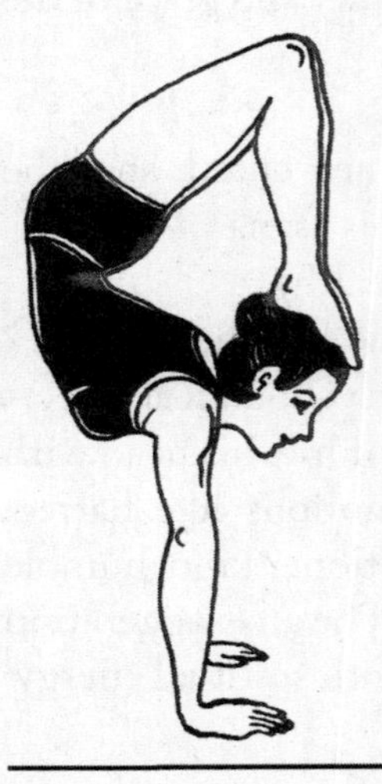

Comment: This asana is comparatively difficult. Those with a flexible spine, strong wrist, who have control over balancing one's body, and those who have accomplished Vrishchikasana, should do this asana.

Method: Stand in Tadasana. Bend forward and place your palms on the ground, in line with your shoulders. Keep your arms absolutely straight.

Then, apply pressure on your hands and lift your legs up. Bend your knees and exhale. Bring your body and legs straight up. Lift up your head and neck. Maintain balance. Stretch your spine and chest. Then, bend your knees and bring your heels to touch the back of your head. Let the toes point in front.

Breathing/time: Hold the position for 10-15 seconds while balancing the body on the palms and the wrists. Breathe normally in the final position.

Note:

- Those practitioners who do Vrishchikasana can come to the final position of the asana, and then straighten up their hands and balance the body on their palms.
- This asana needs strong determination and daily practice.
- In this asana, the entire body including the neck, shoulders, chest, lungs, spine and the abdomen are stretched to the maximum. Therefore, the breathing becomes quick and difficult.

Benefits:

- The lungs expand completely, and hence, work efficiently.
- The spine becomes flexible and strong.
- It enhances the glow on the face, removes wrinkles and brings charm.

- It helps get rid of hair fall, premature graying and dryness of hair.
- The disorders of the abdomen are cured.
- Eye sight is enhanced.
- Negative emotions like anger, pride, and attachment are eradicated and an atmosphere of peace is established in the body.
- The whole body is filled with new life.

Precautions:

- Those with a rigid spine should not do this asana.
- Those suffering from problems like high blood pressure, heart diseases, giddiness, etc. should not do this asana.
- Do this asana under the vigilance of an expert yoga teacher.
- After doing this asana, do forward-bending asanas.

Yoga is a scientific skill. Its objective is to keep the body disease free and to make the energy and power of the soul move in upward direction.

–RJT

Natraja Asana (Lord of the dance pose)

Meaning: 'Nata' means a dancer. Natraja is another name of Lord Shiv. His posture as a dancer (as depicted in the asana) is very famous. The statue of Natraja is one of the most famous and revered statues of South India (Tamil Nadu).

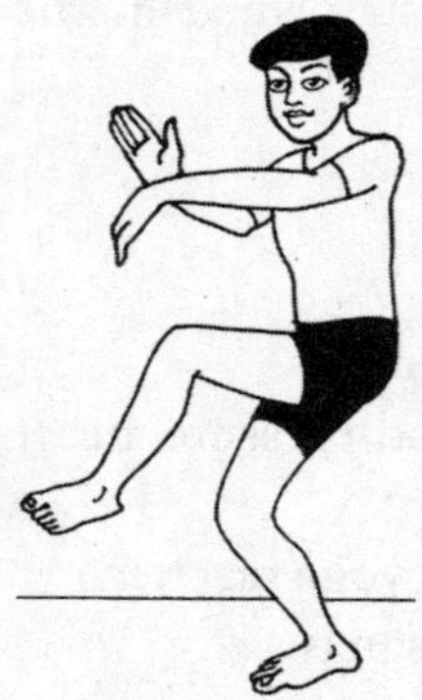

Method 1. Stand straight. Bend your right leg a little and lift your left leg, as shown in the illustration. Then, keep the left hand a little above the left knee, as shown in the illustration. Bend the right hand from the elbow and place it on the left wrist. Make Gyana mudra with your fingers and keep the palm in the blessing position. Keep your gaze fixed in front.

Method 2. Stand in Tadasana. Bend your right leg towards your back. To make it easier, hold the big toe of your right foot with your right hand and slowly raise your leg as high as possible. Maintain balance by shifting the body weight on the left leg. Stretch your right hand in front. Let the palms face down. Keep the fingers close to each other. Let the breathing be normal.

Focus: On Agya chakra. Repeat the same kriya by changing the sequence of the legs and hands.

Benefits:

- The whole body from the legs to the spine is massaged. One gains the practice of balancing the body, and the spine is strengthened by this asana.
- The chest broadened and the body becomes strong.
- In the second method of the asana, along with other benefits, the disorders of the abdominal region are also cured.

Note: Both the above mentioned methods are given here because they are very popular.

Precaution: The second method should only be done by those people who have gained mastery over balancing one's body, have a lot of self-confidence, and a flexible spine.

Vatayanasana (Horse face pose)

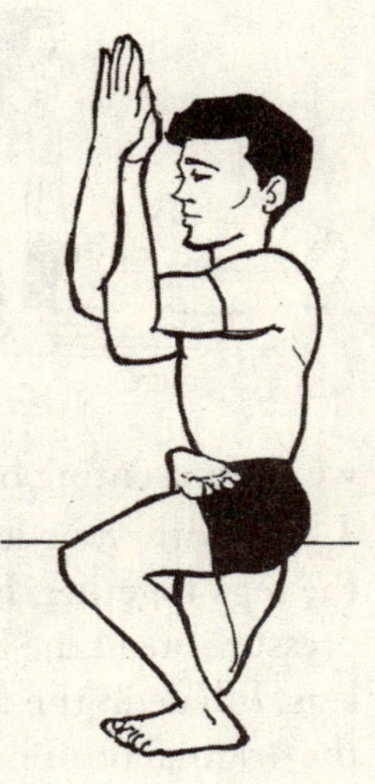

Meaning: 'Vatayana' means a horse. The posture formed in this asana resembles the face of a horse. Hence, it is called Vatayanasana.

Method: Stand in Tadasana. Bend your left leg and place your feet on the right thigh. This is like the Ardha Padmasana position. Then, join your palms in the prayer posture and keep them in front of your chest (some yoga teachers ask to intertwine the hands). Bend your right leg slowly from the knee and bring it down. Try to touch your left knee to the ground. Hold this position as per your capacity. Change the sequence of the legs and repeat the procedure.

Note: Take the support of your hands in the beginning.

Breathing/time: Inhale when you stand on one leg. Hold your breath when you are in the final position and exhale while coming back to the original position. Do it as per your capacity.

Focus: Concentrate on the balance of the body and on the Anahata chakra.

Benefits:

- This is a favourite asana of the yogis because it enhances one's glow and aura. This in turn helps in maintaining celibacy and keeping the materialistic desires under control.
- The ordinary diseases of the buttocks and the thighs are cured.
- It cures arthritis.
- It has a salutary effect on the testicles and the reproductive system.

Tolangulasana (Scale pose)

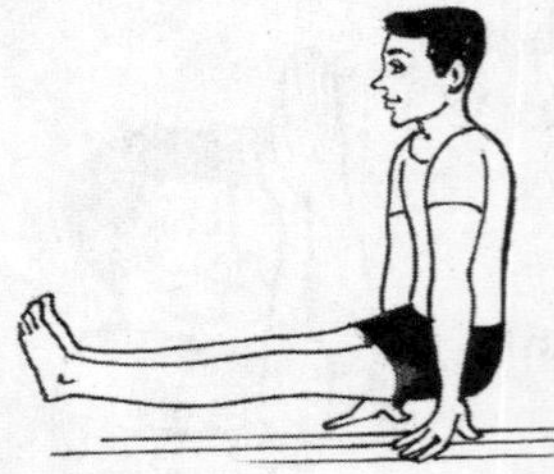

Meaning: 'Tola' means balance; 'Angula' means the palms and the fingers. In this asana, the entire body is lifted up and balanced on the palms and the fingers. Hence, it is called as tolangulasana.

Method: Tolangulasana is taught in two different ways in yoga centres. So, we are presenting both the methods here.

1. Sit with your legs stretched out straight in front. Keep both the legs together. Place your hands by the sides and by applying pressure on all the ten fingers, lift your body up. Do not bend your legs. Inhale in the final position and exhale while coming back to the original position.

Benefits:

- The hands, fingers and arms become strong and firm.
- The disorders of the abdomen are cured.
- The heart gains strength, chest and shoulders become broad and materialistic desires are eradicated.

2. Sit in Padmasana. Place your palms under the buttocks and rest your elbows on the floor. Press them against the ground and apply pressure on them while lifting your body up. When you do this, the weight of the body will be on the buttocks, and it will be borne by the fingers under them. The breathing pattern will be as mentioned in method 1.

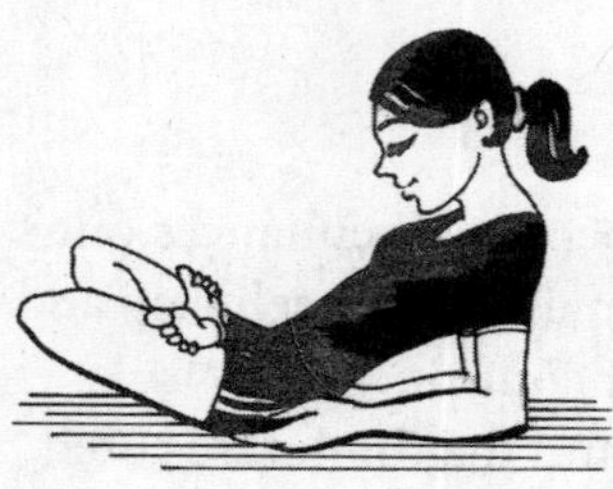

Benefits:

- It gives firmness to the shoulders, back and spine.
- The chest becomes broad and the lungs strong.

Note: Some yogacharyas call the first method Bramhacharyasana; some call it Angushthasana; whereas some yogacharyas call it Tolangulasana.

Mayurasana/Padma Mayurasana/Mayuri Asana (Peacock pose)

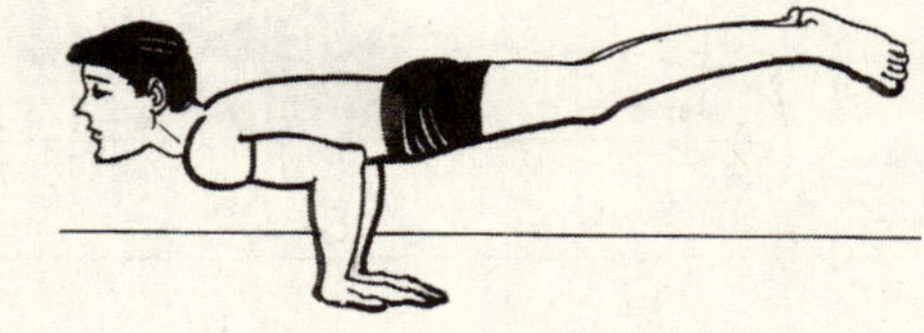

Form: Like a peacock

Method: Sit on your haunches. Let your knees rest on the ground. Place your palms on the ground in front of your toes in such a way that the fingers should point towards the toes. The little fingers of both the palms touch each other. Bend your elbows and try to touch your navel with them. Slowly, shift the whole weight of the body on the hands. Lift your body up, keeping the legs stretched parallel to the ground (You can practice by first lifting one leg and then the other). In the final position, the entire body should be parallel to the ground. After enough practice, try to take your legs further up.

Breathing/time: Inhale while raising the body up. Hold the breath as much as possible in the final position, and exhale while bringing the body down. Do this asana for 5-15 seconds.

Benefits:

- This asana controls obesity.
- It gives strength to the muscles of the hands.
- It gives stability to the whole body.
- It keeps the abdominal region in order, hence, constipation is cured. The digestive power improved. It is said that this asana can even nullify the effect of poison.
- It makes the face glow with rosy cheeks due to increase in blood circulation.

Comment: When this asana is done in the Padmasana posture, it is called **Padma Mayurasana** or **Mayuri Asana**. The benefits of both the asanas are almost the same.

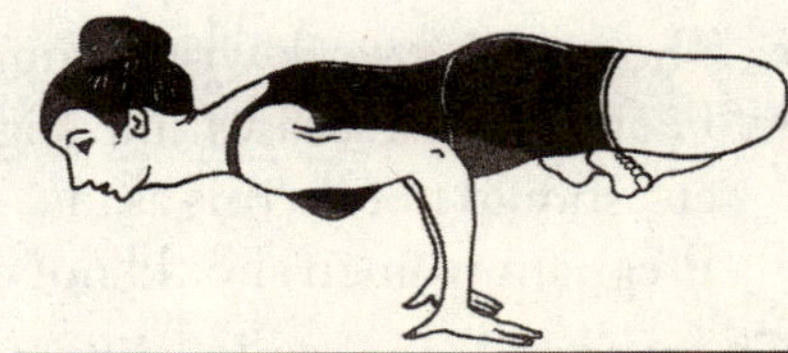

Note: Women should not do this asana forcefully. Some yoga teachers consider this asana as unsuitable for women.

Hansasana (Swan pose)

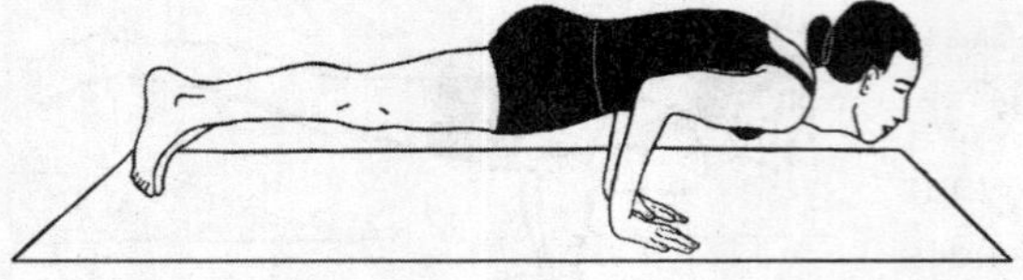

Method: Sit on your knees. Keep your palms on the floor with the fingers pointing in front. Bend forward and place your elbows on the sides of the stomach. Take your legs back, one after the one. Shift your body weight on the elbows and the arms and then lift your legs up. Maintain balance and hold the position for as long as you comfortably can. Then, bring your legs back to the floor and come back to the original position.

Note: Some yogis teach this asana with thin feet touching the ground, which means that they do not let the big toe of the feet be lifted from the floor and the fingers too point towards the feet.

Breathing/time: While performing this asana, hold the breath outside. When you succeed in holding the position well, you can breathe slowly. Hold the breath outside while coming back to the original position. Hold the position as per your capacity and repeat the procedure 3 times.

Benefits:

- It affects all the parts of the digestive system. It cures constipation and expels gas.
- It affects the stomach, pancreas, small intestine, large intestine, liver etc. and protects them from diseases.
- It increases blood circulation and enhances the glow of the face.
- It brings about a balance in life as well.

Precautions:

- Those with a weak wrist should practice it slowly.
- People with diseases like high blood pressure, ulcers, hernia, etc. should not do this asana.
- Pregnant women should not do this asana at all.

Comment: The only difference between Mayurasana and Hansasana is the position of the fingers.

Dvi-hasta Bhujasana (Two hands and arms pose)

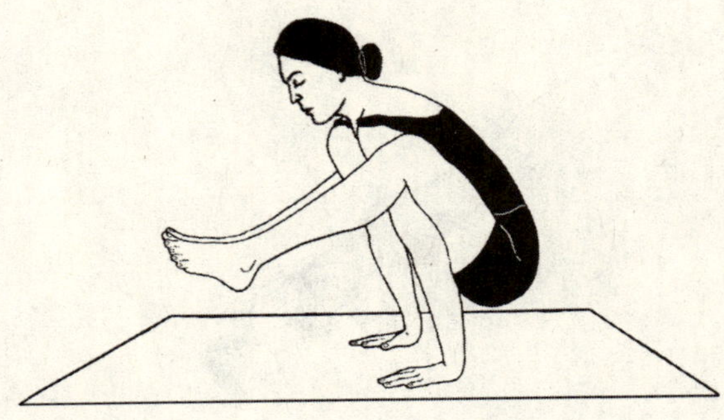

Method: Stand with a distance of about one and a half feet between your legs. Bend your knees and sit down. Place your palms on the floor from between your legs, with your fingers pointing in front. Look in front, and lift up your body, balancing it by shifting the weight on both your arms. Meanwhile, your feet in front.

Breathing/time: Do Antahkumbhaka while forming the asana. Breathe normally in the final position. Exhale while coming back to the original position. Hold the position for 10-20 seconds. Repeat the procedure 2-3 times.

Benefits:

- It strengthens the muscles of the arms, and the shoulder joints become strong.
- It activates the pancreas.
- It activates parts of the digestive system.

Precaution: Be cautious about the balance. Those with a weak wrist should not do this asana.

Note: If you interlock the toes of your feet while doing this asana, it will become **Bhuja Peedasana.**

Bakasana (Crane pose) Variation 2/ Urdhva Prasarita Ekpadasana

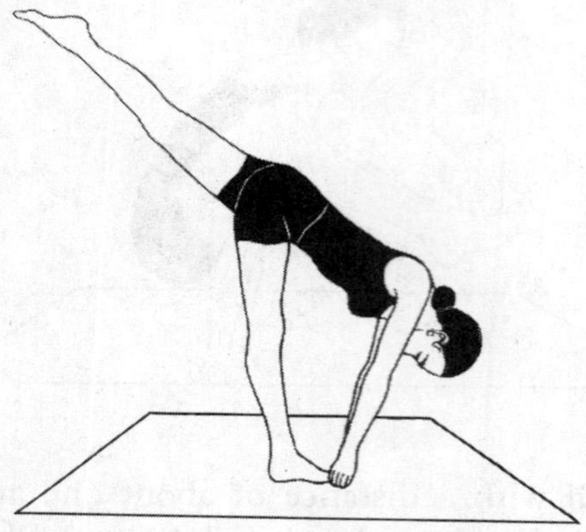

Method: Stand with both your feet together. Take your hands up in such a manner that they touch the ears. Then, bend your waist forward and bring your hands down to hold the big toe of your right leg. Lift your left leg simultaneously and keep it straight. In this position, the left leg and the head will be in one line. Come back to the original position. Finally, repeat the procedure with the other leg.

Breathing/time: Exhale while bending forward. Breathe normally in the final position. Inhale while coming back to the original position. Hold the position for 5-10 seconds and do 3 rounds with each leg.

Benefits:

- One can get all the benefits of Ekpadasana/Veera Bhadrasana.
- It is helpful in curing the disorders of the brain and the head.

Precaution: People suffering from high blood pressure, giddiness and eye disorders should not do this asana.

Padma Parvatasana/Padmasanyukta 'Janusthirasana'/Utthita Padmasana Variation 2/ Gorakshasana (Lotus mountain pose) Variation 1

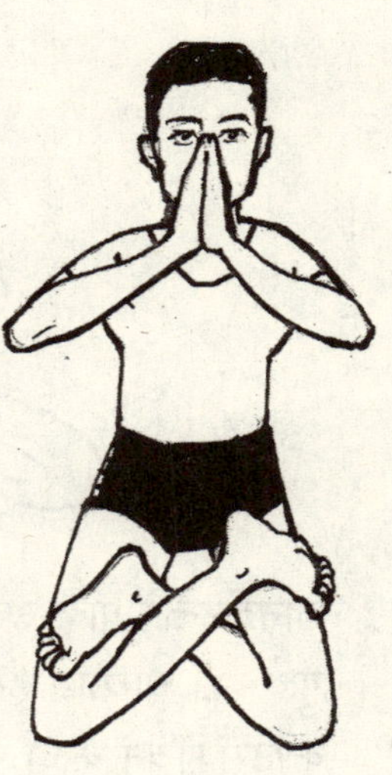

Method: Sit in Padmasana. By taking the support of your hands, bend forward and lift your buttocks. Try to balance your body on your knees. Join your hands in the prayer posture. Keep your waist and spine erect. Slowly and gradually practice this asana. Change the sequence of the legs in Padmasana and repeat it for the same time duration as before.

Breathing/time: Breathe normally in the final position. Practice this asana as per your capacity.

Benefits:

- It increases concentration and cures the disorders related to the brain.
- This asana teaches the practitioner to live a balanced life.
- It fixes vascular defects and gives all the benefits of Padmasana.
- Those who do Gorakshasana do not suffer from pain in the waist.
- It makes the energy move in the upward direction.

Note: The first method is according to the tradition of Shri Iyengar and the second method (given on the next page) is according to Gheranda Samhita. The first method is also called **Parvatasana.**

Precaution: While doing this asana, a lot of balance is needed. Therefore, it is advised to take the support of a wall.

Gorakshasana (Master pose for tantrik yogis or the cowherd pose) Variation 2

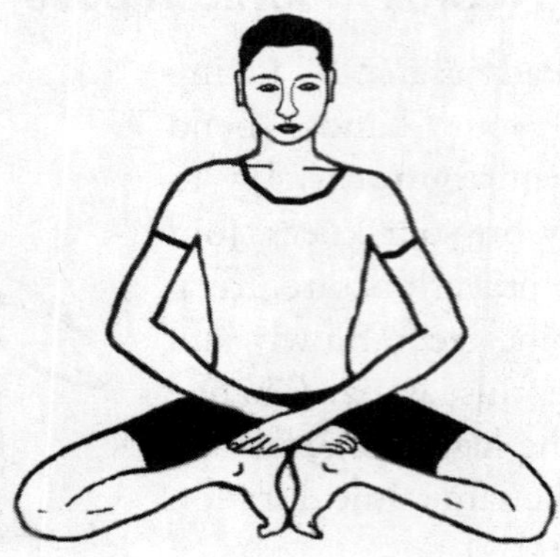

जानूर्वोरन्तरे पादौ उत्तानो व्यक्त संस्थितौ।
गुल फौ चाच्छाद्य हस्ताभ्यामुत्तानाभ्यां प्रयत्नतः।।
कण्ठसंकोचनं कृत्वा नासाग्रमव लोकयेत्।
गोरक्षासनमित्याहुयोगिनां सिद्धिकारणम्। (Gherunda Samhita 2/25-26)

According to Gheranda Samhita: Place your heels between your thighs and knees. Raise them to keep them hidden. Hold your heels with both the hands and contract your neck. Fix your gaze on the tip of the nose. This asana grants mastery over siddhis to yogis.

Benefits:

- It is beneficial for all kinds of neck diseases and ailments.
- When your gaze is fixed on the tip of your nose, you automatically practice Trataka. It cures the disorders of the eyes and make them attractive.
- If this asana is practised daily, it helps calm the feelings of lust and sexual urge. It helps one lead a more balanced life.
- It makes the energy move in the upward direction.
- By practising this asana daily, one can sit in meditation for a long time.

Urdhva Kukkutasana (Upward rooster pose)/ Padma Bakasana (Raised cock pose)

Comment: This asana can be done in two ways.

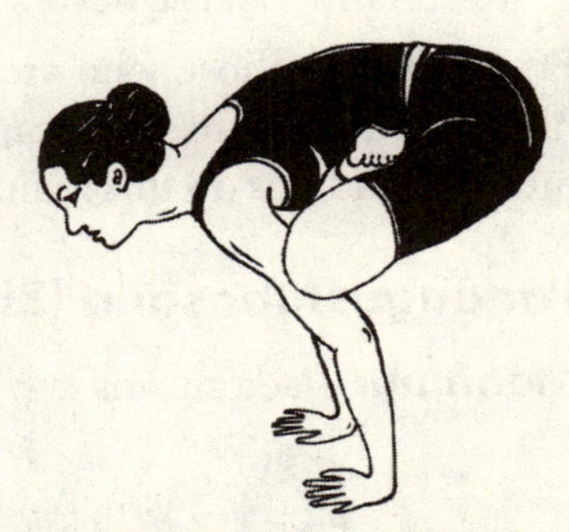

Method 1: Sit in Padmasana. Keep the palms of both the hands on the ground and stand on your knees. By applying pressure on your palms, lift up your body while being in the Padmasana posture. Maintain absolute balance. Increase the time of holding this posture with gradual practice.

Method 2: Recreate the Padmasana Yukta Sheershasana position. Slowly exhale and bend your body down from the waist while keeping the legs in the Padmasana position. Place your knees at the back of your upper arms. Breathe normally while maintaining the balance. Exhale, and with firm hands pull your torso up. Simultaneously, lift your head up. Keep your hands straight and tight. Lift your buttocks from the ground as much as possible. Maintain the balance for a few seconds while breathing normally. Exhale while coming back to the original position. Bend your elbows and rest your knees on the back of the arms. Bend your head down and come into the Padmasana Yukta Sheershasana posture. Release the legs from the Padmasana posture and recreate the Salamba Sheershasana position. Alternatively, sit in Padmasana posture and then open up your legs. Then, rest in Shavasana for some time. Repeat this kriya by changing the position of the legs.

Breathing/time: The breathing pattern is included in the method. Do it as per capacity.

Benefits:

- The hands become strong; the wrist becomes firm by doing this asana.
- The abdominal region and the spine receive optimum benefits.

- It enhances the life force.
- The blood circulation is enhanced in the whole body. Resultantly, all the nerves start functioning efficiently.

Precaution: Those who are heart patients, those suffering from high blood pressure and incapable of doing asanas of the advanced order should not do this asana.

Padangushthasana (Big toe pose) Variation 2

Meaning: 'Pada' means leg; 'Angushtha' means the big toe.

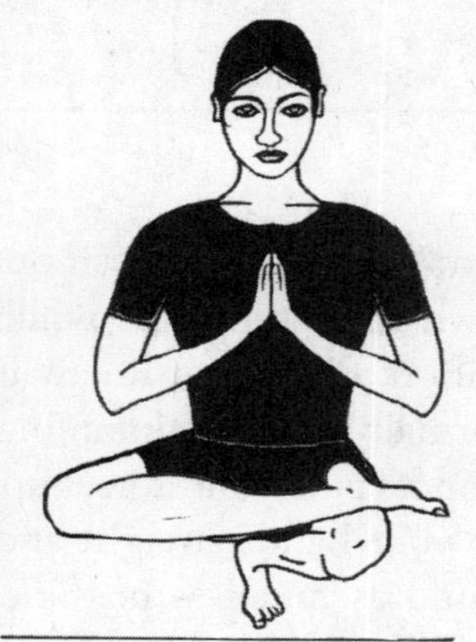

Method: Sit on your haunches with your heels raised. Beginners can take the support of their hands and lift their right leg and place it on the left thigh. Place the heel of the left leg in between your anus and the genital, (Seevni nadi or the perinium) so that the pressure exerted by the heel is accurate. Then, join your hands in the prayer posture and keep them in front of your chest. Repeat the procedure by changing the sequence of the legs.

Breathing/time: Breathe normally and hold the position as per your capacity.

Focus: On maintaining balance and on Mooladhara chakra

Benefits:

- The untimely trembling of feet is cured.
- It gives strength to all the muscles of the legs.
- It is an ideal asana for those who observe celibacy.
- It cures impotency.
- It cures the disorders of the reproductive system.

Precaution: Place the heel only on the Seevni nadi, to put Mooladhara chakra in order.

Janushira Ekpada Skandasana/ Eka Pada Shirasana (One foot to head pose)/ Skandasana (Foot behind the head pose)

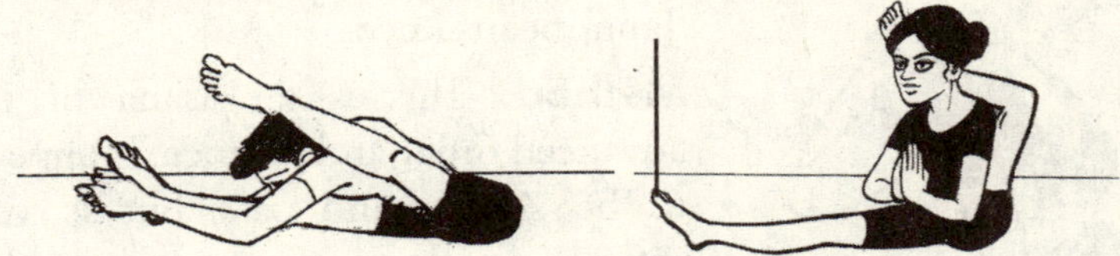

Method: Sit with your legs spread in front. Now, you have to keep one leg on your shoulder. For this, beginners should slightly bend their legs, and hold the ankle of the right leg and take it slowly above the head. Try to keep the calves of the right leg on your shoulder. If you find it difficult, slightly bend your head and torso. Remember to keep the other leg absolutely straight on the ground. Exhale while keeping one leg on the shoulder. This position is called **Ekpada Skandasana**. Now practice Pashchimottanasana in this posture (This position is called **Pada Greeva Pashchimottanasana**.). Exhale and touch the knee with your forehead but the knee should not be bent. Inhale and bring your legs back to the original position. Repeat the asana by changing the sequence of the legs.

Breathing/time: Exhale while bending forward. Inhale while coming back to the original position. Hold the final position for 10-15 seconds; breathe normally.

Benefits:

- The spine receives abundant blood supply and provides more energy and power to the chakras which maintain balance.
- The waist and the buttocks become more supple.
- The disorders related to the reproductive system are cured.
- The body becomes firmer.
- This asana helps in purifying the blood.

Precautions: Those suffering from sciatica, slip disc and hernia should not do this asana.

Note: If before doing this asana or immediately after it, backward-bending asanas are performed, the problems which occur due to this asana are cured.

Sheersha Janusparshasana (Head to knee touching pose)

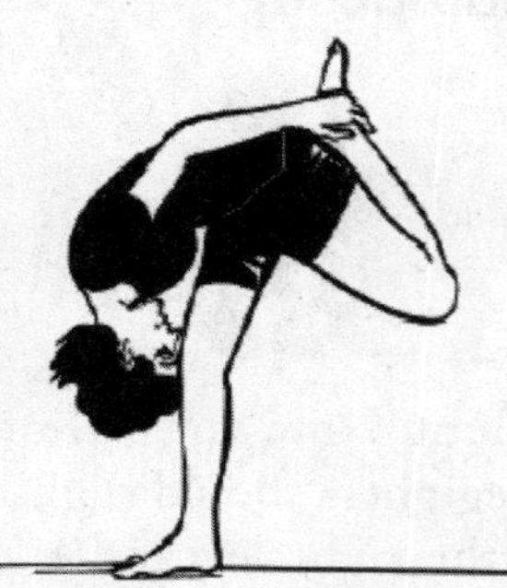

Meaning: 'Sheersha' means head and 'Janu' means knee.

Method: This is an asana of the advanced order and balance. It appears to be simple and easy but is very difficult to execute. Stand in attention position. Bend your left leg backward from the knee and let the heel touch your buttock. Then, bend forward and touch the right knee with your head. Try not to bend your right knee. Repeat by changing the sequence of the legs.

Breathing/time: Be cautious about the breathing pattern. Exhale while bending and inhale while coming back to the original position. Repeat this kriya 4-5 times.

Benefits:

- The air trapped in the body reduces. Practicing this reduces trembling of the body.
- The power of keeping one's balance is enhanced.
- It benefits the spine.
- The thighs become strong by doing this asana.
- It is beneficial for those suffering from joint pains.

Precautions:

- Those suffering from sciatica and slip disc should not do this asana.
- Those suffering from high blood pressure, giddiness and heart diseases should practice this asana patiently.

Ardha Baddha Padmottanasana (Half locked lotus standing and forward bending pose)

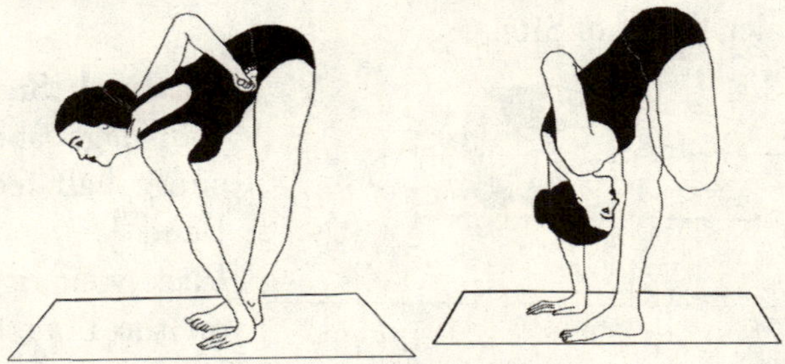

Method: Stand in Samavastha or in other words, stand with both your feet together. Keep your gaze in front. Shift your weight to your left leg. Bend your right leg from the knee using your hand and place it on the left thigh in Ardha Padmasana position. At this stage, the position of the hands can be of two kinds: Either take both the hands to the back and interlock the fingers, or bring the right hand from the back to hold the big toe of the right leg. Then, slowly bend forward and place the left hand on the ground and let your nose touch your knee. Hold this position as per your comfort, then come back to the original position. Relax for some time in this position then, repeat the procedure by changing the sequence of your legs.

Breathing/time: Exhale while bending forward. Breathe normally in the final position. Inhale while coming back to the original position. Hold the final position for 10-15 seconds or as per your capacity. Complete at least two rounds of this asana.

Benefits:

- It activates parts of the abdomen and strengthens the digestive system.
- It cures constipation and gives a light feeling to the body and the mind.
- It cures trembling of the leg and makes them strong.
- It expels the air trapped in the stomach.

Precautions:

- Be patient while trying to maintain balance.
- Pregnant women, people suffering from severe back problems, slip disk, sciatica and those who are mentally weak should not to this asana.

Ashta Vakrasana (Eight-fold body test pose)

This asana is dedicated to sage Ashta Vakra who was the guru of King Janaka, father of Sita.

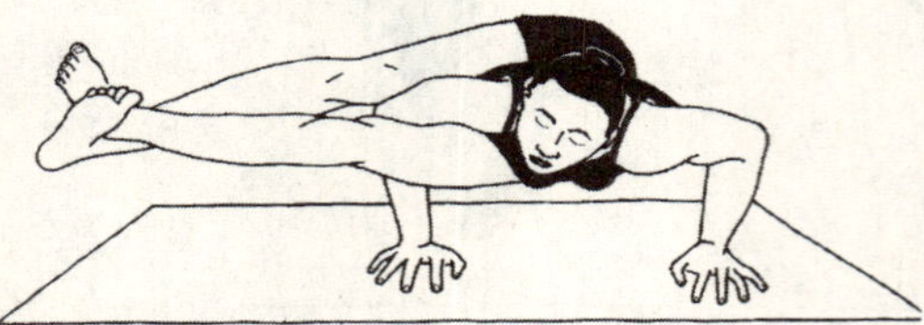

Method: Stand with your legs about one and a half feet apart. Bend your knees. Place your right palm on the floor between your feet and the left palm a little away from the left feet, but in line with the right palm. Place your right thigh on the right elbow in such a way that the back of your thigh is on your elbow. Bring the left leg in line with the right leg and place it next to the right leg. Exhale and lift both the legs simultaneously above the ground. Twist the left foot around the right ankle and lock it (see illustration). Stretch your legs towards the right in a slightly tilted manner. In this way, the right arm will be between the two thighs. Then, slightly bend your right upper arm while keeping your left arm straight. Balance your body on both your hands and bend your elbows to bring the head and the torso parallel to the ground. This is the final position of this asana. Remain in this position for as long you comfortably can. Then, inhale and straighten your arms. Lift up your head and torso. Disentangle your legs and bring them back on the ground. Come back to your original position. Repeat this kriya on the other side too.

Breathing/time: Do Antahkumbhaka while lifting your leg. Breathe normally in the final position. Exhale while bringing the legs down.

Benefits:

- It makes the wrists, arms and shoulders strong and firm.
- It activates the abdominal region.
- It increase the control over our mind and enhances the quality of your life.
- It regularises body's blood circulation.
- It makes the face glow.

Precautions:

- People suffering from ailments of the wrist and shoulders should avoid this asana.
- Concentrate on maintaining balance. This asana should be folowed by asanas of relaxation.

Utthita Tittibhasana (Flying grasshopper)

Meaning: 'Tittibha' is the Sanskrit name for grasshopper.

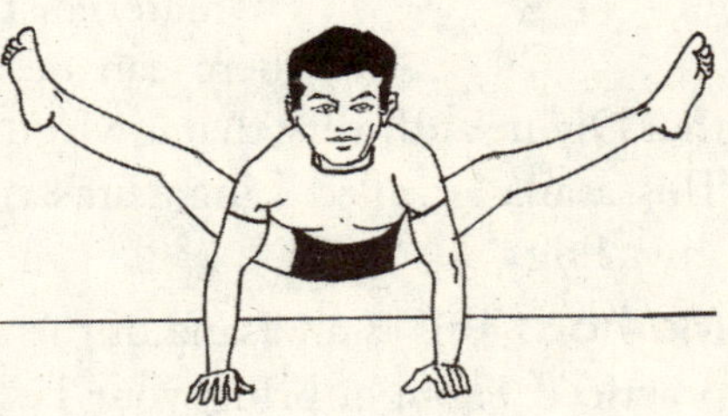

Method: Sit on your mat and stretch your legs in front. Spread your legs apart while keeping your hands on the floor as shown in the illustration. Then, by taking the support of your hands, lift your body from the ground. Keep your legs stretched and do not bend your knees. You will need a lot of practice in order to do this asana perfectly. Therefore, don't be in a hurry to master it.

Breathing/time: Be cautious regarding your breathing pattern. Repeat this asana 4-5 times.

Focus: Concentrate on the energy moving upwards.

Benefits:

- The energy moves in the upward direction in a subtle manner.
- It enhances the self-confidence.
- It gives mental peace.
- The hands get special benefit.
- One does not suffer from trembling legs in old age by practising this asana.
- It strengthens the entire body.

Precautions: Patients of high blood pressure, heart disease and those whose wrists are not so strong should avoid this asana.

Note: This asana can be done by keeping the legs in front as well, but there is no difference in the benefits. This position is called **Dvihasta Bhujasana.**

Lingakarasana (Posture of Lord Shiva)

Comment: 'Ling' is a symbol, an estimate or nature; it is also used to represent Lord Shiv. One needs to use one's wisdom to enumerate the meanings hidden in this term. The entity of Lord Shiv cannot be expressed through anything that is realistic or materialistic in this nature. It is said that there can be no statue or representation of that Divine authority, that is why it is shown as round or elongated. This asana is called Lingakarasan because the body resembles a shiva ling.

Method: This is an asana of the advanced order. Once you have practiced enough, bring your body down to keep the buttocks close to the back and the legs close to the head. In this way, the part of the body from the head to the waist comes parallel to the buttocks, thighs and legs. Further, the buttocks, thighs and legs come parallel to the ground, and the feet stretch beyond the head.

Benefits:

- It is capable of gradually eradicating diseases from our body.
- It is a guaranteed remedy for any kind of trembling in the body.
- It generates flexibility, suppleness and new energy in the body.
- It is helpful in self-realisation.
- After doing this asana, one can do almost all the asanas effortlessly.
- It regularises blood circulation in the abdominal region, lungs, spine, thighs, back, waist, etc.

Precautions:

- It can be accomplished only after a lot of practice. So it should be done under the guidance of a yoga teacher.
- Since the body is bent from the waist so much that the thighs are touch the back, it is possible to accomplish this asana only after a lot of practice.

- Those who have a rigid body and are suffering from high blood pressure, giddiness and heart problems should not do this asana.
- After doing this asana, you must do Pashmittonasana and Pada Hastasana.

Vyaghrasana/Utthita Sheershasana (Supported headstand)

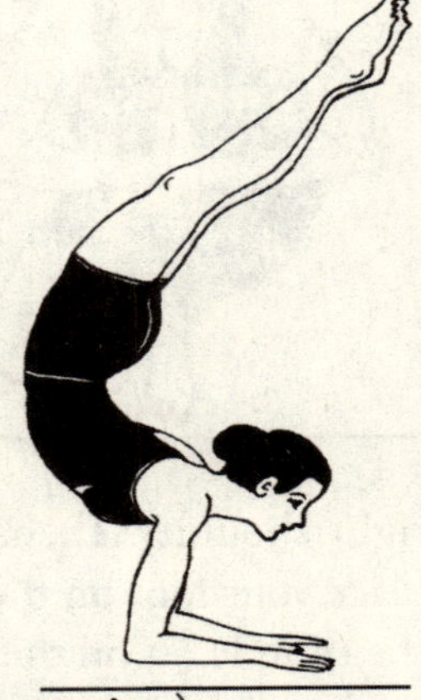

Method: Sit on your knees on the floor. Place your forearms on the floor with your palms flat. Shift the whole weight of your body on the hands. Lift up your body as in Sheershasana, but keep the entire weight on the hands. Lift up your head and try to look in front. Bend your back and keep your legs firmly up.

Breathing/time: Do Antahkumbhaka while lifting your legs up. Breathe slowly in the final position and hold the position for 10-20 seconds or as per your capacity (see illustration).

Benefits:

- It increases blood circulation. It checks hair fall, removes the wrinkles and gives a new glow to the face.
- It improves the eye sight.
- The chest becomes strong. The lungs become healthy.
- The hands, shoulders, spine and waist gain flexibility, suppleness and strength.

Precautions:

- People suffering from high blood pressure, heart diseases and those who are mentally weak shoul avoid this asana.
- Since this is an asana of the advanced order, take the help of a yoga teacher.

Note:

- The first variation of Vyaghrasana has been explained in the earlier pages.
- Some yoga teachers call this asana Pichchha Mayurasana.

Sankhyasana (Posture for concentrating mind)

Comment: This asana can be done in two ways.

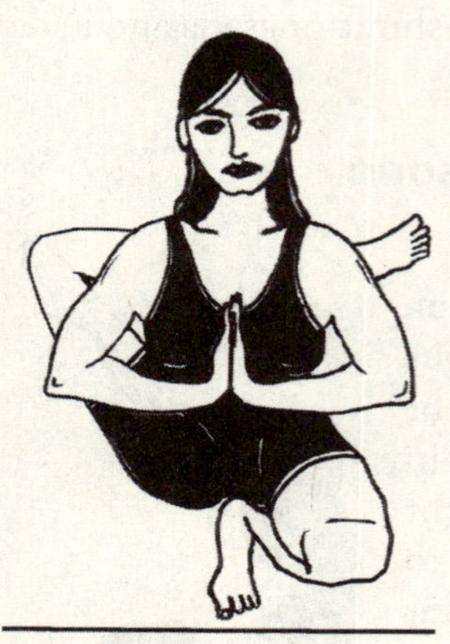

Method 1. Sit in Kagasana (crow posture). With the help of your hands, take your right leg behind the right shoulder and place it at the back. Maintain your body's balance on the toes of your left leg. Let the heel of your left leg be under the right thigh. Keep the hands in the prayer posture in front of the chest. Sit in this posture only according to your capacity.

Method 2. Sit with both the legs spread in front. With the help of your hands, take the right leg behind your right shoulder. Then, slowly pull the other leg closer and firmly place your foot on the floor by bending it from the knees. (While the right leg is on the shoulders, if the left leg is slightly bent from the knees, it becomes easier to do the asana). Join your hands in the prayer posture. Repeat the asana, in both the cases, by changing the sequence of the legs.

Breathing/time: Breathe normally in the final posture. Hold the posture for 5-10 seconds.

Benefits:

- It increases blood circulation in the entire body.
- It also brings about balance in life.
- It benefits the abdominal region, pelvic region and the spine.

Precautions: Since it is an asana of the advanced order, it should be done slowly. You should do it only if you have strong and flexible buttocks and waist.

Dharajasana (Flag posture)/Ekpada Sheersha Sparshasana/Kayotsarga Sthita Ekpada Sheershasana/Urdhva Eka Padtala Sheersha Sparshasana

Note: Some yogacharyas call this asana **Ekpada Sheershasana,** whereas Ekpada Sheershasana is done in many other ways too.

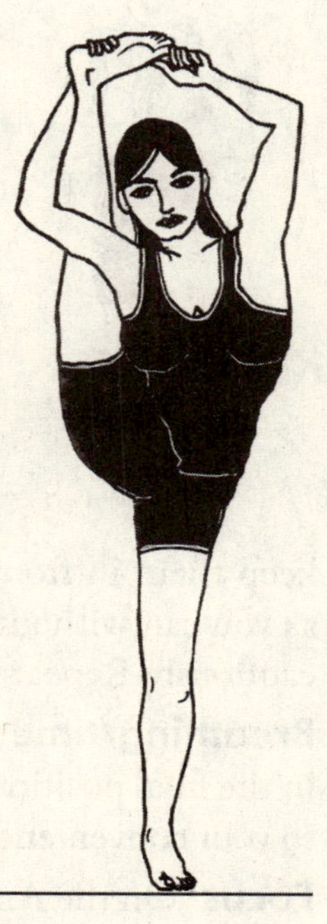

Method: Stand in Samavastha. Since this is an asana of the advanced order, carefully lift up your left leg first upto 90 degrees and then, form an angle of 180 degrees. In this position, the leg will pass your neck and head and the foot will be towards the sky. Taking the support of your hands makes it easier to perform this asana. Do the same procedure by changing the leg. Some practitioners stretch their hands in front while doing this asana.

Breathing/time: Practice Anthakumbhaka while lifting the legs up. Breathe normally in the final position. Exhale while coming back to the original position. Remain in the final position as per your capacity.

Benefits: The muscles of the legs become strong and firm. It sets right the joints of the buttocks and the waist. The muscles of the back and the spine are strengthened. It tones the entire body.

Precautions: Since this asana exerts pressure on the joints of the buttocks and the waist, do it with a lot of patience and gradually, practice more.

Durvasana/Utthita Ekpada Shirasana/Utthita Ekpada Skandhasana (Foot behind the head pose)

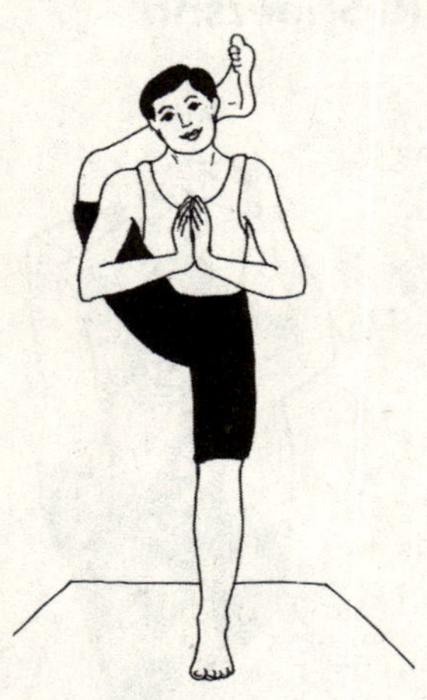

Comment: This asana should be done only by those practitioners who have mastered the asanas of the advanced order.

Method: Sit with your legs spread in front. Keep one leg at the back of your shoulders. Bend the other leg from the knees and sit on your haunch. Then, slowly stand up while maintaining balance (If you are a beginner, you can maintain balance by bending a little, and then stand up.). In the final position, join your hands in the prayer posture and keep them in front of your chest. Hold this position for as long as you can without feeling discomfort. Then, sit down slowly and cautiously. Repeat this asana by changing the leg.

Breathing/time: Inhale when you stand up. Breathe normally in the final position. Inhale while sitting down. Practice according to your convenience.

Focus: On the Anahat chakra

Benefits:

- By doing this asana, life becomes balanced and we learn to be humble.
- It generates us people with self-respect. It makes a person pleasant.
- The untimely trembling of the legs is cured.
- It relieves ordinary back ache and makes the spine flexible.
- It regulates parts of the abdominal region.

Precautions:

- Beginners should take the support of a wall while doing this asana.

- Heart patients and those suffering from sciatica and severe pain in the spine and waists should not do this asana.

Note: In the same asana, when the hands are spread in front, it is called **Yaana Asana.**

Kashyapasana (Pose of Sage Kashyapa)

This asana is dedicated to sage Kashyap, son of Marichi, who was the son of Bramha.

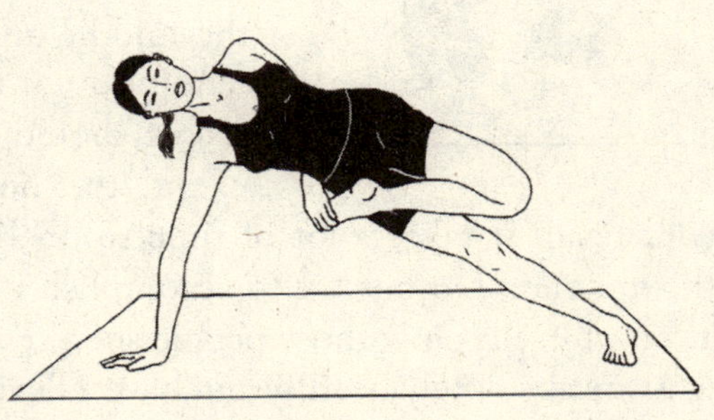

Method: Stand in Tadasana. Bend forward and place both the palms on the floor and take your legs 4-5 feet back. Bend your body in a slanting position towards the right. Balance your body on your right hand and leg. Keep the foot of the left leg on the right thigh in such a manner that it looks like Ardha Padmasana. Bring your left hand in front from the back and hold the big toe of the left foot. This is the final position. Come back to the original position and repeat the procedure on the other side.

Breathing/time: Do Antahkumbhaka while forming the asana. Exhale and hold the big toe of the left foot with the left hand. Breathe deeply in the final position. Exhale while coming back to the original position. Hold the position for as long you can. Do the procedure once on each side.

Benefits:

- It removes the rigidity of the spine.
- It activates all the parts of the digestive system.
- It strengthens the hands and the legs.
- It helps in improving concentration.

Note: Take special care to focus on the balance of the body.

Poorna Shalabhasana (Full locust pose)

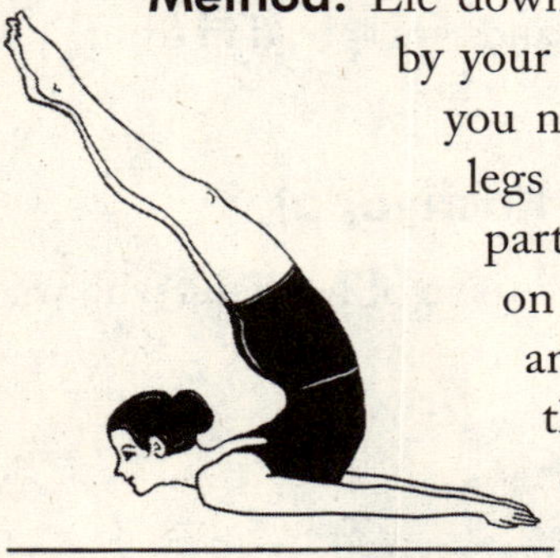

Method: Lie down on your stomach with your hands by your sides and palms facing down. Since you need to bend the spine and raise the legs towards the sky, the hands, upper part of the chest, and the chin will rest on the ground. Lift your legs up to such an extent that your spine bends from the middle and the stomach and the chest do not touch the ground. Your toes should point towards the sky and the heels should be towards your head. It takes a lot of time to do Poorna Shalabhasana in this manner. Do not try to accomplish it completely in the first attempt itself. Only those people should attempt to do this asana who are absolutely healthy and have a flexible spine.

Breathing/time: Practice Antahkumbhaka while taking your legs up and bringing them down. Breathe normally in the final position. Repeat this asana for 5-10 seconds.

Benefits: It gives all the benefits of Shalabhasana. The benefits of Sheershasana and Sarvangasana can also be obtained to some extent.

Precautions:

- Those with a rigid spine should not do this asana. People with kidney problems, weak intestine, ulcers, hernia and high blood pressure should not do this asana.
- Heart patients should definitely not do this asana.
- Only those who can do difficult asanas such as Vrishchika asana, should practice this asana.

Note:

- Some yogacharyas suggest placing the feet on the head to do Poorna Shalabhasana.
- Since this is an asana of the advanced order, do it with utmost care and in the presence of a yoga teacher.

Paryankasana (Couch pose) Variation 2

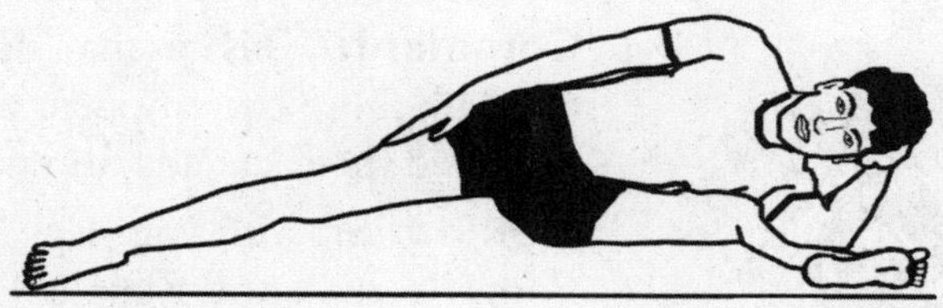

Method: Sit with your legs spread in front. Take your left leg to the left side and slightly bend the knee. Then, bend towards the left and lie down by keeping the left hand on the leg. Support your head by keeping the palm under the head like a pillow. Then, spread the right leg in front and keep the right hand straight on the right leg. Repeat this kriya by changing the leg.

Breathing/time: Inhale while spreading the legs. Breathe deeply but slowly in the final position. Exhale while coming back to the original position. Hold the posture for half to one minute.

Benefits: This asana has a salutary effect on the thighs, waist, chest, spine, back, neck and the digestive system. Hence, all the parts of the body become active and functional.

Precautions:

- This asana should be done only by those practitioners who can do Dvipada Shirasana.
- Those with a flexible and supple body should do it gradually.

Note: The first variation has been explained in the previous pages.

Dvipada Shirasana/Dvipada Skandhasana (Legs behind head pose)

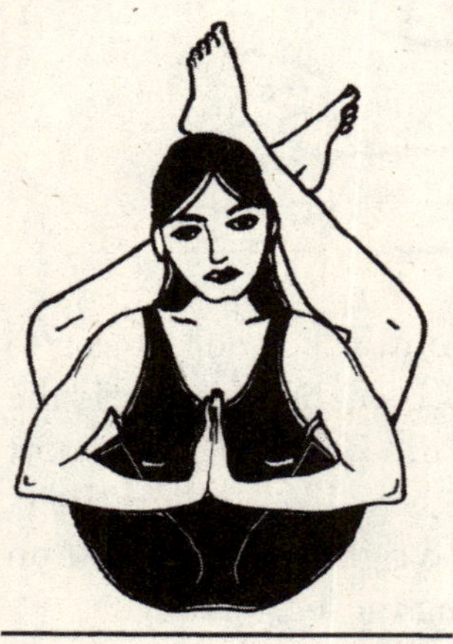

Comment: This asana should be done by those practitioners who have mastered the Eka Pada Shirasana.

Method: Sit with your legs spread in front. Recreate the Ekpada Shirasana position with the help of your hands. Place both legs over your shoulders. Cross over your feet behind your back, but do not do it forcefully. It can be mastered with regular practice. Then, balance your body on your buttocks and join your hands in the prayer posture.

Focus: On Svadhishthana chakra

Breathing/time: Exhale while slowly keeping your legs on the shoulders. Breathe normally in the final position and exhale while you disentangle your feet. Practice it as per your capacity.

Benefits:

- It is very beneficial for men's body and cures many diseases.
- Women can get rid of menstrual problems by doing this asana.
- It rectifies the digestive system and cures diseases like constipation, indigestion, etc.
- It makes the waist and the spine flexible and strong.
- It helps get rid of obesity.

Precautions:

- Beginners should not do it for more than 10/15 seconds.
- People suffering from spine, back or waist problems should not do this asana.
- Pregnant women and people suffering from high blood pressure, sciatica, heart diseases and cervical spondylitis should not do this asana.

Utthita Dvipada Greevasana/Utthita Dvipada Shirasana/Utthita Dvipada Kandharasana/ Utthita Dvipada Skandasana (Dynamic two-legged shoulder pose)

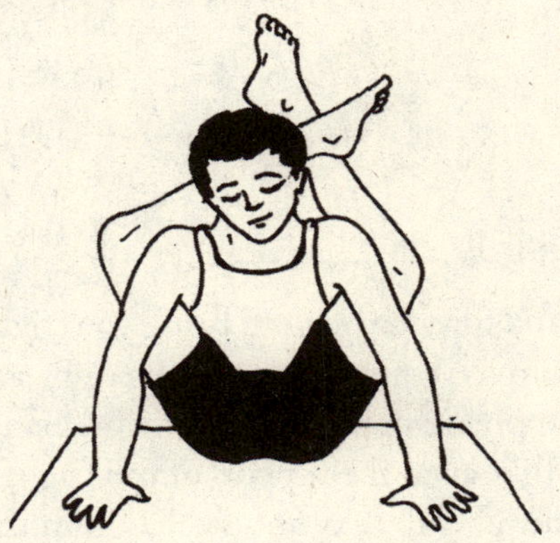

Method: Keep your hands by the sides of your thighs or sit with your legs spread in front. First lift one leg with both the hands and place it firmly on your shoulder. Then do the same with the other leg and cross over the feet like a pair of scissors. Pass both the arms between the thighs and place the palms on the floor. Maintain the balance of the body and gradually lift it on your hands. If you feel tired or unstable, come down slowly and disentangle your legs.

Breathing: Breathe in while raising your body. Breathe normally in the final position and breathe out while coming back to the original position.

Time: 10-30 seconds or as per your convenience

Benefits: It gives all those benefits which are obtained by doing Dvipada Shirasana, Utthita Ekpada Sheershasana and Dvipada Kandharasana.

Note: Only those practitioners who can do Utthita Ekpada Sheershasana/Dvipada Kandharasana or Dvipada Shirasana, should do this asana.

Precautions: Same as Dvipada Shirasana/Utthita Ekpada Sheershasana.

Kaala Bhairavasana (Pose dedicated to Lord Shiva) Variation 2

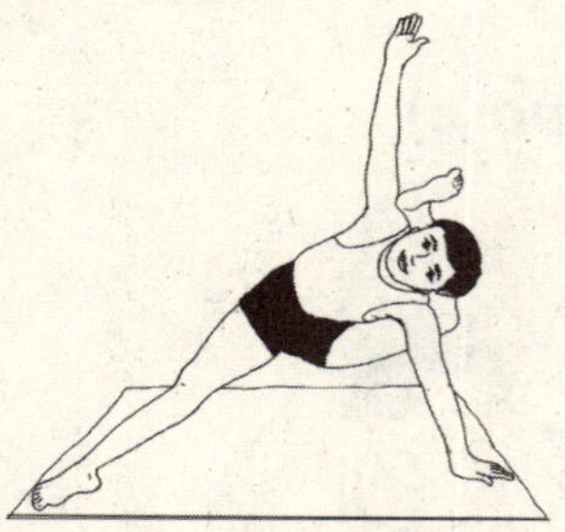

Meaning: It is another name for Lord Shiva.

Method: Sit with both the legs spread in front. Hold the left ankle with both your hands and bring it in front of your chest. Slightly bend your chest and neck in front and place your left ankle behind your neck. Keep both your hands near the buttocks and turn to your left. Bring your right hand on the left side for support. Stretch your right leg to the right side. Exhale and lift up your body by applying pressure on both the hands. Breathe normally, then exhale. Take away the support of your right hand. Then, take the right hand up towards the sky and stretch it. In this way, the entire weight (balance) of the body will be on the right leg and the left hand. Come back to the original position, rest for some time and repeat with the other leg.

Breathing/time: Remain in the final position for about 5-10 seconds and breathe slowly and deeply. Do Antahkumbhaka while coming back to the original position.

Benefits:

- A type of energy is generated in the entire body which activates all the seven chakras.
- The blood circulation in the body gains speed due to which the heart becomes capable of purifying the impure blood.
- It rectifies the nervous system and the Nadis.
- The chest becomes strong and the breathing becomes more complete.

Precautions:

- Those suffering from very high blood pressure should not do this asana.
- If you have any kind of complication in the body, you should not do this asana.

Comment: The first variation of Kaala Bhairavasana has been explained in the previous pages.

Vishwamitrasana (Balancing side angle)

Vishwamitra is the name of a famous sage. This asana is dedicated to him.

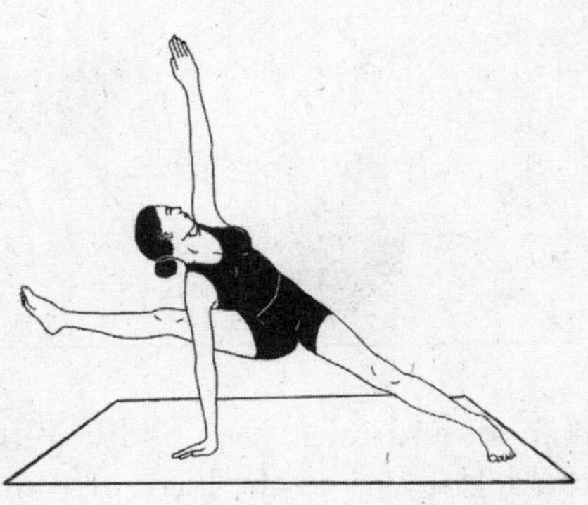

Method: Stand in Tadasana. Bend forward and place your palms on the ground. Place your legs about 4 to 5 feet apart. Exhale. Bring your right leg near the right arm. Place the front part of your right thigh at the back of the right upper arm, and quickly turn your body to the left. Keep the left hand on the left thigh and balance yourself. Then, stretch your left leg to the side. Press your left feet against the floor with the help of your right hand. Lift your right leg up and don't bend it. Take your left hand straight up, turn your head up and look at the left hand. This is the final position of this asana. Come back to the original position. Repeat the procedure with the other leg.

Breathing/time: Practice Antahkumbhaka while lifting your leg. Breathe normally in the final position. Exhale while coming into the original position. Hold the final position for 10-15 seconds. Repeat the asana once on each side.

Benefits:

- One establishes coordination between concentration and balance.
- This asana makes hands and legs strong.
- The entire body becomes firm and strong.
- It makes the abdomen healthy.

Note: Please focus on balancing the body.

Dvipada Kandharasana (Two-legged shoulder pose)

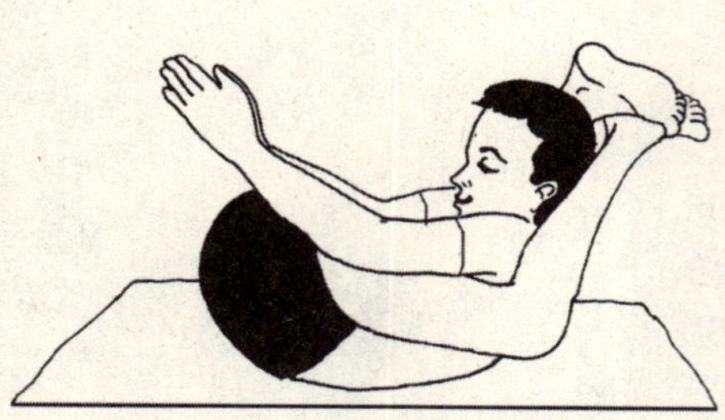

Note: Some yoga gurus call this asana Supta Dvipada Kandharasana.

Method: Before doing this asana, fold a blanket into thick layers because the weight of the body will be on the back and the spine. Lie on the blanket and relax your body. With the help of your hands, take one leg slowly to the back of your head. Then take the other leg also. Now, you have to establish the thighs under the arms. Do it very cautiously. In the final position, cross your feet at the back of your head like a pair of scissors and join your hands in the prayer posture.

Focus: On Svadhishthana chakra

Breathing/time: Exhale while taking the legs behind your head. Breathe normally in the final position and exhale while coming back into the original position. Practice according to your capacity.

Benefits:

- The energy starts flowing upwards. This asana is helpful for those observing celibacy.
- It rectifies the abdominal region, digestive system and the reproductive system.
- It enhances the willpower and self-confidence.
- It makes the muscles of the spine, waist and the back supple and strong.

Precaution: People suffering from severe back ache, sciatica, heart diseases, very high blood pressure, hernia, people with a rigid spine and low self-confidence, as well as pregnant women should not do this asana.

Pranavasana/Yognidrasana/Supta Garbhasana (Reclined foetus pose)

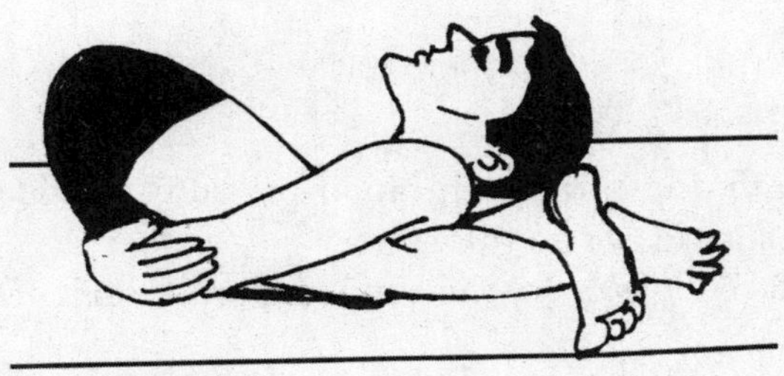

Meaning: 'Yoga Nidrasana'– 'Nidra' means sleep and Yoga Nidra means a state of Samadhi to a certain extent. In this position, the practitioner is neither asleep nor awake. This intermittent position is called yoganidra.

Pranavasan: 'Pranava' means root mantra Omkara.

Method: Place a blanket folded into thick layers on the ground and lie on your back. With the help of your hands, take your right leg and bend it from the knees. Take it to the back and place it under the head. Breathe normally. Exhale. Similarly, take the left leg back and interlock the left ankle and the right ankle. Breathe normally. Lift up your shoulders, take your arms to the back and interlock your fingers. Exhale in the final position. Lift up your chest and stretch your neck backwards. Hold this position for 10-20 seconds while breathing normally.

Exhale while coming back to the original position. Disentangle your hands and loosen up the grip of your legs. Straighten up your legs and rest. Repeat the asana but this time change the sequence of your legs.

Benefits:

- By practising this everyday, the kidneys, liver, spleen, intestine, pancreas, etc. become healthy. The testicles and the urinary bladder become healthy.

- Regular practice makes parts of the abdomen healthy. The practitioners feel happy and light.
- The reproductive organs gain strength and power.
- Negative thoughts stay away and one is inspired to do good work.

Precautions:

- Those suffering from high blood pressure, sciatica and heart diseases should not do this asana.
- Since this is an asana of the advanced order, do it gradually.

Yogabhyasa, simultaneously calms a person down and makes him/her more active.

–RJT

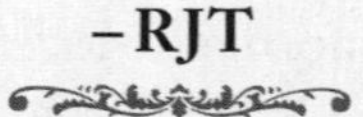

Nadis : Types and Functions

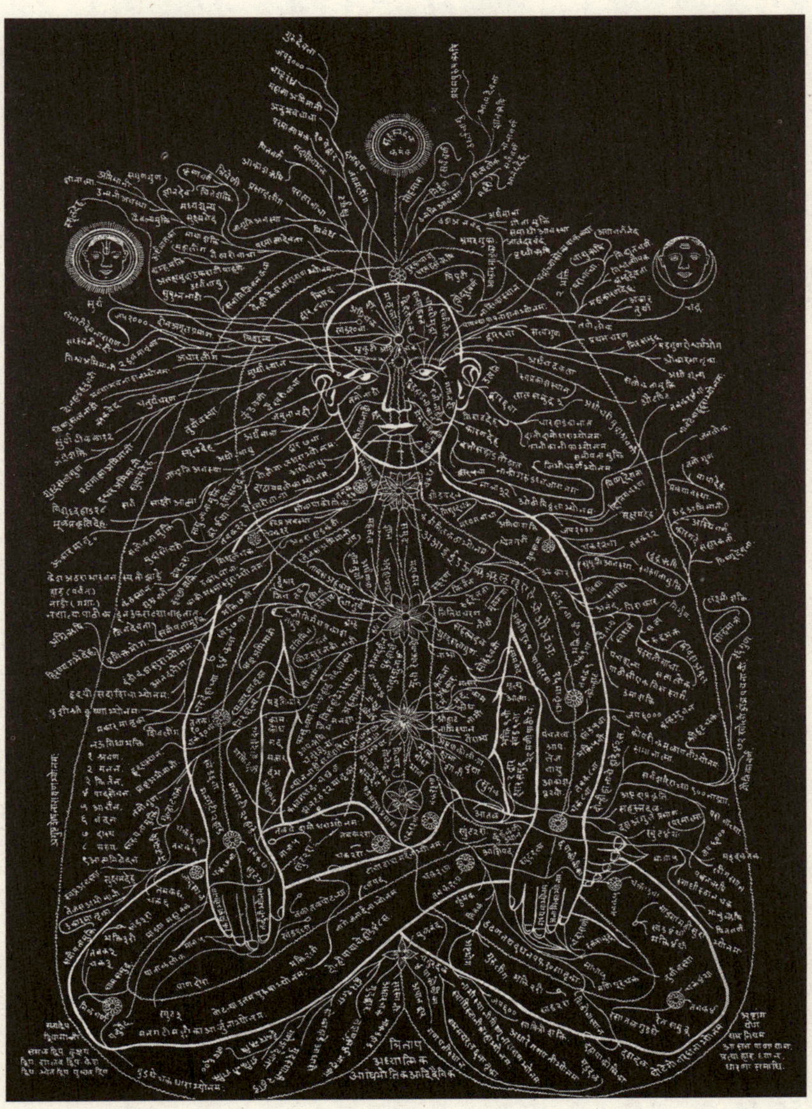

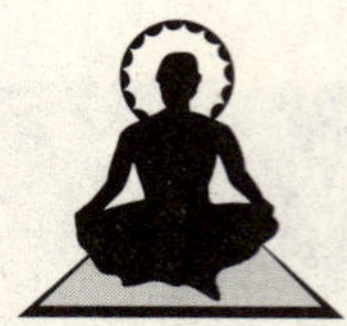

Nadis: Types and Functions

The word 'Nadi' is derived from the word 'Nada' which means a hollow stem of vegetation or grass. It also means sound or wave. The meaning of Nada in the dictionary is given as one or more drains in our body made out of flesh and tissues which carry pure blood from the heart to all the parts of the body. According to modern science, nerves are a group of fibres which carry impulses from one part of the body to the other. Each fibre is an axon of a nerve cell. According to yoga shastra, nadis or arteries circulate in the entire body, carrying with them the air, water, blood and other nutritional substances. These Nadis are used in the process of pranayama.

सार्धलक्षत्रयं नाड्यः सन्ति देहान्तरे नृणाम्।
प्रधानभूता नाड्यस्तु तासु मुख्याश्चतुर्दश।।
सुषुम्णेडा पिङ्गला च गान्धारी हस्तिजिह्विका।
कुहू सरस्वती पूषा शंखिनी च पयस्विनी।।
वारूणालम्बुषा चैव विश्वोदरी यशस्विनी।
एतासु तिस्त्रों मुख्याःस्युःपिङ्गालेडासुषुम्णिका।। (Shiv Samhita 2/13-15)

There are three and a half lakh nadis in our body (72,000 are mostly mentioned), out of which fourteen are main. They are:

1. Sushumna **2. Ida** **3. Pingala** **4. Gandhari**
5. Hastijivha **6. Kuhu** **7. Sarasvati** **8. Pusha**
9. Shankhini **10. Payasvini** **11. Varuni** **12. Alambusha**
13. Vishvodara **14. Yashasvini**

Out of these fourteen, there are three main nadis:

1. Ida **2. Pingala** **3. Sushumna**

Nadis are very minute. Nadi chakras are the centres where many nadis meet throughout the three kinds of bodies: physical, subtle and causal. Scientists and modern doctors disagree with the existence of the subtle and causal but our great sages learnt, understood and explained them in detail. It is written in Varahopanishada that the nadis are spread throughout our body, from the soles of our feet to the crown of our head. The prana, which is the very breath of our existence, is present in them. The soul, which is the abode of power and the creator of the sentient and the insentient universe, resides in the prana.

According to the other Shastras, there are 72,000 nadis in our body, which originate from the place twelve fingers above the anus and the genitals and is right under the navel, which is called the root or base. Most yogis have accepted that their origin is under the navel but there is a dispute regarding the ending of some nadis. According to Kathopnishada and Prashnopnishada, the place of origin of the nadis is the heart, which is the point of dissemination of several thousand nadis.

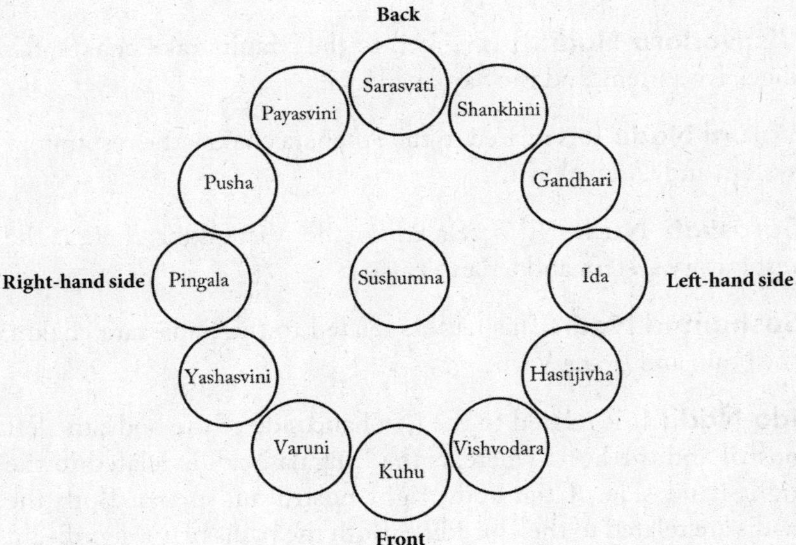

The explanation of the fourteen main nadis is as follows:

The position of the nadis is clear from the given illustration. The Sushumna goes from the centre of the base right till the head. Pingala is on the right and Ida is on the left of Sushumna. The Moon element is in Ida and the Sun element is in Pingala. The Sarasvati and the Kuhu nadis are at the back and the front of the Sushumna respectively. Gandhari and Hastijivha are at the back and front of Ida. Pusha and Yashasvini are at the back and the front of Pingala. Vishvodara is in between Kuhu and Hastijivha. Yashasvini is situated in between Pingala and330runi. Varuni is situated in between Yashasvini and Kuhu. Payasvini is situated between Pusha and Sarasvati and Shankhini is situated in between Gandhari and Sarasvati. Alambusha is in the centre of the base.

According to yoga and Ayurveda, since the nadis are a part of the subtle body, they play an important role in the flow of prana, in its control and in the treatment of diseases.

Alambusha Nadi: It is related to the Mooladhara chakra, anus, Apana Vayu, and the excretory system.

Kuhu Nadi: It is related to the Svadhishthana chakra, reproductive organs, urinary tract and Apana Vayu.

Vishvodara Nadi: It is related to the Manipuraka chakra, the digestive system, and the Samana Vayu.

Varuni Nadi: It is related to the Anahata chakra, the respiratory system and Udana Vayu.

Sarasvati Nadi: It is related to the Vishuddhi chakra, the respiratory system and Udana Vayu.

Sushumna Nadi: This nadi is related to the Sahasrara chakra, the brain and Prana Vayu.

Ida Nadi: It is related to the left-hand side of the body, the left nostril and the heart where as the **Pingala Nadi** is related to the right-hand side of the body, right nostril and prana. Both the nadis are related to the Third Eye. Both the nadis play a significant role in Pranayamas such as Nadi Shodhana, Suryabhedana, Chandrabhedana, and Anuloma-Viloma and in controlling the cool and hot nature of the body.

Shankhini is related to the left ear, **Payasvini** to the right ear, **Gandhari** to the left eye and **Pusha** to the right eye. **Yashasvini** passes through the right hand and leg and through their thumbs. **Hastijivha** passes through the left hand, leg and thumbs.

Diseases emerge due to the imbalance of the flow of prana in the nadis. The treatment of these diseases can be done by massaging and hot fomentation of the related parts of the body.

पद्मासने स्थितो योगी नाडिद्वारेण पूरितम्।
मारुतं धारयेद्मस्तु स मुक्तो नाऽत्र संशय।।

Meaning: The yogi who does Pranayama in the Padmasana posture should have no doubt about his deliverance.

In any kind of Pranayama, while inhaling, visualise:
All the pure energy, divinity, peace and God's light in the universe is entering my body. I am being filled with supernatural energy. I am being purified. My soul is being cleansed. While exhaling, visualise:
My Karmas are being expiated – Anger, Pride, Illusion and Greed are being destroyed.

When we think in this manner, we can obtain manifold benefits.

–RJT

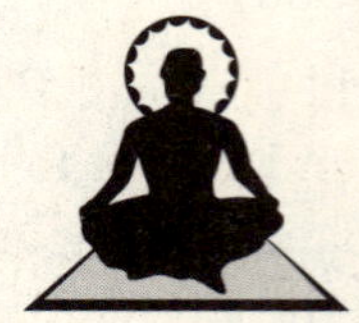

Pranayama

A Significant, Defined, Ideological Perspective

Pranayama has a very special place and significance in Ashtanga Yoga. Various yogacharyas have defined it in different ways with similar meanings. The fourth chant of the Ashtanga yoga says, 'प्राणास्य आयामः इति प्राणायामः', which means that the expansion of prana is nothing else but Pranayama. Daily practice of pranayama enhances the life force tremendously. Maharshi Patanjali has mentioned in the 49th shloka of Sadhanpada:

तस्मिन्सति श्वास प्रश्वास योर्गति विच्छेदः प्राणायामः ।।

Having mastered the asana, when the pace of inhalation and exhalation of breath is interrupted (the normal pace is controlled and balanced by holding the breath), that process is called Pranayama.

Pranayama is made by joining two words – pran+ayam. 'Prana' means 'life force'. It seems that Pranayama is the essence of the entire Ashtanga Yoga. Prana is an energy present in the entire universe at one level or the other. This life force or energy is found in every living being in a very subtle and powerful form. Prana consists of energy, vigour, glow, vitality, and life giving power. 'Ayam' means expansion, scope, regulation, or control. Hence, Pranayama means to expand, prolong, and then control the prana (life force) or breath.

The subject of Pranayama is very vast. It has innumerable possibilities hidden in it. With Pranayama, one can search and discover the internal relation between the body and the brain. Pranayama is not as easy and simple as it appears to be. When one tries to do Pranayama, one realises that it not so effortless, rather a complicated yet meaningful art.

Pranayama is not an imaginary process. It is instantly effective. Many kriyas of Pranayama become subtler and minute progressively.

In present times, humankind has become rather stressful. It seems that it has become difficult to lead a balanced and peaceful life. The worries and diseases affecting the nervous and the circulatory systems are on the rise. Some people are suffering due to psychological reasons while others are suffering due to practical problems. They are trying to take refuge in intoxicants in order to get some peace, but instead of providing peace, it makes their life a living hell. They might forget their sorrows temporarily due to the intoxicants but it is not a permanent solution. The troublesome physical and mental disorders reappear in their lives. We have conducted experiments and seen that by adopting powerful methods such as Pranayama, we can solve many of our problems.

Pranayama is beyond debate. In order to learn Pranayama, we need to have joy in our heart, patience, dedication, guidance of the guru, and cautious efforts; it is these qualities that makes it meaningful.

Expounding the special and significant place of Vayu in Ayurveda, Maharishi charaka has made it clear in the sutra 12/7 of *Charaka Samhita* that Vayu is the one which upholds the body and its faculties. It is of five types – Prana, Udana, Samana, Apana and Vyana – which promotes all physical activities controls and inspires the mind; indulges all the sense organs in receiving their respective subjects; organises the elements of the body, and directs the body. It is the promoter of voice; the inherent nature of touch and sound; the root of the sense organs of sound and touch; the origin of joy and happiness; the igniter of digestive power; the destroyer of diseases; the one that expels the impurities such as sweat, urine and stool from the body and finally, the one which penetrates the physical and the subtle sources. In this way, a favourable Vayu helps in re-establishing our life. It is also said that Vayu is called Matarishva. Vayu is prana. The past, present and future – everything is based on prana. It is written in the second chapter of *Hatha Yoga*:

चले वाते चलं चित्तं निश्चले निश्चलं भवेत्।
योगी स्थाणुत्वमाप्नोति ततो वायुं निरोधयेत्।। (Hatha Yoga Predeepika 2/2)

Meaning: When the Vayu (breath) wanders, or is irregular, the mind is unsteady; when Vayu (breath) become still, the mind also becomes still. When the pranvayu and mind, both become still, the yogi attains the power of stillness of mind. The sadhaka attains stability and lives for a long time. Therefore, yogis should control their pranvayu (breath). It is further said that:

यावद्वायुः स्थितो देहे तावज्जीवनमुच्यते।
मरणं तस्यनिष्क्रांतिस्ततो वायुं निरोधयेत्।। (Hatha Yoga Predeepika 2/3)

Meaning: As long as the Vayu is present in the body, the world considers the creature alive. It considers the departure of the prana (Vayu) from the body as death. Therefore, in order to enjoy a long and healthy life, we should control our breath and do Pranayama.

The writer further says:

शुद्धिमेति यदा सर्व नाड़ी चक्रम मलाकुलम।
तदैव जायते योगी प्राणसंग्रहणेक्षमः।। (Hatha Yoga Predeepika 2/5)

Meaning: When all the nadis perturbed by the impurities are purified and cleansed, the sadhaka becomes capable of holding/accumulating Vayu (breath). Hence one must always do Pranayama.

As mentioned earlier, Prana means life force and Ayama means expansion or scope. Therefore, Pranayama means to first expand or lengthen the breath and then to control it. In *Shiv Samhita*, the art of breathing has been called Pranayama. Maharishi Patanjali has defined the process of sitting firmly in an asana and controlling the process of breathing in and breathing out as Pranayama.

According to the tenth shloka of the second chapter of *Hatha Yoga Predeepika*: The yogi should breathe in (puraka) from the Ida nadi (left nadi), control or hold it (kumbhaka) and then, breathe out (rechaka) from the Pingala nadi (right nadi). Further he/she should again breathe in from the Pingala nadi (do puraka from the right nadi), hold the breath (kumbhaka) and then breathe out (rechaka) from the left nadi. He/she must breathe in the above mentioned Sun-Moon method, which means inhale from the Moon nadi, hold the breath, and exhale from the Sun nadi; then, inhale from the Sun nadi, hold the breath, and exhale from the Moon nadi. In this way, by regularly practising this method of breathing, the faculties of the nadis of the yogis are purified and cleansed in three months.

According to Shri Iyangar, Pranayama is an art and many techniques have been included in it which direct the faculties of breathing with will, rhythm and intensity. This includes the prolonged control and subtle flow of the puraka kriya (breathing in), rechaka kriya (breathing out) and kumbhaka (holding the breath). The puraka kriya stimulates the respiratory system; rechaka expels the polluted and toxic air out of the body and kumbhaka distributes the energy through the body. In these processes, the upper expansion of the lungs and the ribs as well as the horizontal ascent and effect on the related organs are included. Therefore, by breathing in a disciplined way, the mind becomes focused and ultimately the practitioner benefits from it.

Types of Prana (Knowledge about Vayu)

In sutra 12/7 of *Charaka Samhita*, Maharishi Charak has divided Prana into five parts and are briefly explained below:

1. Prana 2. Apana 3. Samana 4. Udana 5. Vyana

1. Prana

It controls the process of breathing, or in other words, it is the process by which we draw the breath in and move our chest. In Pranayama, the Vayu works using internal breath or by the breath which is drawn in.

2. Apana

This functions in the lower part of the abdomen (below the navel area). It controls the excretion of urine, semen and stool. Apana works using external breath.

3. Samana

It activates the abdominal region. It assists in the digestive process. It protects the parts of the abdominal region and makes them function efficiently.

4. Udana

It works in the throat region and takes care of or looks after the voice and the intake of food. Udana drives the energy from the lower part of the spine and directs it to the brain.

5. Vyana

It is present in the entire body. It regulates, rectifies and controls all the activities of the body. It distributes the energy generated by food and breath to the entire body through arteries, nerves, and nadis. Vyana Vayu is necessary for the working of Prana and Apana.

The five types of Prana mentioned above are the medium of transmitting energy from one to another.

Prana is divided into five sub categories (Up-prana), which are:

1. Naga : Reduces the weight of the abdomen

2. Koorma : It protects the eyes from external object through the blinking process; seeing is controlled by Koorma.

3. Krikala : It helps in check external objects which enters the body through the nose or the throat (by actions like sneezing and coughing).

4. Devadutta: It helps bring sleep (yawning).

5. Dhanajaya: It creates phlegm and nourishes the body.

As mentioned above, there are five kinds of prana and five kinds of up-prana. Similarly, our body is divided into three types or forms which surround the soul like a halo. These forms have five mutually intrusive and interrelated Koshas.

1. **Physical body (Sthoola shareera)**
2. **Subtle body (Sooksma shareera)**
3. **Reason body (Karana shareera)**

1. Physical body

It is called the Annamaya Kosha of the body and is thick in appearance.

2. Subtle body

It is made by the Manomaya, Pranmaya and the Vigyanmaya Kosha.

3. Reason body

It is called the Anandmaya Kosha and is the reason for the sadhaka to experience knowledge and awareness.

Stages of Pranayama

Acharyas have explained the stages of Pranayama in four steps:

1. **Aarambha** (Beginning)
2. **Ghata** (Body equated to an earthen vessel)
3. **Parichaya** (Introduction to the self)
4. **Nishpatti** (Completion/accomplishment)

In the first satge of Aarambha, the sadhaka's curiosity and interest in Pranayama is awakened. Initially he/she tries to hurry, and as a result feels tired. Soon his/her body starts trembling and he/she starts sweating due to his/her haste to get quick results. When he/she does it in a systematic manner with patience, the sweating and trembling of the body stops and he/she reaches the second stage called Ghatavastha. The body is compared to a ghata or an earthen vessel. Just as a raw earthen vessel which has not been cultured in the kiln breaks easily, similarly, the body made of five elements disintegrates quickly. However, if it is cultured and heated in the kiln of Pranayama as well as practiced, it gains stability and further moves on to the third stage of Parichaya. In this stage, he/she gets to acquires special knowledge about the practice of pranayama and about himself/herself. Resultantly, he/she is able to identify his/her virtues and vices and understand the reason behind his/her karmas (actions). After this, the sadhak reaches the fourth stage of Nishpatti. This is the final stage of the sadhaka's ultimate state of life. His/her efforts bear successful results. He undertakes actions and acquires various qualities, and finally, gains self-realisation.

Objectives of Pranayama

There are many objectives of Pranayam. One of them is to improve overall health and attain long life. By doing Pranayam, we can control the movement of breath and gain happiness. In Naute, we can see that the birds and animals who breathe fast have a shorter life. We can understand this better from the following table:

1. **Tortoise** : 4-5 breaths in 1 minute, has a life span of about 200-400 years
2. **Snake** : 8-10 breaths in 1 minute, has a life span of about 120-150 years
3. **Human being** : 15-16 breaths in 1 minute, has a life span of about 100 years
4. **Horse** : 24-26 breaths in 1 minute, has a life span of about 40 years
5. **Cat** : 30 breaths in 1 minute, has a life span of about 20 years
6. **Dog** : 30-32 breaths in 1 minute, has a life span of 14-15 years

In this way, it can be proved that by controlling our breath, we can prolong our precious life.

In the text, *Swara Yoga*, the proof of Prana has been explained as the result when the rechaka (exhalation) is of a certain measurement. For example, the normal exhalation (rechaka) of breath is 12 angulas. The normal puraka is 10 anguls. It is 24 angulas while walking, 42 angulas while running and 65 angulas during inter-course. It is 18 angulas during eating and vomiting. Lord Shiv further explains to Mother Parvati that if the yogi can reduce his pace of breathing by one angula, he can attain selflessness. He can attain bliss by reducing his pace of breath by 2 angulas and gift of poetry by reducing his breath by 3 angulas. He can attain mastery over his words if he reduces his pace of breath by 4 angulas, get nava nidhi (the nine kinds of treasures) by reducing his breath by 9 angulas and if he reduces his pace of breath by 11 angulas, he can get rid of even his shadow. He further says that by reducing the pace of breath by 12 angulas, he can attain Hansgati and become capable of enjoying the nectar from the Ganga. This kind of expression enhances the significance of Pranayama more than ever.

Types of Breathing in Pranayama

In order to understand the process of breathing in Pranayama, we should first understand abdominal breathing, thoracic breathing, clavicle breathing and yogic breathing.

1. Abdominal breathing

Lie down in Shavasana, or sit in any meditative posture and breathe normally. Place the right hand on the navel and the left hand in the middle of the heart region. Take a long breath. Immediately, the abdomen starts rising and the heart region on the left starts coming down. Slowly take deep breaths. This time, expand your abdominal region as much as possible, but do not let the heart region expand. Then exhale. The abdomen goes down, and the right hand goes towards the spine. Inhale and exhale in similar manner, but keep your chest and shoulders stable.

2. Thoracic breathing

In this type, the breathing is done totally by expanding the rib cage.

Sit in any meditative posture, or lie down in Shavasana. Focus all your attention on the rib cage and inhale. Take the breath to your rib cage without expanding the abdominal region. Expand the chest area as much as possible and experience the expansion. Be aware of the breath that enters the rib cage. Then, exhale and feel that the rib cage contracting. Rest for a while and do it again. In this way do chest breathing for some time.

3. Clavicle breathing

In this type of breathing, expand the rib cage to the maximum and then take another breath. By doing like this, the muscles of the neck, specially the upper part of the lungs, become active. Then, exhale and release the tension on the neck and empty the rib cage. Bring it back to the original situation. Do this process again.

4. Complete Yogic Breathing

In this type of breathing, the abdominal breathing, the thoracic breathing and the clavicle breathing are done together in a systematic sequence.

Sit in any meditative position, or lie down in Shavasana. Slowly take deep breaths and let the abdominal region expand. Let the breath enter the lungs. Slowly continue to breathe more so that the muscles of the neck experience tension. Be aware and cautious of the muscles of the abdomen, lungs and the neck. Then, gradually relax the muscles of the neck, lungs and the abdomen in this order and exhale. Apply slight pressure on the abdominal region to expel maximum air out of the body. This entire process should be done in one continuous and rhythmic movement and not in a fragmented manner.

Having understood these four types of breathing, you can implement them in your life and understand the significance of Pranayama all the more.

Time and Duration of Pranayama

In the eleventh shlok of the second chapter of *Hatha Yoga Pradeepika*, the time and duration of Pranayama have been explained. The writer says that from the time of sunrise till about two and a quarter hours thereafter is the ideal time to do Pranayama, which means that if the Sun rises at 5.45 a.m., it is best to do Pranayama till 8.00 a.m. If we divide the day into five parts, then in the mid-day, and in the evening, i.e. before and sunset as well as during midnight, one can do 80 Pranayamas in four sets. If one is unable to do four sets, they should do at least three sets. If one does four sets, the total comes to 320 and if one does three sets, it comes to 240 times.

When we consider the above statements, they appear to have been said for exemplary yogis, because one round of Pranayama comprises of Puraka kriya, Antahkumbhaka kriya, rechaka kriya and Bahyakumbhaka kriya. One has to complete 320 such rounds, which is not possible for a common person. Moreover, the environment of the earlier days and that of today is not the same. Yet it is important to do Pranayama. Therefore, if possible, do Pranayama before sunrise when the environment is fresh, energetic and relaxing. If you are unable to do it in the early morning, then it would be better to do it sometime around sunset. Those sadhakas who do chanting of mantras will gain double benefit if they do Pranayama at this time.

Signals, Precautions and Rules Related to Pranayama

In this section, we have mentioned almost all the significant facts related to Pranayama – when it should be done, how it should be done, etc. We are including all the facts by which the readers can gain maximum benefit.

- There should be arrangement for protection from external obstacles such as mosquitoes, flies, and other small insects.
- Pranayama is ideally done by sitting in Padmasana or Siddhasana. Old people or those who are ill can use a stool or chair.

- The place should be clean, free from disturbances and well ventilated.
- The person doing Pranayama should not take *tamasika* things, non-vegetarian food, intoxicating substances, etc. In order to get maximum benefit from Pranayama, they must give up all these things and enhance their beauty, glow and power.
- Do Pranayama joyfully, after yogasana and before meditation, or as per your convenience.
- Try to do Pranayama at a fixed time, place and direction.
- The ideal time to do Pranayama is at sunrise and sunset. In case it is not possible, then there should be a gap of four hours after a meals and before doing the asana. If one wants to eat after doing Pranayama, do so after a gap of half an hour.
- Practice Pranayama by fixing your gaze on the tip of the nose or by keeping your eyes closed.
- Concentrate your mind entirely on the breathing process. This will help in enhancing the power of concentration, memory and mental power quickly.
- Children of younger age should not do kumbhaka.
- Do not do Pranayama in haste. Do not do Pranayama when the lungs are congested.
- Rest in Shavasana after doing Pranayama.
- Pranayama is more beneficial when done after a bath. However, never bathe immediately after doing Pranayama. Wait for at least half an hour.
- If one is under severe mental agony, is mentally and physically upset, discouraged, sad or worried about something, do some light asanas first to calm the mind, then start with Pranayama.
- If Pranayama is not done in the right way, it can cause unrest and create irritation, restlessness and tension. It is reflected on the face as well. Hence, always avoid such wrong practices.

- With regular practice, the nerve fibres of the lungs become supple and Pranayama can be done in the right manner.
- You must empty your urinary bladder and your intestines before doing Pranayama.
- Do not do Pranayama amidst a lot of noise or when you are nervous.
- If you encounter any kind of physical or mental problem during or after Pranayama, you must immediately consult a yoga teacher.
- It is important for a person to have sufficient oxygen in the blood. Pranayama does this job.
- According to the yoga texts, the ratio between puraka, kumbhaka and rechaka should be 1:4:2. This means that the time taken for kumbhaka should be four times the time taken for puraka, and the time taken for rechaka should be two times the time taken for puraka.
- Decide the number of counts for doing Pranayama. Increase the count gradually by following all the directions.
- Some Pranayamas generate heat in the body and some cool it down. Practice as per the situation demands.
- To begin with, two things are very important in Pranayama: One is to keep the mind stable, and the other is to keep the spine absolutely straight. Practice to keep the spine in such a position that it is neither bent too much to the back nor too much to the front. If the spine bends backward, the lungs will expand, and if it bends in front, they will contract. Therefore, it is important that the spine be kept firm and erect.
- Siddhasana, Padmasana, Sukhasana and Swastikasana are ideal for Pranayama.
- Concentration of the mind and maintaining the rhythm of the breath is very important.
- It is written in *Hatha Yoga Pradeepika* that just as a trainer controls and domesticates lions, elephants and leopards by slowly training them, similarly, the sadhaka should gradually

gain control over his breathing. Otherwise the results could be quite opposite to what is desired.

- People suffering from serious ailments as well as pregnant women should first consult a yoga teacher. Those observing fast or who are empty stomach should not do Pranayama or do not do it immediately after.
- If possible, purify the air in the area where you are going to do Pranayama. By burning incense, guggal or a lamp of pure ghee, you can also purify your mind.
- If the asana is not executed properly, the breathing process becomes slow and tolerance becomes low.
- It is written in *Shandilyopnishada*:

  युक्तं युक्तं तजेद्वायुं युक्तं युक्तं च पूरयेत्।
  युक्तं युक्तं च बहनीयादेवं सिद्धि भवाप्नुयात्।।

A new practitioner should do puraka and rechaka very slowly. They should not hurry while doing puraka and rechaka, and practice it slowly. In this way, practicing pranayama will not harm them in any way and they will not have any disease. Even if they have any disease, they will improve their health and attain mastery over yoga.

One can read books and attain knowledge about yoga, but when one practises it, one should do under the guidance of an expert yoga guru.

Benefits of Pranayama

- Pranayama gives one a long life.
- It leads one towards celibacy. In other words, it makes the energy flow in the upward direction, which enhances vitality, glow and power.
- Bramhacharya and Pranayama can be seen as complementing each other because those who do Pranayama with commitment their delusions in the worldly matters are automatically eradicated and their cardinal desires are controlled. Those who observe celibacy can master the Pranayama with ease.

- It destroys the three defects of the bio elements (air, bile and phlegm).
- Pranayama generates life and power in the entire body.
- Pranayama keeps old age at bay. In old age, the breathing process becomes slow and the heart does not receive sufficient oxygen. As a result, the air cells of the lungs contract. Through Pranayama, the sadhaka can regularise the flow of blood and rectify the process of breathing.
- It purifies the impurities in the nadis and makes the body light and swift.
- Pranayama not only gives us physical and mental strength, but also helps in uplifting or awakening of the soul. Therefore, we must make Pranayama a part of our daily life.
- When it is practised in the correct manner, it diverts the mind away from cardinal desires and the sadhaka becomes capable of controlling his/her sense organs.
- If we master the asanas and then do Pranayama, we can get exceptional benefits.
- By doing Pranayama, the digestion power becomes strong. Resultantly, constipation and other such problems do not arise.
- Pranayama has a very strong connection with our nervous system. If the nerves do not function well, the mind is unable to focus. If the nerves are tensed, the mind is also tensed, and till the mind is not at peace or in a receptive state, Pranayama cannot be practiced.
- Pranayama enhances the immunity of the body.
- Through Pranayama, ignorance is destroyed and the light of inner knowledge is awakened.
- In a way, by doing Pranayama we can assist the world be healthy.
- It cures the diseases of the abdominal region. It keeps the digestive system healthy. Hence, constipation is cured. Stool does not stick to the intestine; gas is also expelled from the

body. So, ailments related to gas, like headaches, migraine, premature graying of hair, pain in the joints etc. are cured.

- When the digestive system functions well, the food is digested properly. Hence, all the nutrients present in the food, like vitamins, proteins, and mineral salts nourish our body well. As a result, our body remains healthy till old age. Since a healthy mind resides in a healthy body, in old age, we do not suffer from any kind of mental illnesses or instability. The diseases that often troubles one in old age do not harm those who do Pranayama.
- Since by doing Pranayama, the digestive system, lungs and the heart function well, the whole body gets sufficient oxygen and blood becomes pure. Blood circulation is also regularised. This results in the generation of new energy, new life, and freshness in the body. The body is transformed. Glow and vitality are enhanced. Wrinkles do not appear on the face and the face shines. Eyes become beautiful by doing Pranayama. We always appear to be fresh, and everyone seems to be fresh for us. We find the atmosphere around us happy. Our home, family, neighbours, friends, city, state, country and the world are enlivened by the energy of our body made out of five elements.

Pranayama brings about balance in life and
develops tremendous willpower.

–RJT

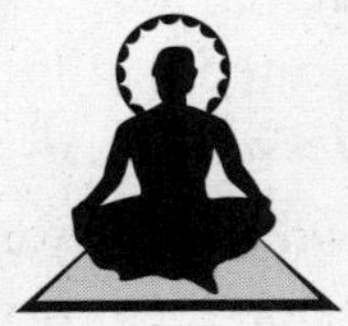

Pranayama

Nadi – Shodhana Pranayama

(Alternate Breathing Technique through Nostrils)

(We have already explained nadi. For detailed information, read the chapter 'Nadi – Types and Functions')

The purification of nadis is called Nadi-shodhana. When there is any kind of blockage in the nervous system of the body, numerous physical ailments start appearing. In many of our texts related to yoga, like *Shiva Samhita, Hatha Yoga Pradeepika, Gheranda Samhita,* etc. Pranayama is suggested for the purification of the nerves.

Factually, the entire credit of the success of Pranayama goes to one's concentration and alertness, but if one can be specially careful about the Nadi-shodhana Pranayama, one can start getting maximum benefits from the other Pranayamas as well. Even though one starts getting the benefits of Pranayama in the beginning itself, firm determination is needed to practice it. It is very essential to direct the energy thus generated with sensitivity, concentration and determination in order to give stability and discipline to the breath, so that the breath, Prana and the brain can be directed towards spirituality. This is a small but significant process of purifying the soul. This is one of the paths that lead to the communion of the Atma with the Parmatma (soul with the supreme).

Amongst all the Pranayamas, Nadi-shodhana Pranayama is the most sensitive, complicated and subtle. When the nerves are purified at the most subtle level, it leads to self-realisation.

To do Nadi-shodhana Pranayama effectively, first and foremost, one has to master the working of their fingers and secondly, one has to develop the sensitivity of their nasal membranes – only then can one do this Pranayama perfectly.

Nadi-shodhana Pranayama or Anuloma Viloma Pranayama (Alternate nostril breathing)

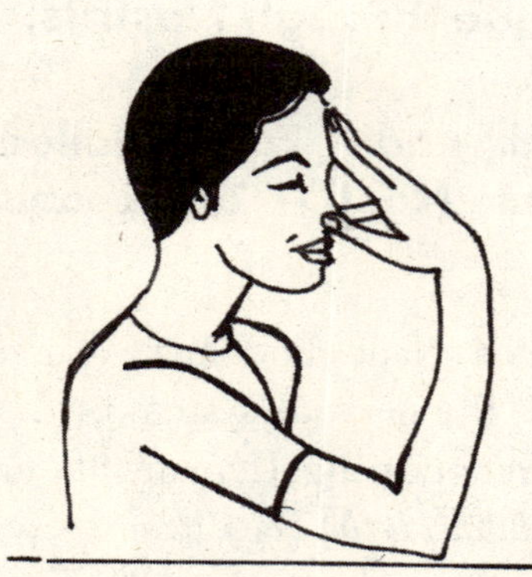

Exercise 1. Method: Sit down in any posture of Sukhasana (Padmasana or Siddhasana), in which you can sit comfortably for at least some time. Keep your spine, neck and head straight in one line. Now, get ready to do Pranayama. Keep your left hand on the left knee. Place the fingers of the right hand in between the brows (right in the centre of the forehead). Keep your shoulders upright. Then, keep the pointer and the middle finger of the right hand in the middle of the forehead (some yoga teachers instruct to keep only the pointer). Keep the thumb on the right nostril and the ring finger on the left nostril. Close the right nostril with the right thumb and inhale (puraka) from the left nostril. Then, exhale (rechak) from the same nostril. Concentrate solely on your breathing. Puraka and rechaka together make one round. Do 10-15 such rounds. Close the left nostril with the ring finger and inhale-exhale 10-15 times as mentioned above.

Precautions: The process of breathing should not be loud. Breathe from both the nostrils with equal rhythm. Do not expand or contract your chest.

Time: Do this kriya for 5-10 minutes.

Note: If you feel tired, do Shavasana. By doing this Pranayama, the nostrils and the fingers get enough practice and helps in gaining maximum benefit from Pranayama.

Puraka = Breathing in, Rechaka = Breathing out

Antahkumbhaka = Holding the breath inside

Bahyakumbhaka = Holding the breath outside

Exercise 2. Do Anuloma-viloma Pranayama in order to further the process of Nadi-shodhana Pranayama.

Method: Sit with absolute alertness in Sukhasana, Siddhasana or Padmasana. Close your right nostril with your right thumb and inhale from your left nostril. Close your left nostril with the ring finger and exhale from the right nostril. Then, inhale from the same side. Close the right nostril with your thumb and exhale from your left nostril. This is one complete round.

While doing this kriya, you should gradually increase the speed of breathing from medium to fast. Do the process as directed at slow, medium and fast pace. As a result, some sound may be generated during this process. You can measure your breathing by chanting *Om* mentally. You can begin with one chant, and then go up to seven. You can begin by doing the Pranayama for 3 minutes and increase it up to 10 minutes. In this method, the rechaka and puraka should be of equal duration.

Precautions: If you feel tensed or fatigued while doing this Pranayama, rest for some time, then when you feel relaxed, you can resume the process.

Comment: The energy of the Mooladhara starts moving in the upward direction.

Exercise 3. Sit in any posture of Pranayama. As mentioned in the above method, close the right nostril and inhale from the left nostril. Close both the nostrils and hold your breath inside (antahkumbhaka). Close your left nostril and exhale from the right nostril. Inhale from the right nostril, hold the breath and exhale from the left nostril. This is one round. While holding the breath, you can chant *Om* in your mind or count to 5. Do 25 such rounds. Later, make the ratio of puraka, kumbhaka and rechaka to 5:10:10. This means that you have to inhale up to 5 counts, hold the breath up to 10 counts and exhale for 10 counts. You can increase the counts with practice. Do this process of inhalation-exhalation and holding the breath with a tension-free mind. Then, consult an expert guru, or judge yourself and increase the ratio. For example, you can make the ratio 1:6:2, then 1:6:4, and then after practice, you can make it 1:8:6. Here, 1:8:6 means that if you inhale for 5 counts, hold the breath for 40 counts and exhale for 30 counts. Do these rounds for 10-15 minutes, or do 20-25 such rounds.

Exercise 4. Comment: Since you have to do Bahyakumbhaka along with Antahkumbhaka in this method, be very cautious and careful. Do this Pranayama in a well ventilated room, with a peaceful atmosphere and a tension-free and joyful heart. The ratio of this Pranayama will be 1:4:2:2, which means that you have to inhale for 5 counts, hold your breath inside for 20 counts, exhale for 10 counts and hold the breath outside for 10 counts. If you increase the time of inhalation, you have to increase the time of the other kriyas in the same proportion. After enough practice, try doing Moola bandha, or Jalandhara bandha at the time of Kumbhaka under the guidance of an expert guru. Don't forget to do Shavasana in the end.

Method: Inhale from the left nostril. Do Antahkumbhaka. Exhale from the right nostril. Do Bahirkumbhaka. Then do it in the opposite manner by inhaling from the right nostril. Do Antahkumbhaka. Exhale from the left nostril. Do Bahyakumbhaka. This is one round. Do 15 such rounds if possible.

Benefits:

- The practice of Nadi-shodhana is the base of all other Pranayamas. Therefore, the better Nadi-shodhana a sadhaka is able to do, the more benefit he/she will be able to derive from other Pranayamas.

- It makes the brain swift, active and sensitive.
- It establishes physical and mental balance, due to which, one does not suffer from any physical and mental ailments.
- The level of Dharna, Dhyana and Samadhi is raised to a higher level.
- The impurities of all the nadis are cleansed and purified, which leads to better results in the present and the future.
- The mind becomes at peace and joyful by doing it.
- One acquires many qualities automatically and falsehood gradually takes leave from your life.
- It is helpful in controlling asthma, diseases related to tonsils and cough, skin problems and blood pressure. It is specially beneficial for migraine and sinus problems.

Vritti Pranayama

Vritti Pranayamas are of two types:

Sama Vritti Pranayama and Vishama Vritti Pranayama.

Sama Vritti Pranayama (Equal breathing)

In Sama Vritti Pranayama, the duration of puraka, rechaka, antahkumbhaka and bahyakumbhaka is the same. In Sama Vritti Pranayama, if the inhalation is for 5 seconds, the antahkumbhaka will also be for 5 seconds. The exhalation will be for 5 seconds and the bahirkumbhaka will also be for 5 seconds.

In this kriya, the duration and the rhythm of the puraka and rechaka should be the same. After regular practice, there comes about a balance between the duration of puraka and the rechaka and between antahkumbhaka and bahyakumbhaka. However, first and foremost you must practice with antahkumbhaka. The ratio between the three kriyas should be 1:1/4:1. So, if you do puraka for 16 counts, you should do antahkumbhaka for 4 counts and complete the rechaka in 16 counts. Gradually, increase this ratio to 16:8:16, and when you thoroughly get used to it, you can increase the antahkumbhaka to 16:16:16.

Gradually introduce bahyakumbhaka. In the beginning, keep the ratio of puraka, antahkumbhaka, rechaka and bahyakumbhaka as 16:16:16:4. Then, gradually increase it to 16:16:16:8. When you master this ratio, you can increase it to 16:16:16:16. In this way, the ratio of Sama Vritti Pranayama should be gradually increased.

Vishama Vritti Pranayama (Unequal breathing)

Since this is very irregular in nature, the sadhaka should have very strong lungs and nadis to practice this Pranayama. In this Pranayama, the duration of puraka, antahkumbhaka, rechaka and bahyakumbhaka are all different. Due to the difference in ratio, it is difficult to practice.

Begin with puraka, antahkumbhaka and rechaka kriya in the ratio of 8:16:8. Gradually increase the ratio to 8:24:8 and then increase it to 8:32:8. Once you get used to this ratio, move on to make it 8:32:10, then 8:32:12, then 8:32:14, and then 8:32:16. When you gain absolute mastery over this, you can begin doing bahyakumbhaka in the ratio of 8:32:16:2, then 8:32:16:4, 8:32:16:6, and then 8:32:16:8. These four ratios form one round of Vishama Vritti Pranayama.

In the beginning, the sadhaka will have problem in regularising the rhythm between puraka, antahkumbhaka and rechaka. Initially he/she will run short of breath and will start panting, but with regular practice over a long period of time, it will become simpler.

An ideal ratio for Vishama Vritti Pranayama will be this: if you inhale for 8 seconds and do antahkumbhaka for 32 seconds, do rechaka for 16 seconds and bahyakumbhaka for 8 seconds, the ratio will become 8:32:16:8, or in other words, it will be 1:4:2:1. When you get accustomed to this ratio, you can do it in the opposite order. Do puraka for 16 seconds, antahkumbhaka for 32 seconds and rechaka for 8 seconds. In this way the ratio will be 16:32:8 (2:4:1). When you add bahyakumbhaka to it, you can follow the ratio 16:32:8:4, then 16:32:8:6 and then, 16:32:8:8.

You can follow different durations. For example, puraka for 32 seconds, kumbhaka for 16 seconds, rechaka for 8 seconds and bahyakumbhaka for 4 seconds. This way the ratio will be 32:16:8:4.

The time of Vishama Vritti can differ in different ratios. For example, it can be 8:16:32:4, 16:32:4:8, 32:16:4:8, or 4:8:32:16. There can be many permutations and combinations in Vishama Vritti Pranayama.

Precautions: This is a very strict rule that till you master it, you should do this Pranayama under the guidance and vigilance of an expert yoga teacher. Vishama Vritti Pranayama is specially full of danger. Please do not attempt to do it without guidance.

Vishama Vritti Pranayama can cause tension in the brain. Due to increase in the speed of the flow of blood in the arteries, it can cause high blood pressure and uneasiness.

Types of Pranayama

The following types of Pranayama have been mentioned in Gheranda Samhita:

सहितः सूर्यभेदश्च उज्जायी शीतली तथा ।
भस्त्रिका भ्रामरी मूर्च्छा केवली चाष्टकुम्भकाः ।। (Gherunda Samhita 5/46)

1. **Sahita-kumbhaka**
2. **Surya Bhedi**
3. **Ujjayi**
4. **Sheetali**
5. **Bhastrika**
6. **Bhramari**
7. **Moorchchha**
8. **Kevali**

These are the eight kumbhaka pranayamas.

Sahita kumbhaka is of two types:

A. Sagarbha **B. Nigarbha**

In Sagarbha kumbhaka, beeja mantra is used, and in Nigarbha kumbhaka, beeja mantra is not used during practice.

(A) Sagarbha kumbhaka (breathing with Counting): Maharishi Gheranda has said that one should sit in Sukhasana posture facing North or East and meditate on the red faced

Bramha who represents Rajoguna. Inhale from the left nostril and chant beeja mantra 'Am' sixteen times while inhaling. After inhaling and before kumbhaka, do Uddiyana Bandha. Then, focus on the dark-complexioned Lord Vishnu who represents Satoguna and chant the beeja mantra 'U' sixty-four times while doing kumbhaka. Meditate on the fair-complexioned Shiva, who represents Tamoguna, and chant the beeja mantra 'M' thirty-two times while doing rechaka from the right nostril. Then, do puraka from the right nostril, followed by kumbhaka and then rechaka from the left nostril, by following the same pattern as mentioned above. Practice doing Anuloma Viloma without using the thumb and the ring finger.

(B) Nigarbha Kumbhaka (Breathing without counting): In this Pranayama, beeja mantra is not chanted. For Pranayamas with puraka, kumbhaka and rechaka there are units (matras) ranging from one to hundred vowel counts. It follows that the best or excellent Pranayama has twenty matras, medium has sixteen matras and the ordinary or that of low quality has twelve matras. In the same way, Pranayama has three parts. In the Pranayama of low quality, sweat is given out of the body, in the medium Pranayama, the spine trembles and in the best or highest quality Pranayama, the sadhaka rises above the earth and is able to move in the sky. In this way, sweating, trembling of the spine and rising above the ground, all the three are indicators of having mastered different siddhis. The practice triggers the power to move in the sky, to fight diseases and to awaken the kundalini. The practice of Pranayama makes the heart blissful and one becomes happy in life.

Surya-bhedana Pranayama (Right nostril breathing)

Significance: In this Pranayama, all the purakas (inhaling) are done from the right nostril and all the rechakas (exhaling) are done from the left nostril.

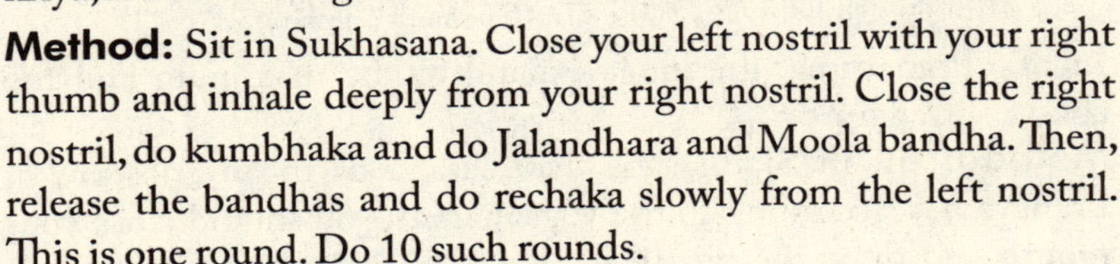

During puraka kriya, the life energy flows through the Pingala nadi (Surya nadi, Jamuna nadi) and during rechaka kriya, it flows through the Ida nadi (Moon nadi, Ganga nadi).

Method: Sit in Sukhasana. Close your left nostril with your right thumb and inhale deeply from your right nostril. Close the right nostril, do kumbhaka and do Jalandhara and Moola bandha. Then, release the bandhas and do rechaka slowly from the left nostril. This is one round. Do 10 such rounds.

Comments: The duration of kumbhaka should be gradually increased. It is written in *Hatha Yoga* that you should hold your breath in kumbhaka till you start sweating. It is not possible in the beginning, so do the kriya with a lot of wisdom.

Benefits:

- It strengthens the digestive system, because the right swara (inhaling from the right side) assists in digestion.
- It increases the warmth or heat of the body. Air and phlegm are brought under control by this Pranayama.
- It cures skin disorders.
- It removes wrinkles. It increases the glow of the face.
- It clears the sinus and cleanses them.
- Its regular practice is beneficial in cases of low blood pressure.

Precautions:

- Patients of high blood pressure should not do this Pranayama.
- Do not do this Pranayama in summers as much as possible.

Ujjayi Pranayama (Psychic breath/Victorious breath)

नासाभ्यां वायुमाकृष्य मुखमध्ये च धारयेत।
हृद्गलाभ्यां समाकृष्य वायुं वक्त्रे च धारयेत।।
मुखं प्रक्षाल्य सम्वन्द्य कुर्याज्जालन्धरं ततः।
आशक्ति कुम्भकं कृत्वा धारयेदविरोधतः।
उज्जायी कुम्भकं कृत्वा सर्वकार्याणिसाधयेत्।
न भवेत्कभ रोगश्च क्रूरवायुरजीर्णकम्।।
आमवातः क्षयः कासो ज्वरः प्लीहा न विद्यते।
जरामृत्युविनाशाय चोज्जायीं साधयेन्नरः (Gherunda Samhita 5/70-73)

In this Pranayama, the lungs expand to the maximum and the chest is lifted up.

Method: Sit in Siddhasana, Padmasana or in any posture of Pranayama. According to the yogacharyas, you should close your mouth and draw the breath in slowly from both the nostrils. It should move through your throat with a sound and fill up your body up to the heart. Do kumbhaka for sometime without any feeling of stress. Then, exhale from the left nostril. When you draw the breath in, expand your chest.

Comment: When you draw your breath in, contract the glottis so that a slight sound is heard. Then, let the air circulate in the mouth, do Jalandhara bandha without any feeling of restlessness and hold your breath as much as you comfortably can.

Time: As per your convenience/as per your capacity

Benefits:

- It enhances the digestive power. It helps attain all goals.
- It destroys phlegm.
- It increases the power of concentration and enhances the retention power of the mind.
- It is beneficial for people suffering from insomnia, mental worries and depression.
- It also cures dysentery, tuberculosis, fever, spleen, harmful air etc.
- According to *Gheranda Samhita*, if we master this kumbhaka, we can overcome old age as well as death.

Sheetali Pranayama (Cooling breath)

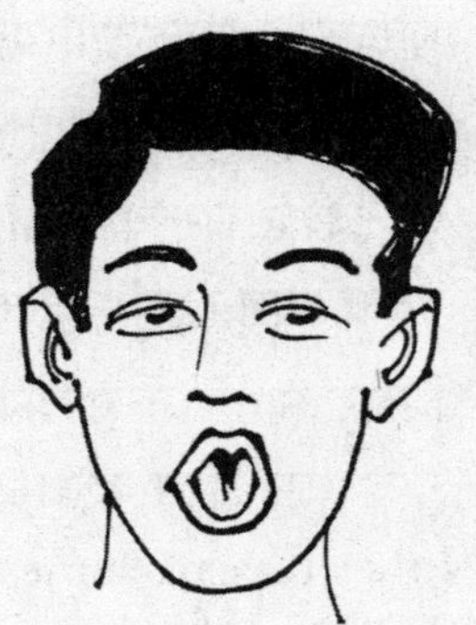

Method: We can lower the temperature of the body by doing this Pranayama, that is why it is called Sheetali Pranayama. Sit in Siddhasana or Padmasana. Place both your hands on your knees. Keep your spine, neck and head straight in one line. Bring your tongue out of your mouth and fold it length-wise in such a manner that it appears like a drain. Do puraka in this position. Breathe in slowly and fill up your lungs. Do antahkumbhaka, take your tongue back inside the mouth and close it. Lower your head and do Jalandhara bandha. Do kumbhaka with or without Moola bandha for five to seven seconds. Release the bandha and do rechaka. This is one round. Repeat this Pranayama for five to ten minutes (do rechaka from the nose).

Benefits:

- This Pranayama makes the heart happy and destroys the problems caused by bile.
- It activates the liver and the spleen.
- It quenches thirst.
- It brings down high blood pressure.
- It purifies the blood.

Precautions: Those suffering from low blood pressure, chronic constipation and excessive cough should not do this Pranayama.

Bhastrika Pranayama (Breath of fire)

भस्त्रिका लोहकाराणां यथाक्रमेण सम्भ्रमेत्।
तथा वायुं च नासाभ्यामुभाभ्यां चालयेच्छनैः।।
एवं विंशतिवारं च कृत्वा कुर्याच्च कुम्भकम्।
तदन्ते चालयेद्वायुं पूर्वोक्तं च यथाविधि।।
त्रिवारं साधयेदेनं भस्त्रिकाकुम्भकं सुधीः।
न च रोगो न च क्लेश आरोग्यं च दिने दिने।। (Gherunda Samhita 5/76-78)

Note: Bhastrika means bellows. In this Pranayama, the speed of inhaling and exhaling is very fast and forceful. During inhaling and exhaling, a certain sound is generated which is compared to the sound of the bellows of an ironsmith.

Meaning: Just as the ironsmith fills the bellows with air, similarly, you have to draw your breath in through your nose and slowly move it in your stomach. You have to do this twenty times and then, hold the breath by doing kumbhaka. You have to expel the air out through your nostrils just as the ironsmith does. This is called Bhastrika kumbhaka. This should be done three times regularly. If you do this, you will not suffer from any disease and gradually, your health will improve.

First method: Sit in Padmasana. Close your right nostril and breathe in rapidly from the left nostril and with the same speed, exhale. Repeat this twenty times. Then, do this process using the right nostril. In this process, the rechaka and puraka should be done in the same rhythm. The expansion and contraction of the abdominal region should be easy and even. This is one round. Do three rounds. Then, do Jalandhara bandha and Moola bandha.

Second method: Sit in Sukhasana. In this method, you have to inhale forcefully from both the nostrils and then exhale forcefully. Do this process twenty times. Then do antahkumbhaka and practice Jalandhara bandha and Moola bandha (as per your convenience). This is one round. Do this process three times.

Comments:

- Keep the pace of your breathing slow, medium and fast as per your health condition.
- While exhaling, keep your thoughts good and pure, and while inhaling, visualise that you are expelling all the disorders of the mind out of your system.
- Those who are suffering from blood pressure problems and heart diseases should not do this Pranayama at fast pace.
- Rest after each round.
- Be absolutely alert. Those who have weak lungs should not do this Pranayama.
- Stop the moment you feel tired or restless.

Time: 5-10 minutes according to the diseases you are suffering from

Benefits:

- The foreign and toxic elements are expelled out of the body, the blood is purified and one becomes healthy by doing this Pranayama.
- The lungs become strong, and hence asthma and tuberculosis are cured by doing this Pranayama.
- It is beneficial for diseases of the throat, and it expels cough out of the body.
- It destroys the excess phlegm, air and bile and helps awaken the kundalini.
- The various parts of the abdominal region, liver, spleen and the digestive system become active by doing this Pranayama.
- It is also helpful in cases of sinus and tonsils.

Onkara Jaapa/Udgeetha Pranayama (Breathing while chanting of *Om*)

Method: Sit down in any asana of meditation and close your eyes. Take a deep breath and chant Om loudly. Do this 5-11 times.

Benefits: It works as a remedy for mental disorders. By doing this Pranayama, the mind becomes calm and stable; the problems of the voice are rectified; one experiences bliss and gets rid of insomnia and nightmares.

Bhramari Pranayama (Breathing bee technique)

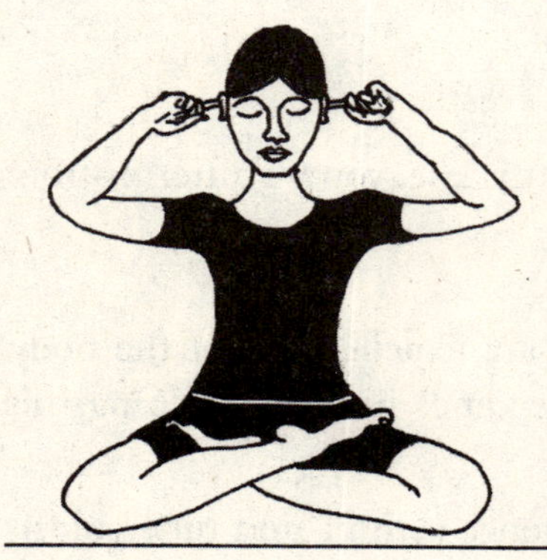

Meaning: 'Bhramara' means a bumble bee. This Pranayama is called as the Bhramari Pranayama because while doing rechaka, a sound resembling the sound of a bumble bee is generated.

Method: Sit down in Padmasana, Siddhasana or Sukhasana. Inhale from both the nostrils. Close both your ears with your index fingers. If you want, you can do kumbhaka for some time. Then, humming like a bumble bee, slowly do rechaka. Do five to ten rounds.

According to *Gheranda Samhita*, when it is past midnight and the sound of all the creature is silenced, the sadhaka should go to a lonely place and close his ears with his hands and practice puraka and kumbhaka. Try to listen to the internal sounds from the right ear. You will first hear the sound of cricket, then of a flute, then the thundering of clouds, a sistrum, humming of a bee, huge bells, gong of the clock, clarion, battle siren, kettledrum, percussion drum (mridang), etc. You will notice that the sounds start echoing in the Anahata. It is an amazing sound. The illumination that one sees during this is none other than the Bramha or the Lord

Almighty. When one's heart get immersed in this light, one is able to get the Parama Pada of Lord Vishnu. In this way, when you master Bhramari Pranayama, you can master Samadhi. Shri Gheranda says that Dhyana is eight times superior to Japa, Tapa is eight times superior to Dhyana, music (divine sound Anhana) is eight times superior to Tapa, and nothing is superior to this divine music (the divine sound).

Comment: When you do this Pranayama at a fast pace, the sound generated is that of a male bumble bee, and when done slowly, the sound generated is that of a female bumble bee. Both give a lot of joy and bliss.

Focus: On Agya chakra

Comment:

- While humming you can chant the Pranava Mantra *'Om'*.
- Close your mouth, but do not join your teeth.
- This can also be done with Shanmukhi mudra.
- While humming, other sounds may also be generated. So be very careful.

Benefits:

- It makes the voice melodious and clear.
- It cures insomnia.
- It gives spiritual benefits.
- It helps overcome mental disorders like irritation, anger, impulse, tension, etc.
- It is beneficial for high blood pressure patients.
- It is also beneficial for the patients of heart diseases.

Note: Some sadhakas do this kriya by closing their ears with the thumbs, with their index fingers on the forehead, middle finger on the eyes, ring finger near the nose and the little finger near the mouth.

Murcha Pranayama (Swooning breath)

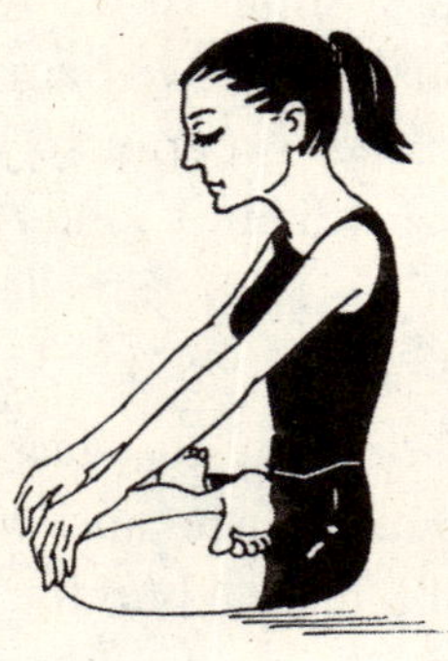
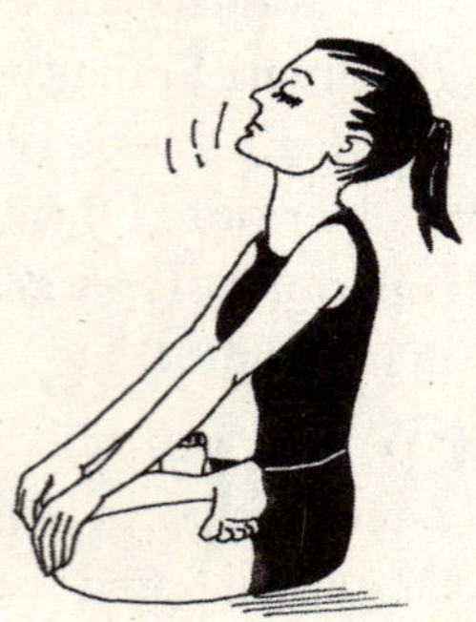

Method: Do this Pranayama in Padmasana or Siddhasana so that you can maintain stability. Keep both your hands on your knees. Close your eyes and take your head back (form an angle of almost 45 degrees). Inhale from both the nostrils and do antahkumhaka. Give up all your mental worries, bring your head down and do rechaka. Even though your eyes are closed, try to focus between your brows. Be very alert regarding your body and mind. Repeat this exercise at least 5 times or as per your convenience.

According to *Gheranda Samhita*: First of all, sit joyfully and do the above mentioned kumbhaka. Drive out all the materialistic and cardinal desires from your mind and focus between your brows. This is called Moorchchha kumbhaka. While doing this kumbhaka, you can experience bliss.

Benefits:

- It gives relief to people who are mentally upset, or whose brain has become inert.
- It is beneficial in cases of headaches and related diseases.
- It is helpful in awakening the kundalini and in doing meditation.
- It develops the brain and cures all the mental problems.

Precautions: People who are suffering from high blood pressure, heart diseases, fits, giddiness and mental disorders should do this Pranayama slowly and with patience.

Kevali Pranayama (Holding the breath)

According to *Gheranda Sambita*: According to Maharishi Gheranda, every creature unknowingly chants the alphabet 'Ham' every time they breathe out, and chants the alphabet 'Sah' (So) every time they breathe in. In this way, every creature takes in 21,600 breaths in every 24 hours. The letter 'Ham' represents Shiva and the letter 'Sah' represents Shakti, which is called as the 'Ajapa naama Gayatri' and this 'Hams', which when read in the reverse becomes 'Soham', is chanted by every creature unknowingly.

The air moves through the passage between the anus and the genitals, and between the heart and the nostrils. Maharishi Gheranda says that the physical body measure up to 96 angulas and the speed of the breath which habitually goes out of the body is 12 angulas. While singing, it becomes 16, 20 while eating, 24 while walking, 30 while sleeping, 36 during intercourse, and becomes much more in other works which demand hard work (Different acharyas have given different measures according to their understanding.).

Yogis have said that when the pace of the breath becomes less than its natural speed, one's life span is prolonged, and when it becomes more than 12 angulas, the life span reduces. As long as the prana vayu exists, one does not die. In the practice of kumbhaka, this prana vayu is the main aspect. Keep the body stable and do ajapaajapa while doing Kevali kumbhaka (Pranayama). One is blessed with long life by doing Kevali Pranayama. This means that when you complete 21,600 japas, the speed of your breath reduces and the heart is filled with joy.

Draw in the breath from the nostrils and do kumbhaka. On the first day, do this 64 times. Kevali kumbhaka should be practised eight times in eight parts of the day (8 x 8 = 64). Practice it in the morning, afternoon and evening in equal measures. In this way, till you master the Kevali kumbhaka, continue to increase the measure by five counts along with the ajapaajapa gayatri.

According to *Hatha Yoga*: Sit in Svastikaasana. Without inhaling and exhaling, hold your breath as it is. This is called Kevali kumbhaka.

> रेचकं पूरकं त्यक्त्वा सुखं यद् वायुधारणम्।
> प्राणायामोऽयमित्युक्तःस वै केवल-कुम्भकः।।

Some acharyas consider Stambhvritti Pranayama and Kevali kumbhaka as one.

> कुम्भके केवले सिद्धे रेचक-पूरकवर्जिते।
> न तस्य दुर्लभं किंचित त्रिषु लोकेषु विद्यते।।

Nothing remains unattainable when you master the art of controlling rechaka and puraka and doing only kumbhaka. Everything becomes within reach. Yogis are of the opinion that when you master 'Sahita Kumbhaka', in which kumbhaka is done with rechaka and puraka, 'Kevali kumbhaka' becomes easy to perform and success comes sooner.

Benefits:

- It is written in *Hatha Yoga Pradeepika* that there is nothing in this world which one cannot achieve after mastering Kevali kumbhaka.
- When you master the art of holding and directing the prana vayu as per your own wish, you can even attain high positions of authority.
- It grants divine vision.
- It grants stability in meditation.

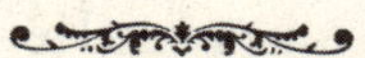

Pranayama gives us good health and
a lively disposition.

–RJT

Chandra-bhedana Pranayama (Breathing with left nostril)

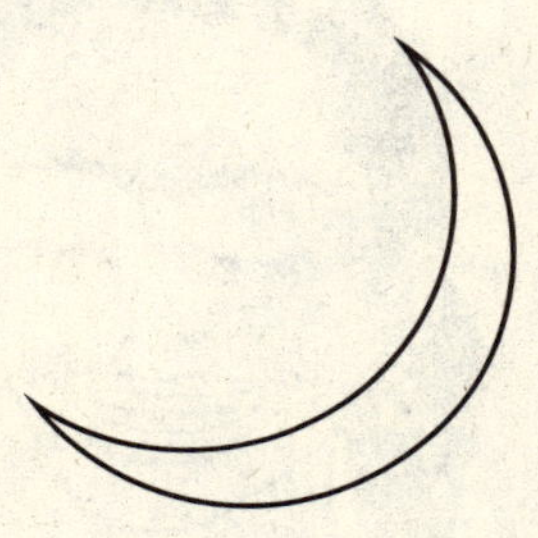

Method: All the kriyas of this Pranayama are opposite to those of Surya-bhedana Pranayama. Sit in Sukhasana. Inhale (do puraka) from your left nostril. In this puraka kriya, draw in the breath slowly, deeply, and carefully. Then, close both the nostrils. Do Jalandhara bandha and Moola bandha along with kumbhaka. Hold, as much as you comfortably can. Release the Bandha and do the rechaka kriya (exhale) with the right nostril. This is one round. Do 10 such rounds and increase the duration of kumbhaka gradually.

Note: In this Pranayama, all the purakas are done from the left nostril and the rechaka are done from the right nostril.

Comment: Do not do both the Pranayamas (Surya-bhedana and Chandra-bhedana) on the same day.

Benefits:

- It makes the body cool and keeps the heart happy.
- It calms the bile.
- It is beneficial in summers.
- It helps control anger and gives mental peace.
- It reduces stress.
- It is helpful in enhancing the retention power of the mind.
- Those suffering from high blood pressure should practise this regularly and gain its benefits.

Precautions:

- Those suffering from low blood pressure should not do this Pranayama.
- As far as possible, do not do this Pranayama during winters.

Seetkari Pranayama (Hissing breath)

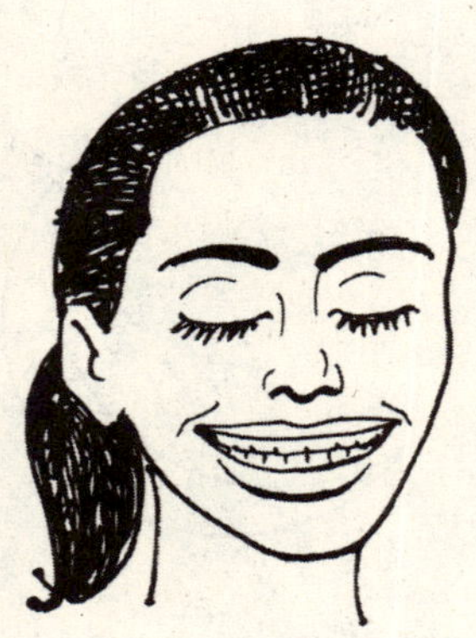

Method: This is similar to Sheetali Pranayama, but the position of the tongue is different. Turn your tongue backward in such a manner that the tip of your tongue touches the upper part of the glottis. Then, join the upper and the lower denture and spread your lips wide to the sides. Inhale deeply with a s…s…s… sound and let the breath fill your lungs. Do Jalandhara bandha and close your mouth. Hold it for some time. Then, release the bandha and do rechaka from the nose. This is one round. Do 8-10 rounds.

Comment: This can also be done without the bandha.

Benefits:

- It keeps the body cool when done during summers.
- It gives all the benefits of Sheetli Pranayama.
- It is beneficial in diseases of the throat, mouth and nose.
- Those who have bile imbalance must do this Pranayama to gain benefit.
- It normalises high blood pressure.

Note: This Pranayama is a type of Sheetali Pranayma. This also keeps the body cool.

Precautions:

- Those suffering from low blood pressure should not do this Pranayama.
- Those with imbalanced air (vaata) should not do this Pranayama.

Kapalbhati Pranayama (Body cleansing technique/Frontal brain cleaning breath)

Meaning: 'Kapal' means head and 'Bhati' means shine or illumination/aura. The Pranayama which illuminates the forehead or the brain is called Kapalbhati Pranayama.

Method: This Pranayama is like Bhastrika Pranayama. In this Pranayama, the speed of inhalation is slow, and the exhalation is done forcefully. Inhale normally, and focus on the exhalation. In other words, exhale forcefully. Inhale normally and exhale in quick successions (Some wise men talk of practising this Pranayama with bandhas. Please consult an expert teacher before doing so). Close your eyes and focus on Agya chakra. You will experience freshness and strength.

Precautions:

- Those who are suffering from cataract (or any disease of the eye), pus in the ears, or any other such disease should not do this Pranayama.
- Patients of high blood pressure, heart diseases, giddiness, gastric ulcers etc. should use their wisdom and do this Pranayama slowly.

Benefits:

- This Pranayama gives a lot of freshness, peace and happiness.
- It is beneficial in diseases related to the brain.
- It destroys diabetes and constipation.
- It reduces obesity.
- It balances the body weight.
- It cures many incurable diseases.
- It is beneficial in diseases such as cancer.
- Due to the forceful expelling of the breath, the diaphragm expands and contracts, which in turn benefits the entire abdominal region, and the kidneys, pancreas, stomach, liver, spleen, uterus, etc. start functioning efficiently.

Notes:

- Some learned men consider this as a kriya of Pranayama, while others consider this as a part of the Shatkarma Kriya. To know more, please see the chapter on Shatkarma.
- For a normal person, the rechaka count up to 120 per minute is considered satisfactory. Alternatively, one can do it for 3 minutes to 15 minutes depending on the physical condition of a person or the disease one is suffering from.

Comments:

- For better benefits, do Kapalbhati under the guidance of a guru, for a longer duration. If you feel giddy, or experience any discomfort, discontinue, and do Shavasana. Also consult a yoga teacher.
- When you exhale, you should imagine that all the disorders and diseases of your body – fear, ignorance, anger, pride, illusion, greed and sorrow – are being expelled out of your body and you are becoming physically, mentally and spiritually happy.

Pranayama removes obstructions in the subtle areas of the body and makes the Prana flow harmoniously in the nadis by rectifying them.

–RJT

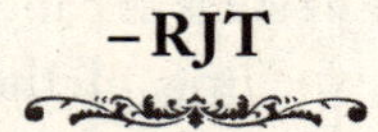

Plavini Pranayama (Breathing technique while floating)

अन्तः प्रवर्तितोदारमारुतापूरितोदरः ।
पयस्यगाधेऽपि सुखात्प्लवते पद्मपत्रवत् ।। (Hath Yog Pradipika 2/70)

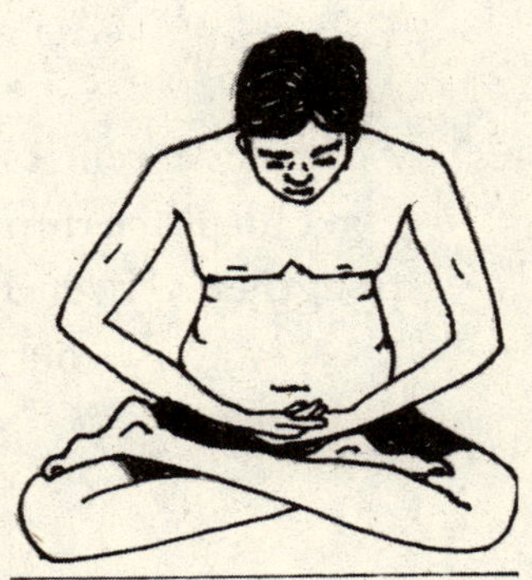

Meaning: 'Plavana' means to swim or go down. By mastering this Pranayama, the sadhaka can easily swim in water.

Method: Sit in Sukhasana and inhale from both your nostrils. Fill up so much air in your stomach that it blows up like a balloon and gets tensed. Do kumbhaka as per your capacity and gradually breathe out from your nostrils. This is one round. Repeat it as per your capacity.

Benefits:

- By practising this Pranayama, the sadhaka can float on water like a log.
- It rectifies parts of the digestive system and cures constipation.
- It does not let the Samana and Apana Vayu become imbalanced.

The practice of Pranayama regularises the flow of prana in the entire body.

–RJT

The nerve centres, glands and nadis of our body get life force through Pranayama. They also get strengthened by it. Thus, they provide good health to our body and mind.

– RJT

By initiating yoga into the soul, troubled by the illusion of attachment and hatred, the mind, words and body connect by one vayu (Harmony is established and they are balanced.), and by this vayu, this machine called the body, indulges in its functions.

– Acharya Poojyapada Swami

Samadhi Tantra Gatha No. 103

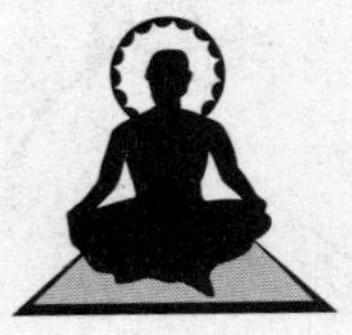

Mudra

A Perspective

Our ancient sages have given a lot to humankind. There must have been some laxity in our capacity to receive; otherwise, today the entire world would have been following our footsteps. The sages unveiled many secrets. They taught us many skills and imparted understanding about various faculties of knowledge. Among those skills is the science of mudra. Mudra is considered profounder and more subtle than asana and Pranayama. Its effects are so deep and far reaching that the capacity of our entire life giving energy can be made even sharper and more internal. The weaknesses, diseases and fatigue which affect its functioning are removed or cured. By using these mudras, one can develop a better personality and enjoy the peak of spirituality in life.

Twenty-five Mudras are mentioned in *Gheranda Samhita* which give unlimited benefits, but we shall chiefly discuss those mudras which are more popular and in use. The benefits of the other mudras can also be obtained from these mudras. All these mudras are easy and would subsequently prove to be meaningful to us.

1. Mahamudra (Great seal/Great psychic attitude)

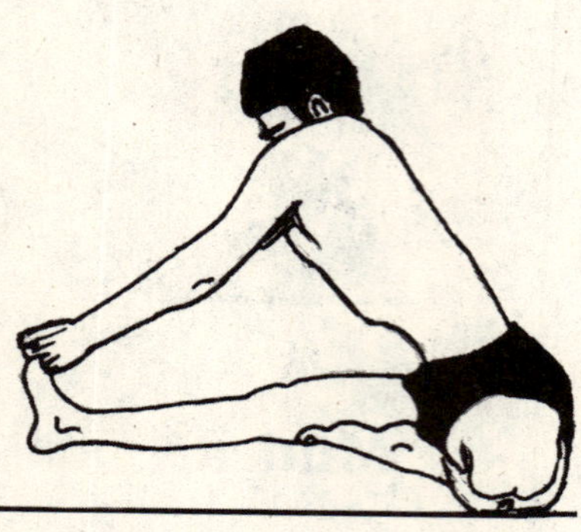

Method: Sit joyfully on your mat and spread your legs in front. Bend your right leg from the knees and place the heels under the anus. Then, bend forward and hold the big toe of the left leg with both the hands. Breathe deeply. Do Moola bandha and Jalandhara bandha. Do kumbhaka and try to make the energy flow in the upward direction. Focus on the kundalini chakras and release the Bandhas. Slowly do rechaka. Repeat the procedure by bending the right leg. Do 3-5 rounds.

Benefits:

- It cures the diseases of the abdomen like poor digestion, acidity, indigestion, constipation, etc.
- It destroys piles and diabetes.
- It is excellent for meditation and is helpful in awakening the kundalini.
- It cures enlarged spleen and tuberculosis.
- It is a good remedy for chronic fever.

Note: To know more, please see Mahamudrasana.

2. Mahavedha Mudra (Great piercing posture)

Method: Place the heel of the right leg at the Seevni nadi (Perinium) in between the anus and the genitals. Spread the left leg in front. Bend forward and hold the big toe of the left leg with both the hands. Inhale. Fix your gaze in between your brows. Do Tribandha (Jalandhara bandha, Moola bandha and Uddiyana bandha). Focus on your energy.

Concentrate on the chakras from the Mooladhara to the others in the upward direction. Hold the position as per your capacity. Then, gradually release the Uddiyana bandha, Moola bandha and finally, Jalandhara bandha, and bring your gaze back to normal. Do rechaka slowly.

Comment: In some places, while sitting in the above mentioned position, we must gently hit our buttocks against the ground, a few times after doing the bandhas. But this should be done only after one has mastered the asana.

According to *Gheranda Samhita*: Moola bandha and Maha bandha are of no consequence without Mahavedha. First practice Maha bandha; then, hold the breath by doing kumbhaka with Uddiyana bandha. This is called Mahavedha. The yogis who do Mahavedha everyday, along with Maha bandha and Moola bandha, become the best among yogis. Old age and death stay away from them, or in other words, their body undergo a total transformation.

Benefits:

- One attains mastery over many siddhis automatically.
- Wrinkles do not appear on the body; the person always remains young.
- It cures trembling limbs, and keeps the hair from turning grey.
- The life force starts flowing in the Sushumna and the person practising Mahavedha attains the state of Samadhi.

Note: To know about Maha bandha, please see the chapter on bandha.

3. Khechari Mudra (Tongue lock)

Method: Upturn your tongue and take it back to touch the throat cavity, while keeping the mouth closed. This mudra is called the Khechari mudra. It is not easy to touch the throat cavity with the tongue. Therefore, there are three methods to increase the length of the tongue: Chhedana, chaalana and dohana.

Chhedana: The tongue is attached to the lower jaw by a thin nerve fibre, that is why it becomes difficult to take the tongue back to the throat cavity. To loosen it, you should rub the nerve fibre everyday with a huge chunk of rock salt, or if possible, get a surgery done. In a few days, with practice, you will be able to take the tip of your tongue back into the throat cavity.

Chaalana and dohana: Hold the tongue with the thumb and the index finger or with a fine cloth. Then, turn, move and pull it. This is called chaalana kriya.

Apply some butter or ghee and pull the tongue with both the hands, just as you milk a cow. Pulling the tongue in this manner is called dohana. Out of these, you must follow what is most comfortable to you. Do it under the guidance of a guru. Gradually, your tongue would become so long that it would reach above the nose, in between the brows.

Precautions: Do not try to do the above mentioned exercises in haste. Otherwise, the result could be fatal. Do not do it without the guidance of an expert teacher.

Comment: If you observe celibacy, the chances of success is enhanced.

Benefits: When this mudra is mastered, one is able to savour the nectar that drips from Bramharandhra. When the tongue enters the throat cavity, the paths of Ida, Pingala and Sushumna open up. This creates a situation for Samadhi. By drinking the nectar, one can even win over death (prolong one's life). One is not troubled by sleep, laziness hunger and thirst.

Note: We have seen sadhakas who, with regular practice, have elongated their tongues so much that they have succeeded in touching the throat cavity with the tip of their tongue.

4. Vipareetkarni Mudra (Inverted pose)

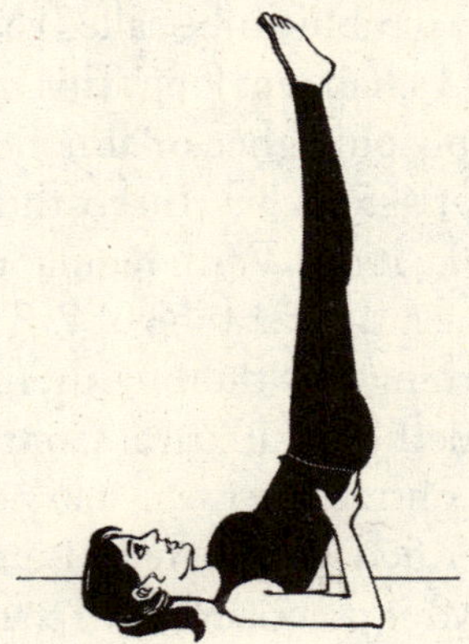

Method: According to *Gheranda Samhita*, the Surya nadi is at the root of the navel and the Chandra nadi is at the root of the palates. When the Surya nadi consumes all the nectar present in the body with its heat, the person dies. That is why, Surya should be lifted up and Chandra should be brought down. This is called Vipareetkarni mudra. To do this, you should follow the method of Sarvangasana. With a little effort, you will be able to apply Moola bandha and Uddiyana bandha. In *Gheranda Samhita,* acharya says that after doing puraka pranayama when you do kumbhaka and hold the breath as per your capacity, the kriya is called Vipareetkarni mudra.

Precaution: Those suffering from high blood pressure and heart diseases should not do this mudra.

Benefits:

- The sadhaka who does this mudra everyday wins over old age and death.
- With regular practice of this mudra, the appetite increases and digestion improves. So, one should keep a check over the amount of food they intake.
- When this mudra is done with the focus on the chakras, the aura, glow, vitality, and strength get enhanced.
- It also gives stability.

5. Vajroli Mudra (Thunderbolt mudra)

Method: Take a special rubber tube called catheter of 4-5 number, which is about one and a half feet long. This rubber tube is inserted into the urethera. Apply pure ghee or almond oil at the beginning of the tube up to about 4-5 inches. Insert this tube slowly into the urethera. If it hurts, take it out. With regular practice, once you get used to it, you can take a thicker tube of 7-8 number and practice inserting it. After learning this thoroughly, insert the tube and lift up your intestine by doing nauli kriya. Contract the Mooladhara and pull the air in by contracting the urinary tract. Then, try to pull in water and milk (purified and treated). Later, these elements are excreted with urine. After practising with the rubber tube, practise with a silver tube.

Comment: Do this only under the vigilance of an expert guru.

Benefits:

- The energy starts flowing in the upward direction.
- Celebacy is protected.
- One gets mental peace, joy and spiritual benefits.
- The sadhaka remains young till his death.
- The sadhaka's body starts emitting fragrance.
- This mudra provides nectar to the sadhaka and makes him a great yogi.

Mudras gradually lead a person towards the upliftment of the soul as well as towards purity.

–RJT

6. Yoni Mudra/Shanmukhi Mudra (Womb experience)

Method: Sit in sukhasana. Place both your hands on your face in such a manner that the thumbs are on the ears, the index fingers are on the eyes, middle fingers are on the nostrils and the ring and the little fingers are above the lips. Draw the breath in by Kaki mudra and infuse it with the Apana vayu. You should then awaken the kundalini and take it till the Sahasrara by focusing on the chakras or by chanting 'Ham Sah' mantra. While doing this mudra, you should imagine that you are becoming one with Shiva by awakening Shakti, and experiencing bliss while becoming Poorna Bramha. This is called Yoni mudra.

Benefits:

- This is a rare mudra. One can expiate many of his/her sins by doing this mudra *(Gheranda Samhita)*.
- The aura, strength and vitality of the body are enhanced by doing this mudra.
- The body becomes disease free by doing this mudra.
- This mudra grants a fresh youthful phase.
- When one practises this mudra with full concentration, he/she can hear subtle sounds.

The objective of all the approaches of yoga is one:
To enhace physical health, mental peace and
to make the awareness move in the upward direction.

–RJT

7. Shaktichalini Mudra (Energy conduction)

Method: According to Gheranda Samhita, as long as the kundalini – lying asleep in the Mooladhara, coiled up in its three and a half wraps – continues to be asleep, a person remains in the state of ignorance. Therefore, until you achieve absolute knowledge, you should continue to strive to awaken it. Just as a door cannot be opened without unlocking it, similarly, the Bramharandhra cannot be opened without awakening the kundalini. Look for a lonely place. Take a soft cloth, 1 metre long and 4 angulas wide. Tie it around your waist, covering the navel. Smear some ash on your body and sit down in Siddhasana. Then, draw the prana (air) in and infuse it with apana. Contract your anal region by doing Ashvini mudra. When kumbhaka is done in this manner, the kumdalini, which is in the form of a snake, awakens and starts rising up. After doing Shaktichalini mudra, do Yoni mudra.

Benefits:

- With daily practice, one can attain mastery over many siddhis including Vigraha siddhi.
- All kinds of mental and physical ailments are cured by doing this mudra.
- One experiences bliss by doing this mudra.

If you are healthy, do Pranayama to maintain your
good health and if you are unhealthy,
do Pranayama to become beautiful and healthy.

–RJT

8. Tadagi Mudra (Stick pose)

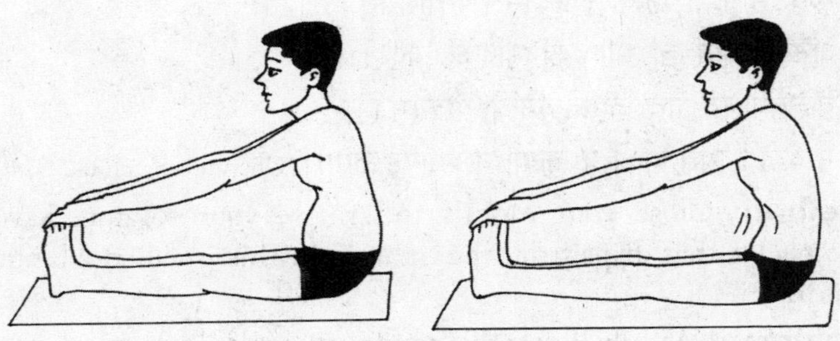

उदरंपश्चिमोत्तानं कृत्वा च ताड़ागाकृतिः।
ताड़ागी सा परामुद्रा जरा मृत्युं विनाशनी ।। (Gherunda Samhita 3/73)

Meaning: Sit in Pashchimottanasana and blow your stomach as if it is filled with water. This is Tadagi mudra. By practising this, you can attain victory over old age and death. Sit in Pashchimottanasana. Hold the toes of your feet with your hands, but don't bend forward. Draw the breathe in and blow your stomach out as much as possible. Hold the breath as much as you can. Then, slowly do rechak. While doing rechaka, contract your stomach in to look like a deep pond. Some yogis move the air like waves while doing kumbhaka.

Benefits:

- All the diseases related to the abdomen are cured by doing this mudra.
- The stomach becomes supple and the digestive system works efficiently by doing this mudra.
- One gains victory over old age by doing this mudra.

9. Manduki Mudra (Frog gesture)

मुखं संमुद्रितं कृत्वा जिह्वामूलं प्रचालयेत।
शनैर्ग्रसेदमृतं तां माण्डुकीं मुद्रिकां विदुः।।
वलितंपलितं नैव जायते नित्य यौवनम्।
न केशे जायते पाको यः कुर्यान्नित्यमाण्डुकीम्।। (Gherunda Samhita 3/74-75)

Method: Close your mouth and rotate your tongue. Savour the nectar that drips from the Sahasrara. This is called Manduki mudra.

Comment: While doing this mudra, one should concentrate on the Sahasrara to enjoy spiritual bliss.

Benefits:

- It prevents hair fall and premature greying of hair.
- One remains young forever by doing this mudra.
- The body becomes beautiful and begins to glow, all the diseases are destroyed by doing this mudra.
- This mudra establishes a balance between the air, bile and phlegm in the body.

10. Ashvini Mudra (Horse gesture pose)

आकुंचयेद् गुदाद्वारं प्रकाशयेत् पुनः पुनः।
सा भवेदश्विनीमुद्रा शक्ति प्रबोधकारिणी।।
आश्विनी परमा मुद्रा गुह्यरोग विनाशनीं।
बलपुष्टिकरी चैव अकालमरणं हरेत्।। (Gherunda Samhita 3/82-83)

Method: Sit in Sukhasana without any stress or tension. Close your eyes and do puraka. Hold your breath and contract your anal muscles repeatedly. Do this as per your capacity. Then, do rechak as per your convenience.

Comments: You can also do this with normal breathing.

Benefits:

- It eliminates the fear of untimely death.
- All the diseases of the anal region are automatically cured by doing this mudra.
- It is helpful in awakening the kundalini.
- It gives physical and mental benefits.

11. Pashinee Mudra (Folded psychic pose)

कण्ठपृष्ठे क्षिपेत्पादौ पाशवद् दृढ़बन्धनम्।
सा एव पाशिनी मुद्रा शक्ति प्रबोधकारिणी।।
पाशिनी महती मुद्रा वयःपुष्टि विधायिनी।
साधनीया प्रयत्नेन साधकैः सिद्धिकांक्षिभिः।। (Gherunda Samhita 3/84-85)

Method: Take both your legs up behind the neck and interlock them firmly. This mudra, which awakens the kundalini, is called Pashini mudra.

Comment: Do it under the vigilance of an expert teacher.

Focus: On Vishuddhi chakra

Benefits:

- It increases strength, the body becomes healthy.
- It grants siddhis. One can accomplish Ashta siddhis.
- It gives mental peace and happiness.

12. Kaki Mudra (Crow's beak)

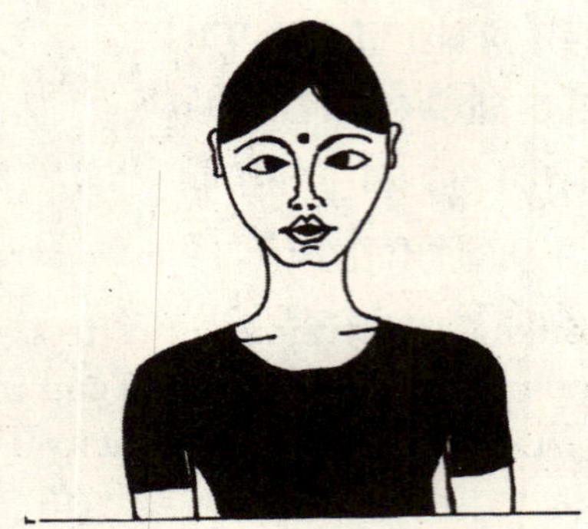

काकचन्चुवदास्येन पिवेद्वायं शनैः शनैः।
काकी मुद्रा भवेदेषा सर्वरोग विनाशनी।।
काकी मुद्रा परा मुद्रा सर्वतन्त्रेषुगोपिता।
अस्याः प्रसादमात्रेण काकवन्नीरुजो भवेत्।। (Gherunda Samhita 86-87)

Meaning: Slowly draw in air by pouting the lips like the beak of a crow. By doing this, all kinds of diseases are cured. This is called Kaki mudra. By practising this, the sadhaka becomes disease free like a crow.

Maharishi Gheranda says that this mudra should be kept a secret.

Comment: In this mudra, one has to inhale from the mouth and not from the nose, but while exhaling, one should close the mouth and exhale from the nose.

Benefits:

- It destroys all diseases.
- It keeps the body cool.
- It is beneficial for the patients of high blood pressure.
- It rectifies the digestive system and cures constipation.
- It gives mental peace.
- It normally cures many other diseases.

Precaution: Those suffering from low blood pressure should not do this mudra.

13. Matangini Mudra (Elephant seal)

कण्ठमग्नेजले स्थित्वा नासाभ्यां जलमाहरेत्। मुखान्निर्गमयेत्पश्चात् पुनर्वक्त्रेण चाहरेत्।।
नासाभ्यां रेचयेत्, पश्चात कुर्यादिवं पुनः पुनः। मातङ्गिनी परा मुद्रा जरामृत्यु विनाशनी।।
विरले निर्जने देशे स्थित्वा चौकाग्रमानसः। कुर्यान्मातङ्गिनी मुद्रां मातङ्ग इव जायते।।
यत्र यत्र स्थितो योगी सुखमत्यन्तंमश्नुते। तस्मात सर्व प्रयत्नेन साधयेत् मुद्रिकांपराम्।
(Gherunda Samhita 3/88-91)

Meaning: Stand in neck-deep water. Draw in water from your nose and expel it from your mouth. Then, take in water from your mouth and expel it from your nose. Again draw in water from your nose and expel it from your mouth. Repeat this kriya many times. This is Matangini mudra.

Benefits:

- Once this mudra is mastered, there is no fear of old age and death.
- One can become as powerful as an elephant by mastering this mudra.
- One can attain all kinds of happiness by doing this mudra.

14. Bhujangini Mudra

वक्त्रं किच्यित्सुप्रसार्य चानिलं गलया पिवेत्। सा भवेद् भुजङ्गी मुद्रा जरामृत्युविनाशिनी।।
यावच्च उदरे रोगमजीर्णादि विशेषतः। तत्सर्वनाश्येदाशु यत्र मुद्रा भुजङ्गिनी।।
(Gherunda Samhita 12/93)

Meaning: Open your mouth wide, and draw the air in. Do it in such a way that the throat experiences the force of the air. This is called Bhujangini mudra.

The above mentioned method should be done by sitting in Siddhasana, Padmasana, or Vajrasana.

Benefits:

- It keeps old age and death at bay.
- The disorders related to the abdominal diseases are cured.
- It cures indigestion. The digestive system becomes strong by doing this mudra.
- The diseases of the throat are cured by this mudra.

15. Yoga Mudra (Gestures of yoga)

Method: Sit peacefully in Padmasana and close your eyes. Take your hands back and hold the big toes of the legs with them. Exhale and slowly bend forward. Touch the ground with your forehead. Remain in this position for 10-15 seconds. Breathe normally. Then, inhale and come back to the original position.

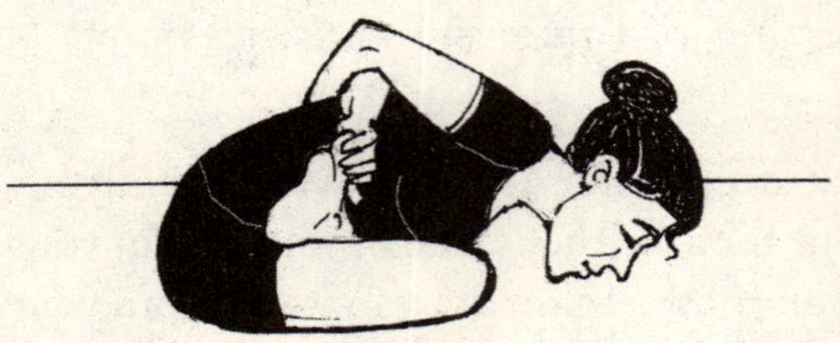

Direction: Face East or North for spiritual reasons.

Focus: It is ideal for awakening all the chakras. But special focus should be on the Mooladhara and the Agya chakras.

Benefits:

- It activates the digestive system.
- It cures constipation.
- It gives spiritual benefits.
- It totally benefits the spine.

Comment: Practice gradually to execute the full asana. If you find it difficult, you can interlock your hands at the back in the beginning.

Note: For more information, see the Yogmudrasana part as well.

If you want to create a new heaven for yourself,
you should adopt yogavidya.

–RJT

16. Bramha Mudra (Moving inward)

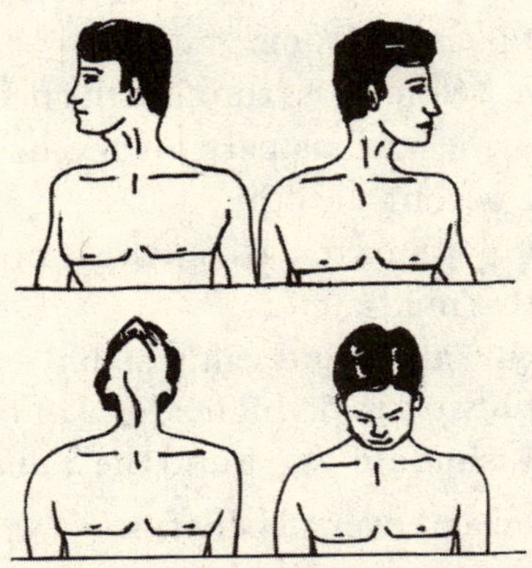

Appearance: Like the four faces of Bramha

Method: Sit in the posture of meditation (Padmasana or Sukhasana). Keep your spine and torso straight and close your eyes. Keep your hands on your knees in Gyana mudra or China mudra. To do this mudra with a calm attitude, hold your head firmly in front. Then, gradually turn your head to the right. The turning should be so slow that it takes at least two and a half minutes to come in line with the right shoulder. Maintain a count or keep a track of the number of breaths you take. After keeping it still for about one fourth of a minute (about 15 seconds) start turning the head towards the left. The head should take about five minutes to come in line with the left shoulder. After holding it stable for about one fourth of a minute, start bringing your neck back to the first position taking two and a half minutes. After keeping it stable for about half a minute, slowly start taking your head back, in two and a half minutes. Again, hold the position for 15 seconds and bring it back in front and place it on the sternum in five minutes. Hold this position for 15 seconds and then bring the head back to the original position in two and a half minutes. In this way, the entire process of turning the head in all the four directions should take 21 minutes. This is one round of Bramha mudra. The rate of breathing in this mudra will be slower than the normal rate.

Benefits:

- By alternatively stretching and relaxing the nerves of the neck, they become supple and strong.
- The cranial nerves, which pass through the neck, get a thorough massage. Hence, the various parts of the head like eyes, ears, nose, tongue etc. become healthy.
- The unwanted growth of tonsils, inflamation and swelling are cured by doing this mudra.
- It helps in keeping the mind calm, stable and focused. Thus, one can successfully try to do higher level of meditation.
- It activates the Vishuddhi, Agya and the Sahasrara chakras.

Mudra: Conclusion and over all benefits:

- The practice of mudra fulfills all the desires.
- It keeps old age and death at bay.
- It is confidential and difficult to achieve even for the gods. It should not be revealed to atheists and notorious and undeserving people.
- This knowledge should be passed on to true devotees, thoughtful and calm minded people.
- It cures all diseases. Regular practice can protect your modesty.
- It activates the power of digestive.
- The person who practises this mudra wins over old age and death. He/she does not fear fire, water and air.
- It cures twenty types of diseases like diseases related to breath, spleen, leprosy, phlegm, etc.
- It purifies the blood.
- It calms the air, bile and phlegm.

Yoga is not something to be flaunted. Rather, it is a science to be adopted for the sake of its benefits.

–RJT

Hasta Mudra Vigyana

(The Science of Hand Gestures)

Our body is a treasure house of innumerable secrets. Whatever knowledge we have today is only one percent of the knowledge granted to humankind by the Supreme power. If we manage to acquire even a fraction of this one percent, we become proud. And sometimes, this pride goes up to such an extent that it takes the form of arrogance. We are unable to balance ourselves and our life goes haywire. In order to bring this balance back, the Maharishis of the ancient times established certain principles and taught us many scientific skills. Those scientific skills exist in this world in many forms. One such skills is Hasta Mudra Vigyana. Through these mudras, we can bring back and imbibe the energy that goes out of our body, and gain multiple benefits. Our body is made out of five elements of nature. Whenever there is an imbalance, our body becomes prey to diseases. In order to control the elements, we need to learn how to utilise the Hasta Mudras. Additionally, we can elevate our lifestyle with the help of these mudras by tapping into the physical, mental and other subtle powers and thereby controlling and rectifying many unknown events that take place within our body.

The five fingers of our hands represent the five elements. The thumb represents the fire, index finger represents air, middle finger

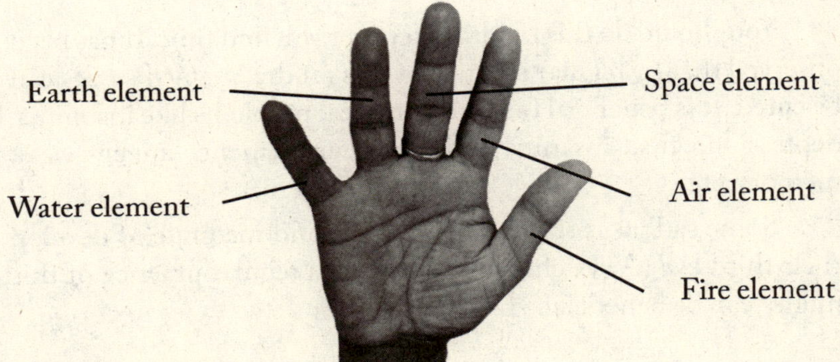

represents space/ether, ring finger represents earth and little finger represents water. Through the various mudras, we can establish balance among the elements in our body and rectify any natural disorder that may have occurred due to their imbalance. Thus, we can regain our health through mudras.

When we join the tip of any finger with the thumb, half the disorders of the related element are balanced. If we join the thumb to the base of a finger, the element related to that finger starts increasing. If we press the tip of a finger with the first part of the thumb, the related element starts decreasing.

In this way, whether physical or mental, we can cure many ailments by using these mudras. Here we are elaborating on a few of the main mudras.

1. Gyana Mudra (Knowledge pose)

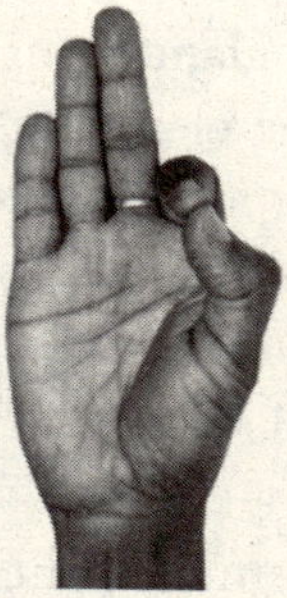

This Mudra is very popular. It is simple and very effective.

Sit in any asana such as Padmasana, Ardha Padmasana, Siddhasana or Sukhasana. Keep your hands on your knees and touch the tip of your thumbs with the tip of the index finger. The rest of the fingers should be kept straight. In this posture, when your palms face up, it is called China mudra, and when they face down, then it is called Gyana mudra. (Nowadays, people have started doing Gyana mudra while walking, standing, and watching TV).

You should do this mudra whenever you find time. It has been observed that by regular practice of this mudra, many diseases can be cured. It is beneficial for many physical problems like insomnia, depression, fits, insanity, irritation, excitement, anger, weak memory, etc.

Some sadhakas sit in Gyana mudra and meditate to develop their third eye (Agya chakra). In this way, regular practice of this mudra can be beneficial.

2. Vayu Mudra (Balancing the air gesture)

Many kinds of diseases emerge if the air element is in excess in the body. For example, trembling of the hands and legs, paralysis, arthritis, headache, heart problems, etc. All these disorders can be cured by doing **Vayu mudra**.

Bend your index finger and place it at the base of the thumb, as shown in the illustration. Keep the thumb over the index finger and apply a little pressure. Keep the other three fingers straight. This mudra removes the imbalance of the air element in the body and keeps it in check.

3. Shunya Mudra/Akasheeya Mudra (Sky Gesture)

By doing this mudra, disorders like pain in the ears, loss of hearing and other diseases of the ears can be cured.

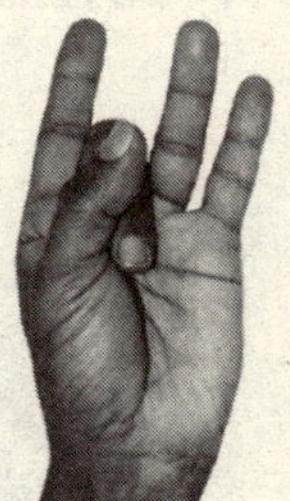

Bend the middle finger and place it at the base of the thumb, as shown in the illustration. Keep the thumb over it and apply a little pressure. Those who are suffering from disorders caused due to the imbalance of this element should do the mudra with both the hands to gain more benefit.

4. Surya Mudra (The Sun gesture)

The ring finger represents the earth element. According to the science of palmistry, the ring finger shows the impact of the Sun in our life. It also assists in the flow of energy in our body.

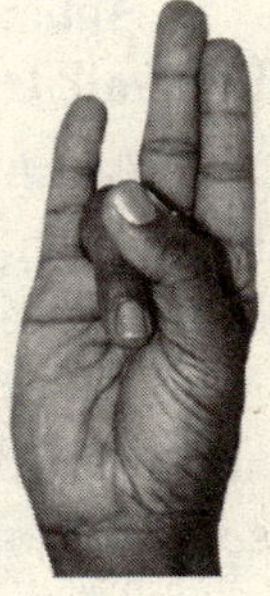

Bend the ring finger and place it at the base of the thumb, as shown in the illustration. Keep your thumb over it and apply a little pressure. This is Surya mudra. By doing this mudra, obesity and heaviness can be reduced. Any Agya chakra can be activated by touching it with the ring finger.

5. Varuna Mudra (Water gesture)

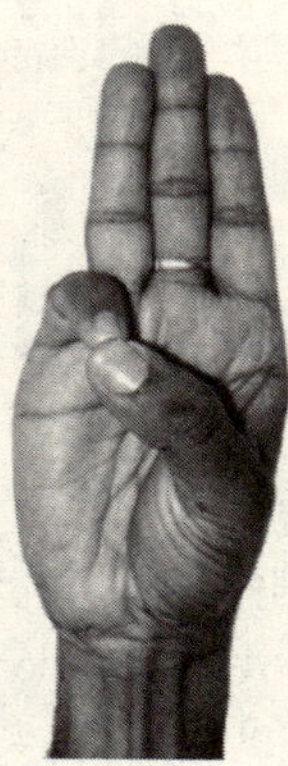

This Mudra represents the water element. When there is a deficiency of water element in the body, diseases like disorders of the blood, dryness, etc. start emerging. In order to cure such diseases, we should do Varuna mudra.

To do Varuna mudra, let the tip of the little finger touch the tip of the thumb, as shown in the illustration.

6. Surabhi Mudra (Wish-fulfilling gesture)

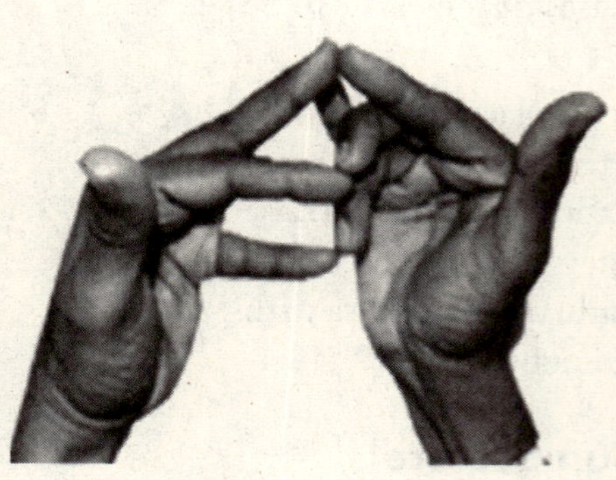

This yogic mudra is believed to be very mysterious. Almost all the sadhakas must do this mudra. It cures the diseases caused in our body by the imbalance of air, bile and phlegm. By regularly doing this mudra, a person can quickly gain physical and spiritual benefits.

Acharyas opine that it is very difficult to explain this mudra in detail. It has many secrets hidden within it.

As shown in the illustration, touch the ring finger of one hand with the little finger of the other hand and the little finger of the first hand with the ring finger of the other hand. Touch the middle finger of one hand with the index finger of the other hand and the index finger of the first hand with the middle finger of the second. Both the thumbs will remain open.

7. Prithvi Mudra (Earth gesture)

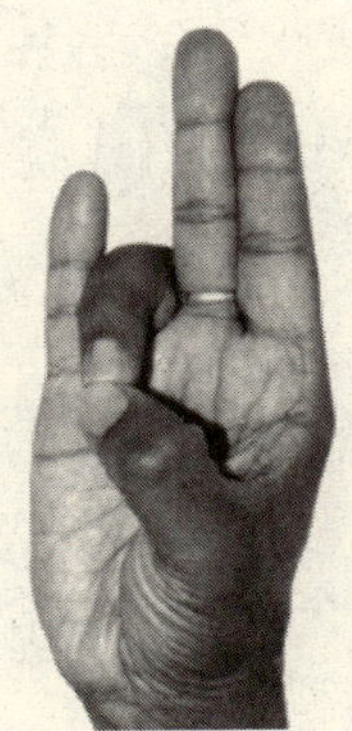

By doing this mudra, one can establish balance among all the mineral elements of the body. It maintains the body weight and keeps the body glowing.

Touch the tip of the ring finger with the tip of the thumb, as shown in the illustration. This is Prithvi mudra.

8. Apana Mudra/Mrita Sanjeevani Mudra (Purification gesture)

It is believed that the stomach should be soft and the blood should be warm. If you are suffering from constipation and the food is putrefying in your stomach, you can suffer from many diseases. If you do Apana mudra, you will be relieved of the imbalance of air in the body, and it will become beautiful and attractive.

With regular practice, the air can be controlled and balanced and the functions related to the air are carried out efficiently. The harmful air and the stool trapped in the body are easily released and the digestive system starts functioning well.

Form the mudra as shown in the illustration. Do it for at least 15-45 minutes. For maximum benefit, do Prana mudra along with Apana mudra.

9. Prana Mudra (Energy gesture)

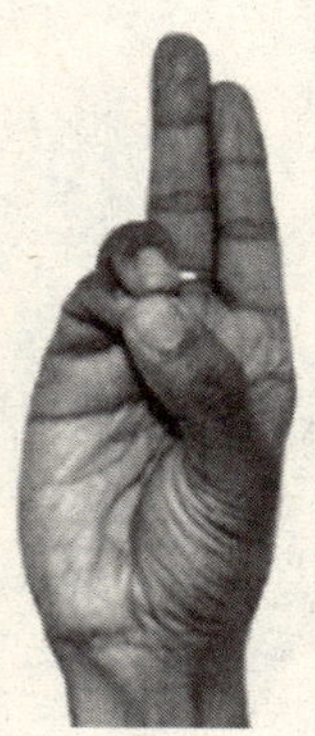

This mudra is actually a life giving mudra, because when we do it, the energy starts flowing through our body. The weakest of people can do this mudra and overcome the deficiency of proteins and vitamins in the body and enjoy good health. Eye disorders can be cured by doing this mudra. As a result, the number of the eye can be reduced, or, one can totally get rid of spectacles.

The Prana mudra helps all the systems of the body to function efficiently. Touch the tip of the ring finger and little finger with the top part of the thumb, as shown in the illustration.

10. Linga Mudra (Phallus gesture)

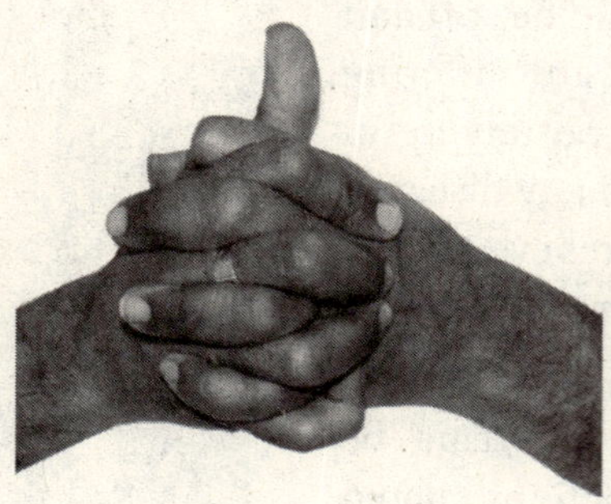

This Mudra is used to increase the heat in the body. You can use this mudra to keep your body warm in winters and gain many other benefits. Chronic colds can be cured by doing this mudra.

Interlock your fingers and point one thumb towards the sky, as shown in the illustration. Within a few minutes of doing this, you will feel the heat even in winters.

To conclude, what is common in all the mudras is: Patience, perseverance and faith. Without these factors nothing will work. Hence, you can gain the maximum benefit by keeping the mentioned facts in mind.

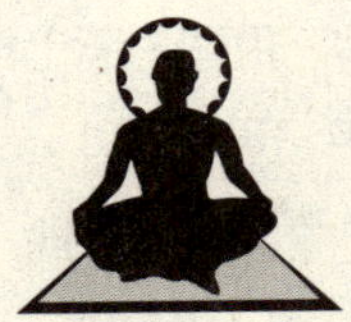

Bandhas

Their Types and Benefits

The literal meaning of 'Bandha' is to tie, to join with each other, to tighten up or to control.

In the processes explained in this section certain faculties or parts of the body are held tightly by holding the pranavayu, or breath. These bandhas help us in diverting our strength towards the inner self and assist us in doing pranayama. When the energy starts flowing in body of the sadhaka by doing the pranayama process, the sadhaka prevents its outflow with the help of these bandhas. These bandhas help in distributing the energy generated by pranayama in the internal organs of the body. These bandhas are also practised to awaken the kundalini. The function of the bandhas is to remove the impurities from the internal organs and make them cleaner and more functional. By applying the bandhas, the organs become stronger. They sort of get massaged. Bandhas instigate specific nadis and make them more efficient. They purify the blood. By applying bandha, all those glands of the body which obstruct the flow of Prana through the chakras, open up. During the process of bandha, the flow of energy gets directed by the Sushumna nadi. Practitioners of the higher level experience this during their Samadhi. One can gain special benefits by doing bandha and mudras along with pranayama. Since kumbhaka (antahkumbhaka and bahyakumbhaka) and bandhas are important for doing pranayama, one must increase one's capacity to do kumbhaka.

Here, we shall mainly explain five kinds of bandhas:

Moola Bandha (The root lock)

पार्ष्णिना वामपादस्य योनिमाकुञ्चयेत्ततः।
नाभिग्रन्थिं मेरुदण्डे सुधीः संपीड्य् यत्नतः।।
मेढ्रं दक्षिणगुल्फेन दृढबन्धं समाचरेत्।
जराविनाशिनी मुद्रा मूलबन्धो निगद्यते।।
संसारसागरं तर्तुमभिलषति यः पुमान्।
सुगुप्तो विरलो भूत्वा मुद्रामेतां समभ्यसेत्।।
अभ्यासाद्बन्धनस्यास्य मरुत्सिद्धिर्भवेद्ध्रुवम्।
साधयेद्यतस्तर्हि मौनी तु विजितालसः।। (Gherunda Samhita 3/6-9)

Meaning: Moola means root, beginning, base, foundation or earth. In yoga, Moola bandha is related to the Mooladhara chakra, which is situated in between the anus and the genital.

Method: Sit in Siddhasana or Padmasana. Keep your palms on your knees to come to a meditative position. Keep the spine straight, close your eyes, and relax your body. Focus on Mooladhara chakra.

Breathe in, and do antahkumbhaka. Simultaneously, do Jalandhara bandha. Contract your anal muscles and your genitals and draw them upwards (You must have seen how a cow and other animals draw their anus in after defecating.). Similarly, pull your Mooladhara region upward. This is the final position of Moola bandha. Hold this position as per your capacity. Relax the lower part of the body, lift up your head and exhale. This process can also be done with bahyakumbhaka. Repeat 5-10 times as per your convenience.

Note: While sitting in any asana, ensure that the heels apply pressure on the anus.

Comment: If you do this bandha incorrectly, there are chances of you developing physical weakness and impotency. If you practise Ashwini mudra, you can master Moola bandha sooner.

Benefits:

- It is helpful in awakening the kundalini.
- It helps the energy flow in the upward direction. As a result, the glow of the face, strength and vitality of the body are enhanced and even old people start looking young while building the capacity to work like them.
- The disorders of the reproductive organs are cured.
- With the regular practice of Moola bandha, the prana, apana, naada and bindu merge together and you gain mastery over yoga. You become one with the Supreme.
- It also gives all the benefits of Jalandhara bandha.
- It helps in practising celibacy.
- Disorders related to the anus, like piles, protruding of the anus, etc. are cured.

You should never feel discouraged, hopeless or distressed in life because you have the divine energy, called the soul, within you. It is the embodiment of profound vision, profound knowledge, profound happiness and profound strength. So, go ahead and identify it, and transform your life.

–RJT

Uddiyana Bandha (The abdominal lock)

उदरे पश्चिमं तानं नाभिरूर्ध्वं तु कारयेत्।
उड्डीयानं कुरुते यस्मादविश्रान्तं महाखगः।।
उड्डीयानं त्वसौ बन्धौ मृत्युमातंगकेसरी।
समग्राद बन्धनाद्ध्येतदुड्डीयानं विशिष्यते।।
उड्डीयाने समभ्यस्ते मुक्तिः स्वाभाविकी भवेत्।। (Gherunda Samhita 3/12-13)

Meaning: 'Uddiyana' means to fly. By doing this kriya, the energy rises from the lower body and starts flowing to the upper part of the body. In other words, when the energy enters the Sushumna and starts flowing upwards, it is called Uddiyana bandha.

Method: Stand in attention position. Keep a distance of about one or one and a half feet between your legs. Bend your knees a little and bend forward while you place your hands on the knees. Do a prolonged rechaka and do bahyakumbhaka. Do Jalandhara bandha and place your chin on the sternum. Then, pull your stomach in as far as possible towards your back. This is the final position of Uddiyana bandha. Practice as per your convenience. Then, bring your stomach to its original position and release the Jalandhara bandha. Do puraka and repeat. This is also called Shaktichalana Pranayama.

Benefits: According to Dattatreya Yoga, by doing this bandha, even the old can become young. Uddiyana bandha is the best bandha. The muscles of the heart get a good massage. The various parts of the abdominal region become soft and the digestive power becomes strong. This bandha is compared to a lion who can gain victory over an elephant representing death. It removes wrinkles from the face and enhances its glow.

Comment: Do this bandha 5-10 times on an empty stomach.

Note: This bandha can also be practised in sitting postures (Padmasana/Siddhasana).

Jalandhara Bandha (The chin lock)

कण्ठसंकोचनं कृत्वा चिबुकं हृदये न्यसेत्।
जालन्धरेकृति बन्धे षोडशाधारबन्धनम्।।
जालन्धरमहामुद्रामृत्योश्च क्षयकारिणी।
सिद्धो जालन्धरो बन्धो योगिनां सिद्धिदायकः।
षण्मासमभ्यसेद्यो हि स सिद्धो नात्र संशयः।। (Gherunda Samhita 3/10-11)

Literal meaning: 'Jaala' means a net or a network.

Method: Sit in Padmasana, Siddhasana, Svastikasana or Bhadrasana. Keep your back, neck and head straight. Place your hands on your knees. Take in a long breath (puraka) and do antahkumbhaka. Bend your head and press it against the upper part of your chest (in between the collar bones – sternum). Lift up your chest so that the chin can easily touch the sternum. Do not press the neck, or push it down. Relax the muscles of your neck. Keep the sternum and head in one line. Do normal kumbhaka for as long as you comfortably can. Relax your body and lift up your head. Exhale slowly. This is called Jalandhara bandha. Repeat it 5-10 times.

Comment: It is mentioned in the religious texts that the nectar which drips from the thousand petal led lotus of Sahasrara, located at the crown of the head, falls directly on the navel and is burnt by the fire present in the Manipuraka. Hence, by practising Jalandhara bandha, the sadhaka can preserve the nectar, savour it, and live a long life.

Effect: It also presses the Ida and Pingala nadis and helps the pran flow through the Sushumna (Saraswati nadi).

Benefits: It relaxes the brain, destroys pride and arrogance, and purifies the intellect. It activates the Vishuddhi chakra. It cures the disorders of the throat and makes the voice melodious. It destroys depression, worry, tension, anger, irritation etc. It enhances concentration and sharpens the memory. It keeps the entire body disease free.

Note: This Bandha can also be done in standing posture.

Mahabandha (The great lock)

वामपादस्य गुल्फेन पायुमूलं निरोधयेत्।
दक्षपादेन तद्गुल्फं संपीड्य यत्नतः सुधीः।।
शनकैश्चालयेत्पार्ष्णि योनिमाकुञ्चयेच्छनैः।
जालन्धरे धरेत्प्राणं महाबन्धो निगद्यते।।
महाबन्धः परो बन्धो जरामरण नाशनः।
प्रसादादस्य बन्धस्य साधयेत्सर्ववाञ्छितम्।। (Gherunda Samhita 3/14-16)

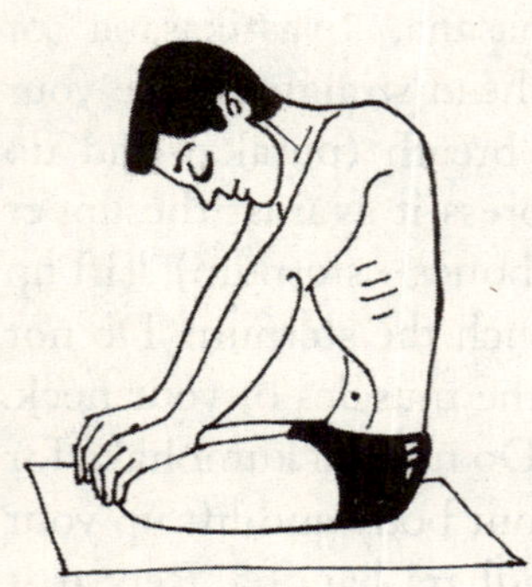

Method: You may sit in any meditative posture, but preferably sit in Siddhayogi asana. In this bandha, all the three bandhas have to be performed simultaneously. Exhale and first perform Jalandhara bandha, followed by Uddiyana bandha and finally, Moola bandha. Remain in this position as per your convenience. Then, gradually release the bandhas in this order: Moola bandha, followed by Uddiyana bandha and finally, Jalandhara bandha. Gradually breathe in and after coming back to the original position, repeat the process. You must perform this bandha only after you have practised all the three bandhas properly.

Benefits:

- One gets all the benefits of the above mentioned bandhas.
- It is wonderful for awakening the kundalini.
- It helps preserve vitality.
- The mind reaches a state of bliss through this bandha. As a result, one automatically attains many Siddhis.
- Like the confluence of Ganga, Jamuna and Saraswati, the three nadis also meet and function in coordination and harmony in this bandha.

Jivha Bandha (The tongue lock)

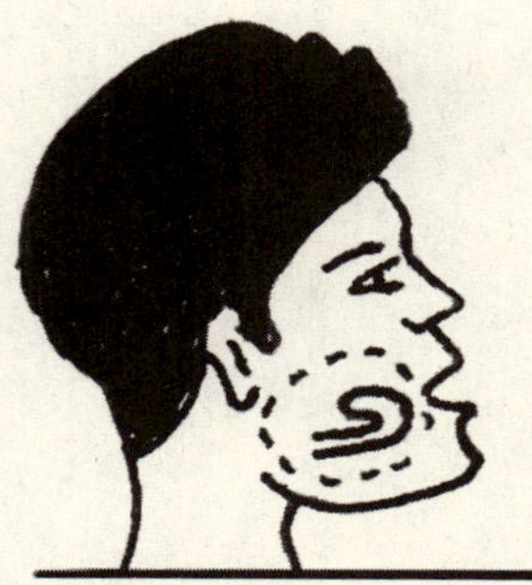

Method: Sit in any meditative posture (Padmasana/Siddhasana) and keep your spine and torso straight. Close your eyes. To do this bandha in a calm and peaceful manner, open your mouth, upturn your tongue and take it to the glottis. After practising it well, the tongue can be taken to the hollow of the throat, and then in the throat.

Benefits:

- It is helpful in the preliminary practice of the Khechari mudra mentioned in Yoga and Tantra Shastras.
- It is helpful in awakening the Lalana chakra.
- It is helpful in controlling or winning over the taste and other senses of desire.
- It is helpful in Pratyahara.

Our own good health can be beneficial for the good health of the world.

–RJT

All the kriyas of yoga vidya not only function to unite the Atma with the Parmatma, but also works to free us from the shakles of our karmas.

–RJT

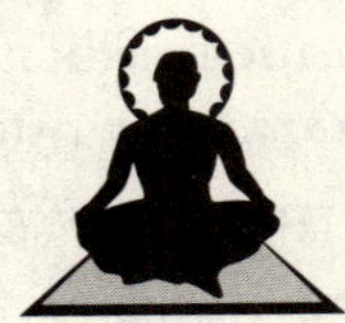

Hatha Yoga (Shata Karma)

India is the only country where the sages have explained numerous ways to attain self-realisation. An individual takes birth according to his past karmas and eventually dies. It is on the basis of these karmas that each individual has different feelings and thoughts. The yogacharyas were aware of this philosophy beforehand. They were of the opinion that if they told people about the common path of experiencing God, they will not be able to understand, because all of them think differently, and their physical condition were also different. If one wants to achieve something in life, first of all one should be in good health. There is a very popular saying that a healthy and disease free body is the greatest blessing one can have. This has been written after a lot of forethought. This is the reason why those great souls gifted the philosophy of yoga to us so that we could be physically healthy and the same practice could help us make our lives beautiful; and finally, we might reach that level of self-realisation where one ends the vicious circle of life and death and attains salvation.

Maintaining the same ideology, they taught us many skills related to yoga. Out of those skills, one is called Malshodhana Shatkarma.

Maharishi Gheranda writes:

षट्कर्मणा शोधनं च आसनेन भवेद्दृढ़म्।
मुद्रया स्थिरता चैव प्रत्याहारेण धीरता।।
प्राणायामाल्लाघवं च ध्यानात्प्रत्यक्षमात्मनः।
समाधिना निर्लिप्तं च मुक्तिरेव न संशयः।। (Gherunda Samhita 1/10-11)

By doing Shatkarma, the body is cleansed. It becomes firm by doing asanas. Mudras grant stability and pratyahara leads to patience. Pranayama makes the body light and swift. Dhyana leads to self-realisation and by focused meditation, one can undoubtedly attain salvation. In *Hatha Yoga*, it is written that:

मेदः श्लेष्माधिकः पूर्व षट्कर्माणि समाचरेत्।
अन्यस्तु नाचरेत्तानि दोषाणां समभावतः।
धौतिर्वस्तिस्तथा नेतिस्त्राटकं नौलिकं तथा।
कपालभातिश्चैतानि षट् कर्माणि प्रचक्षते।।
कर्मषटक्मिदं गोप्यं घटशोधनकारकम्।
विचित्रगुण संधायि पूज्यते योगिपुंगवैः।। (Hath Yog Pradipika 2/21-23)

Meaning: The acharya says that those who have excessive fat and phlegm in their body, should first do Shatkarma. In other words, those who have excessive phlegm, suffer from cold (too much phlegm is expelled from the nose and mouth), and those who are obese should do Shatkarma, which remove the impurities from the body, in order to cleanse it. But those who are not obese and do not have excessive phlegm need not do Shatkarma. The following are the types of Shatkarma:

1. Dhauti **2. Vasti** **3. Neti**
4. Trataka **5. Nauli** **6. Kapal-bhati**

The great scholars have expounded these six ways of doing Shatkarma. These Shatkarmas are confidential. They cleanse the body and generate unusual qualities in it. The yogis praise these Shatkarma and explain that if these are not kept confidential, others will also start following them and the uniqueness of the yogis will no longer be accepted. The objective of Shatkarma is to grant excellence to the yogis. It is written in *Gheranda Samhita*:

धौतिर्वस्तिस्तथा नेतिः लौलिकी त्राटकं तथा।
कपालभातिश्चेतानि षट्कर्माणि समाचरेत।। (Gherand Samhita 1/2)

Meaning: In order to cleanse your body, you should do these six karmas – dhauti, vasti, neti, lauliki, trataka, and kapal-bhati.

Dhauti (Internal Cleansing)

Dhauti is explained in detail in Gheranda Samhita. It is of four types:

1. Antardhauti **2. Dantdhauti**

3. Hriddhauti **4. Moolshodhana**

1. Antardhauti (Internal)

Antardhauti means cleansing of the internal parts of the body. For this we use water, air and cloth. Antardhauti is also of four types:

(A) Vatsara **(B) Varisara**

(C) Agnisara **(D) Bahishkrita**

(A) Vatsara Dhauti (Cleansing with air)

Form your lips like a crow's beak and slowly draw in air. After having taken in enough air, hold it in your stomach and rotate it. Then, slowly expel the air out. This is called Vatsara dhauti.

Benefits: It enhances the digestive power. The disorders related to the abdomen are destroyed and body is cleansed by doing this dhauti.

(B) Varisara Dhauti (Shankha-Prakshalana) (Cleaning the elementary canal)

This kriya is also called kayakalpa kriya. It is very important and significant. The meaning of Varisara dhauti is 'wash with water'. By doing this kriya, the sadhaka gets a new youthful look. The body becomes completely healthy and glowing.

Method: Drink water from your mouth till it fills up to your throat. Then, move it inside the abdominal region and expel it from your anus. This Varisara dhauti is very confidential and beneficial in cleansing the body. If this kriya is done regularly and carefully, sadhakas can make their bodies look like the bodies of divine beings.

Explanation: There are many popular methods of doing this kriya. Since this kriya cleanses the entire internal structure of the abdominal region, one should do some preliminary preparations. Those practitioners who wish to gain absolute benefits from this kriya should do these preparations two to three days in advance.

We assume that this kriya is mostly done by yogic practitioners. As it is, their food habits are very simple. However, it would be better if you eat simple and light food two to three days before you do Shankha-prakshalana. You should give up eating chilies, spices, sour food, oily food, heavy food and should not eat up to the full capacity of the stomach. This makes it easier to cleanse the body. Before and after Shankha-prakshalana, you should eat the following things: Moong dal khichadi, rice khichadi, ghee etc. which are easy to digest and light on the system. The sadhaka who pays attention to his stomach always enjoys good health. The kriya of Shankha-prakshalana is also important because it purifies the stomach. Food particles, undigested food and faecal matter stick to the stomach and putrefies, due to which the muscles of the abdominal region become weak and are not able to absorb the nutritive elements from the food. Resultantly, the blood becomes impure and one develops disorders caused due to air. The nadis become impure and as a result, one is unable to enjoy complete health.

Our intestine is shaped in a twisted form, like a shankha or conch. Just as the conch is cleansed by pouring in water from one side and pouring it out from the other to make it function better, similarly, by taking in water from the mouth and expelling it from the anus by a special technique, our body prepares itself to do yoga sadhana. This kriya is known as Shankha-prakshalana.

Shankha-prakshalana (Deep colon cleansing)

Method. Variation 1. Nowadays, different kinds of Shankha-prakshalana are being taught in different yoga centres (depending on the condition of the sadhaka). We shall describe the more popular types of kriyas.

Take clean filtered water in a bucket (sieve it through a cloth so that no impurities remain) and heat it till it is lukewarm. Make it salty by adding salt. Then, sit in Kagasana (crow posture).

Drink the first two glasses of water quickly. Then, under the guidance of a guru, do the following asanas in the given order: Tiryaka Bhujangasana, Tiryaka Tadasana, Kati Chakrasana and Udarakarshana. Do each asana eight times. Then, drink two glasses of water and repeat the above mentioned asanas. Again drink two glasses of water and repeat the asanas. Go to the toilet. If you do not feel like passing motion, then drink two more glasses of water. This time you will definitely feel like passing motion. Initially, the stool will be solid, then it will become a little watery. After passing motion, drink water again and repeat the asanas. This time the motions will be very watery and yellowish. Drink water once again. This time the motion will be as clear as water. It is not necessary that your stomach will become absolutely clear. You might have to repeat the asanas many times. When the motion is absolutely clear like water, you can be assured that your stomach has been cleared of all the filth. Then, drink four more glasses of water and do Kunjara kriya. Throw out all the water by vomiting and do Jala Neti. After one hour, eat moong khichadi with a lot of pure ghee.

Variation 2. As in the first variation, heat clean water till it is. Add enough salt and squeeze two lemons in it. Mix well.

Drink two glasses of water and do the following five asanas in the given sequence, four times each: Bhujangasana, Dvi-parshvasana, Pavanmuktasana, Vipareetkarni asana and Hastpadasana. Continue to drink water and do the asanas till you feel like passing motion. After drinking four to six glasses of water and doing the asanas two-three times, you will definitely feel like going to the toilet. Go to the toilet immediately. Initially, the stool might be very solid. After that drink two more glasses of water and do the asanas. If you do not feel like going to the toilet, drink two more glasses and repeat the asanas. This time the motion will be watery.

You must continue the kriya till the motion is as a clear as water. When the motion is clear like water, you can assume that your digestive system has been cleared of all impurities, because clear water comes out when there is no impurity sticking inside the system. After this, do Kunjara Kriya. Drink four glasses of water and through Kunjara Kriya, throw out the water stored in the stomach. Then, do Neti Kriya.

Variation 3. Sometimes, five asanas are done in Shankha-prakshalana. The asana added in this sequence is Tadasana. Their sequence will be as follows: Tadasana, Tiryaka Tadasana, Kati Chakrasana, Tiryaka Bhujangasana, Udrakarshanasana. The rest of the procedure is the same as mentioned above.

Note: In all the three variations, the only difference is the practice. Rest of the kriyas are like the first Shankha-prakshalana, and the benefits are also the same.

Laghu Shankha-prakshalana (Short colon cleansing)

Method: As mentioned in the above method, take salty lukewarm water. Since it is best to do it in the early morning hours, do it only at that time. Drink two glasses of water (half a litre). Do eight rounds of each of the asanas mentioned in the first method. If you do not feel like passing motion, drink two more glasses of water and repeat the set of asanas. If you still do not feel like passing motion, drink two more glasses and repeat the asanas. This time you will definitely feel the pressure. Go to the toilet immediately.

Comment: Since in this kriya, you do not have to drink water and do the asanas till the water comes out clear, or till the intestine is thoroughly cleansed, you don't have to be extra careful while doing Laghu Shankha-prakshalana.

Precaution: After going to the toilet, put a gap of at least one hour before eating anything. Those suffering from high or low blood pressure or any kind of abdominal disorder should do it under the guidance of an expert teacher.

Note: Those who suffer from constipation, they can do this kriya twice a week and gain its benefits.

How Do the Asanas Work in the Shankha-prakshalana Kriya: A Scientific Approach

The Shanka-prakshalana kriya is done with a lot of patience and alertness. Taking water in from the mouth and expelling it from the anus is a scientific method. When we sit in the crow posture and drink salty lukewarm salt water, it gives a kind of fomentation to the throat, food pipe and the stomach, and cleanses them. When we do the first asana, Triyaka Bhujangasana, we inhale and turn to the right and left sides, pressure is exerted on the stomach and it activates the pyloric valve. The water moves quickly from the stomach to the small intestine. When we do Triyaka Tadasana, we interlock our fingers and stretch our arms up while inhaling, and turning sideways. This exerts pressure on the small intestine from the sides and on the diaphragm from the top. Resultantly, the water in the small intestine is pushed down into the large intestine. In Katichakrasana, we keep our feet apart and turn sideways from the waist while keeping the arms parallel to the ground. Hence, when we inhale and turn sideways, pressure is exerted on the large intestine and the water and the filth are further pushed into the part of the body which holds the excreta. Since the part which holds the excreta, or the rectum is at the lower part of the food canal, pressure is exerted on it by doing Udarakarshanasana. We sit in the crow posture, inhale and keep our hands on the knees, and then we bring the left knee down near the right foot and press the right knee against the stomach. We then repeat the kriya by changing the legs. Udarakarshana exerts pressure on the rectum due to which the faecal matter and water start coming out. By doing the above mentioned asanas repeatedly, first the solid stool and then the semi-solid stool come out and finally, only water comes out of the body. This kriya has to be done till clear water comes out of the body. Sometimes, the urge to pass motion does not arise. In that case, we should do Udarakarshanasana in the toilet itself.

Kunjala: About 15 minutes after doing Shankha-prakshalana, you should drink warm water without salt and then do Kunjala kriya, followed by Jala Neti. It would be better if you do not take a bath after this. Take rest in a closed room.

Diet: About one hour after the Shankha-prakshalana kriya, you should eat khichadi made out of green moongdal and rice without salt turmeric etc. About 50 grams of ghee should be added to it to cure the dryness caused by repeatedly taking salty water and to grease the inner walls of the system.

Ayurvedic Yoga: Instead of water, if we use a decoction made by boiling black pepper, figs, gulbanafsha dondachoorna, tulsi leaves, black cardamom, ginger, jaggery, black munakka etc. together, it would be more beneficial.

Shankha-prakshalana: A Scientific Reason

If we take a look at our body and consider which part of our body affects it the most, which part gives nourishment to the entire body, and for which part does a person slog the whole day to earn money, the answer would be the same – stomach. A person does everything for the sake of their stomach and it is this stomach that controls and directs the entire body.

Now that we know that it is because of this stomach that our body becomes ill, why should we put unhealthy things into it? Or in other words, why should we eat things which would eventually harm us and hamper the organisation of the entire abdominal region? Why should we eat things which could cause thousands of diseases? They cause constipation, they cause the faecal matter to stick to the walls of the intestine and putrefy, causing harmful gases, germs, microbes etc. If we observe carefully, very few diseases are caused due to outside elements. A person makes way for thousands of diseases from within own body.

The Shankha-prakshalana kriya does not allow the filth to stick to the walls of the intestine. So, germs do not develop and harmful gases are not formed. When the intestine is clear, the appetite improves and our digestive system is able to absorb all the vitamins and proteins from our food. Therefore, our body gets proper nourishment. The body becomes well-toned and develops immunity. As a result, the germs outside the body become ineffective. We become completely healthy, our brain functions better, memory becomes sharper and eyes become clear. The face starts glowing and body develops properly. Our blood remains pure. Negativities and disorders like anger, lethargy, fatigue, laziness etc. stay away from us. The three elements of air, bile and phlegm remain balanced, hence disorders caused due to their imbalance also do not occur.

In this way, we can see that the Shankha-prakshalana kriya is absolutely scientific with clear benefits. Hence, we must do Shankha-prakshalana kriya at least once or twice in our life time and gain benefit from it.

Gurudev Yogacharya Phoolchand Yogiraj has expounded the significance of Shankha-prakshalana in his poem.

कुन्जल/गजकरणी के लिए

बंधु निशदिन शोधिये देह मलिन मलद्वार, जिनसे बहता रहे अतिघृणित अपावन सार।
घृणित अपावन सार देह में व्याधि बढ़ावे, मल संचय मान नित्य षट्कर्म करावे।
कहते 'योगीराज' स्वास्थ्य का मर्म यही है, देह शुद्ध हो जाए वात कफ पित्त सही है।

शंख-प्रक्षालन के लिए

देह ताप अनुसार ही पानी गर्म कराय, ख़ाली पेट पिलाइये सेंधा नमक मिलाय।
सेंधा नमक मिलाय पंच आसन करवाए, आसन के उपरांत पुनः शौचालय जावे।
कहते योगीराज अंत गजकरणी करिए, नेति क्रिया कराय पेट का पानी हरिए।

लाभः

वायु घटे गर्मी घटे चर्म रोग मिट जाए, जठराग्नि को तेज़ कर कफ़ को देय नशाय।
कफ़ को देय नशाय अजीरण शीघ्र पछारे, खांसी रोग विनशाय नाड़ियाँ सभी सुधारे।
कहते 'योगीराज' शक्ति कुंजर सी लहिये, कुंजर क्रिया कराय सदैव निरोगी रहिए।
तन शुद्धि आलस हटै बवासीर मिट जाए, चर्म रोग इत्यादि भी कभी न टिकने पाए।
कभी न टिकने पाय भगन्दर व्याधि नशावे, तन पुरुषत्व बढ़ाय ओज अरु आभा आवे।
कहते 'योगीराज' रक्त रस वृद्धि करीजै, उचित रीति अपनाय शंख प्रक्षालन कीजै।

Benefits of Shankha-prakshalana:

The many benefits of Shankha-prakshalana are as follows:

- It is the only process which cleanses the entire body from the mouth to the anus.
- It removes worms from the stomach and the harmful amoeba from the intestine and makes fresh digestive juices to flow in the digestive system, thereby giving it a totally new and healthy form.
- If the above mentioned procedure is followed, an obese person can lose about 3 to 4 kilos in a week and a thin person can generate new energy in his/her body.
- All the diseases related to the abdominal region are destroyed, whether they are related to air, bile, or phlegm. Hence, it is an effective remedy for tridoshas or the ailments caused due to the three bio-elements.
- It gives a new form to the body and makes it youthful. It cures skin diseases.
- The so-called incurable diabetes can be gradually and completely cured completely by doing this kriya regularly. It also puts an end to laziness and lethargy.
- After doing this kriya, one feels light and absolutely healthy. Also, one is able to maintain total mental well-being.
- Any kind of headaches can be cured completely by doing this kriya.
- The eyes become beautiful, big, attractive, and disease free by doing this kriya.
- The face becomes beautiful, and glowing by doing this kriya.
- It cures the impurities of the blood. It also cures the foul smell of the mouth.
- One can get special benefits from asana, pranayama, mudra, bandha, dhyana and awakening of kundalini after doing Shankha-prakshalana.
- This kriya is wonderful for the body. It enhances its vitality.
- It is beneficial for piles and fistula.

Precautions while doing Shankha-prakshalana:

- Till one week after doing Shankha-prakshalana, one should not drink milk or eat anything made out of milk, chilly, spices, sour things or any kind of heavy food.
- After doing Shankha-prakshalana, you must do Kunjala kriya and Jala neti so that the total cleansing of the abdominal region and the nose is undertaken.
- Do not take bath immediately after doing Shankha-prakshalana. At least on that day, do not take bath with cold water. After this kriya, take rest, but do not sleep.
- Do not do any heavy work after doing this kriya.
- Do light exercise for one week. Do not do advanced or difficult yogasanas.
- Those suffering from low blood pressure or high blood pressure should not do this kriya.
- Those suffering from very severe abdominal disorders should not do this kriya.
- Pregnant women should not do this kriya.

(C) Agnisara Dhauti (Fire purification)

नाभिग्रन्थिं मेरुपृष्ठे शतवारं च कारयेत। अग्रिसारमिद्यं धौतिर्योगिनां योगसिद्धिदा।।
उदरामयजं त्वकत्वा जठराग्रि विवर्द्धयेत्। एषा धौतिः परा गोप्या देवानामपि दुर्लभा।
केवलं धौतिमात्रेण देवदेहं भवेद्ध्रुवम्।। (Gherand Samhita 1/19-20)

Meaning: To do Agnisara Dhauti, hold the prana vayu in kumbhaka and pull your navel back to the spine. By doing this, all the diseases of the stomach are destroyed. This kriya is very confidential and difficult to accomplish even for the devas. By doing this kriya, the body becomes beautiful like that of the devas.

Method: Sit in any suitable asana in which it would be easy to perform this kriya, like Vajrasana, Padmasana, Siddhasana, etc. Keep your spine erect. Take a long deep breath and exhale from the mouth completely. Do bahyakumbhaka and contract the stomach to touch the inner part of the spine. Expand and contract your stomch in and out with great speed. Do this 10-15 times or as per your capacity. Then, slowly inhale and relax. Once again repeat this kriya. While doing this kriya, the abdominal region expand and contract. In this way all the parts of the abdomen get sufficient exercise making them work efficiently and increasing their working capacity.

Comment: Do this kriya 3-4 times on an empty stomach and under the guidance of a guru.

Precaution: Those suffering from heart diseases, high blood pressure, rigid diseases of the abdomen and asthma etc. should not do this kriya.

Benefits: All the parts of the abdominal region get a thorough massage. So, they work efficiently with increased capacity. Both the digestive power and the digestive system become strong. Abdominal disorders are destroyed, so the whole body remains healthy. The glow and vitality of the body is enhanced. The sadhaka starts looking beautiful by doing this kriya.

(D) Bahishkrita Dhauti (Blowing out)

काकीमुद्रां शोधयित्वा पूरयेदुदरं मरुत।
धारयेद्र्धयामं तु चालयेदधोवर्त्मना।
एषा धौतिः परा गोप्या न प्रकाश्या कदाचना।। (Gherand Samhita 1/21)

Method: Pout your lips like a crow's beak and draw in breath till it fills up your stomach. Hold this air for one and a half hours in your stomach. Then, move it down the intestines and out from the anus. Bahishkrita dhauti is very confidential.

Comments: This kriya is very difficult to perform. Therefore, always do it under the guidance of an expert guru.

Benefits:

- It cleanses all the nadis.
- The body remains young by doing this dhauti kriya.
- New energy is generated in the body.
- It destroys the disorders caused by the air.

Prakshalana Karma (Intestines cleansing)

नाभिमग्रजले स्थित्वा शक्तिनाड़ीं विसर्जयेत्।
कराभ्यां क्षालयेन्नाड़ीं यावन्मलविसर्जनम्।।
तावत्प्रक्षाल्य नाड़ीं च उदरे वेशयेत्पुनः।
इदं प्रक्षालनं गोप्यं देवानामपि दुर्लभम्।।
केवलं धौतिमात्रेण देवदेहो भवेद् ध्रुवम्।
यामार्ध धारणाशक्ति यावन्न धरयेन्नरः।
बहिष्कृत महद्धौतिस्तावच्चैव न जायते।। (Gherand Samhita 1/22-24)

Meaning: Stand in navel-deep water and draw out your Shakti nadi (long intestines). Wash it with your hand till all the filth is cleared. Then, draw it in again. This prakshalana kriya is very difficult and not easy to perform even for the Gods. By doing this Dhauti kriya, the body becomes God-like.

Comments: This dhauti is very difficult. It should be done under the guidance of a guru who is himself very adept in it. Do not do it simply by reading about it in the books or by following what someone else has said. One important thing to remember is that 'it is not easy to perform for Gods' means that even very great knowledgeable and wise men do not know about this kriya. 'God-like body' means that the aura, vitality, glow and strength of the body are enhanced to such an extent that one starts looking like a deva or God.

One should necessarily do above mentioned dhauti kriya only under the guidance of an expert guru, with a lot of patience and only when one has had enough practice.

2. Danta Dhauti (Teeth cleansing)

दन्तमूलं जिह्वामूलं रन्ध्रं च कर्णयुग्मयोः।
कपालरन्ध्रं पंचैते दन्तधौतिर्विधीयते ।। (Gherand Samhita 1/25)

Meaning: Danta dhauti is of five kinds:

1. Danta mool: To clean the root/base of the teeth.
2. Jihva shodhana: To clean the root/base of the tongue.
3. Karna dhauti: To clean the right ear.
4. Karna dhauti: To clean the left ear.
5. Kapalrandhra prakshalana: To clean the crown of the head.

1. Danta Moola Dhauti

Use a good quality tooth paste/tooth powder to clean the teeth. A yogi should clean his teeth everyday in order to keep himself free of diseases.

2. Jihva Shodhana Dhauti

By doing Jihva shodhana, one can win over old age and death as well as destroy many diseases. Hence, one must elongate their tongue and do Jihva shodhana.

Put your index, middle and ring finger in your mouth and gently clean the base or root of the tongue. If you do it slowly and gently, it will destroy the disorders of the phlegm. Then, apply some butter and gently pull your tongue. This will help elongate your tongue. By doing Jihva shodhana, the phlegm is destroyed; all the related nadis are purified, and the tongue always remains clean and soft.

3. Karna Dhauti

This is the third type of Danta dhauti. Clean the ear holes everyday with your index and middle finger. If you do this every day, you will be able to hear naada, the cosmic sound. The ears also get cleansed, and germs do not breed inside them; the possibilities of ear-related diseases are minimised.

4. Kapalrandhra

The crown of the head is called kapalrandhra. Pat it gently with your right hand after pouring some water on it. Phlegm disorders are destroyed by doing this kriya. All the related nadis are cleansed and purified, and the sadhaka attains divine vision. This kriya must be done in the morning, after lunch and in the evening.

3. Hrida Dhauti (Cardiac cleansing)

हृद्धौतिं त्रिविधां कुर्याद्दण्डवमनवाससा ।। (Gherand Samhita 1/35)

Meaning: There are three kinds of Hrida dhauti – Danda dhauti, Vamana dhauti and Vasana dhauti – which cleanse the heart.

Danda Dhauti (Cleansing with a stick)

Method: Take the inner stalk of a banana plant or the soft stalk of a turmeric plant, or a smooth bamboo stalk. Insert it in the easophagus and slowly and gently, push it down and then, slowly pull it out. Do this repeatedly. Danda dhauti destroys all the impurities of phlegm and bile and cures restlessness. It destroys all heart diseases.

Comments:

- The stalk of the banana plant is commonly used.
- Do it under the guidance of an expert guru.

Vamana Dhauti (Cleansing of the stomach)

भोजनान्ते पिबेद्वारि-चाकण्ठं पूरितं सुधी:
उर्ध्वां द्रष्टिं क्षणं कृत्वा तज्जलं वमयेत्पुनः ।
नित्यमभ्यास योगेन कफपित्तं निवारयेत् (Gherand Samhita 1/38-39)

Meaning: After meals, a sadhaka should drink water till his throat. Then, he should look up for some time and vomit all the water. This kriya destroys phlegm and bile.

Vamana kriya is of two kinds. The first is done on an empty stomach. It is called Kunjala or Gajkarani kriya. The second is done after meals. It is called Vyaghra kriya or Baghi kriya.

1. Kunjala Kriya/Gajkarani Kriya (Stomach cleansing)

Method: Take about two litres of lukewarm water and add two teaspoon of salt in it. Choose a place where you can vomit comfortably. Then, quickly drink at least six glasses of water, and if you can, then drink even more (Do not drink it slowly). When you will feel like vomiting, bend your head forward or make a right angle from your waist. Open your mouth, and gently rub the root of your tongue with your index and middle finger. When you do this, you will start vomiting. All the water in your stomach will quickly come out. To empty your stomach, repeat the process of rubbing the root of the tongue with your fingers. When the stomach is clear, the water that will come out will also be clear.

2. Vyaghra Kriya or Baghi Kriya (Cleansing like a tiger)

Method: In this kriya, the undigested food is thrown out of the stomach through vomiting.

About half an hour after meals, drink 5-6 glasses of prepared water or as much water as you can. Then, as mentioned in the above method, throw out the water and the undigested food by vomiting. If you feel that the stomach is not clear, drink water again and throw it out by vomiting. Then, do Jala neti kriya.

Precautions:

- Do not do the vomiting kriya forcefully. Prepare yourself mentally for the process.
- The entire stomach is emptied after this kriya. So, do not eat anything till at least 30 minutes after doing this kriya.
- Those suffering from low blood pressure, high blood pressure, heart problems, severe peptic ulcers and hernia should stay away from this kriya and consult a guru.

Benefits:

- By doing this kriya, ailments like acidity and ulcer do not occur.
- Bile is brought under control by doing this kriya. It is very effective in headaches and migraine.
- Since all the undigested and bad food is thrown out, one gets rid of foul smell of the mouth by doing this kriya.
- One gets rid of heaviness, constipation, and the feeling of vomiting due to indigestion by doing this kriya.

- It activates parts of the abdominal region. So, the disorders related to digestion are cured.
- It helps one get rid of gas.
- It is beneficial for cough and cold.
- It enhances the eyesight.

3. Vasana Dhauti/Vastra Dhauti (Cleansing with a cloth)

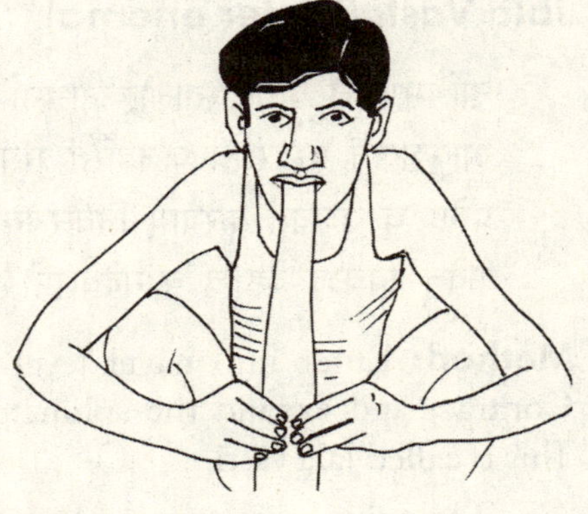

In this kriya, one has to swallow a thin soft cloth. The practice of slowly pulling the cloth out is called Vastra Dhauti.

Method: Take about 2 inches wide and 8 feet long fine cotton cloth. Swallow it slowly. When the first end of the cloth reaches the stomach, gradually pull the cloth out.

Do this kriya in silence in the morning, on an empty stomach. By doing this kriya, tumour, fever, enlarged spleen, leprosy, and disorders of bile and phlegm are destroyed. One gains physical strength, happiness and health.

4. Moola Shodhana/Ganesh Kriya (Rectum cleaning)

If the stomach is not clear, the apana vayu does not flow freely. Therefore, it is important to do Moola shodhana.

To do this kriya one must clean the rectum with soft turmeric root or with one's own fingers. Using a wet middle finger, gently clean the inside walls of the rectum. The apana vayu starts flowing freely when this kriya is done.

By doing Moola shodhana kriya, the hard stool accumulated in the anus is removed and the disorders caused due to gas are also cured. Indigestion is cured and appetite is enhanced by doing this kriya. The body starts glowing and one gets a well-toned healthy body like the Gods.

Vasti (Enema)

जल वस्तिः शुष्कवस्तिर्वस्ति च द्विविधौ स्मृतौ।
जल वस्तिं जले कुर्याच्छुष्कवस्तिं सदा क्षितौ ।। (Gherand Samhita 1/45)

Vasti karma is of two kinds: Jala vasti and Shushka vasti. Jala vasti is practised in water and Shushka vasti is done on the ground.

Jala Vasti (Water enema)

नाभिमग्रजले पायुन्यस्तालोत्कटासनः।
आकुञ्जनं प्रसारं च जलवस्तिं समाचरेत्।।
प्रमेहं च उदावर्तं क्रूरवायुं निवारयेत्।
भवेत् स्वच्छंद देहश्च कामदेवसमो भवेत्।। (Gherand Samhita 1/46-47)

Method: Enter into navel level water and sit in Utkatasana. Contract and expand the sphincter muscles of the anal region. This is called Jala vasti.

To do this kriya, take water in a huge vessel, or stand in a river or pond with water reaching up to your navel. Sit in Utkatasana and contract and expand the sphincter muscles of the anal region like horses and other animals do while excreting. Initially while doing this, only a small amount of water enters the rectum, but with practice, the quantity of water increases. The stool sticking to the inner walls of the intestine comes out along with the water. This cleans the internal organs. Since filth comes out of the body while doing this kriya, it should be done in running water.

Benefits:

- It destroys urinary disorders.
- It cures abdominal diseases.
- It cures disorders of the wind.
- The body becomes cleansed and glowing like the bodies of Gods through this kriya.
- The nadis too get purified by doing this kriya.

Shushka or Sthala Vasti (Dry enema)

वस्ति पश्चिमोत्तानतो चालयित्वा शनैरधः। अश्विनी मुद्रया पायुमाकुंचयेत्प्रसारयेत्।।
एवमभ्यासयोगेन कोष्ठदोषो न विद्यते। विवर्द्धयेज्जठराग्निमामवातं विनाशयेत।।
(Gherand Samhita 1/48-49)

Method: Contract and expand the sphincter muscles by doing Ashvini mudra. Doing Vasti kriya while sitting in Pashchimottanasana is called Sthala vasti. By doing this kriya, air, bile and phlegm are destroyed; the gastric fire is enhanced; constipation and diarrhea are cured.

Neti (Nasal cleansing)

वितस्तिमानं सूक्ष्म सूत्रं नासानाले प्रवेशयेत् ।
मुखान्निर्गमयेत्पश्चात् प्रोच्यते नेतिकर्मकम्।।
साधनान्नेति कार्यस्य खेचरी सिद्धि माप्नुयात्।
कफ़दोषा विनश्यन्ति दिव्य दृष्टिः प्रजायते।। (Gherand Samhita 50-51)

Comment: There are five types of neti: Jala neti, Sutra neti, Dugdha neti, Ghrita neti and Tela neti.

Jala Neti (Nasal cleansing with water)

Method: To perform this, take a container which has a nozzle. Fill some lukewarm water in it and add a little salt. Bend your head to the right and insert the nozzle of the container into your left nostril (Keep your mouth open so that you can breathe.). Pour the water slowly into the left nostril. The water will come out of the right nostril. If it doesn't, bend your head further towards the right. The process of water coming out is natural. Pour all the water from the container. Then, breathe out forcefully as you do in Bhastrika Pranayama. The nostril gets cleansed by doing this kriya. Do the same process with the right nostril by bending your head to the left. After doing the kriya, clean your nostrils.

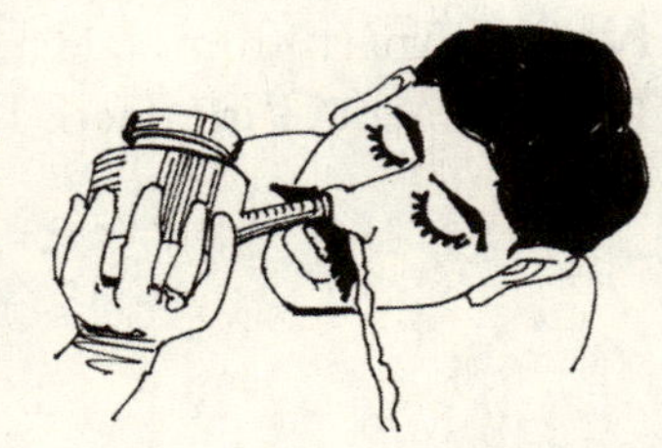

Sutra Neti (Nasal cleansing with a thread)

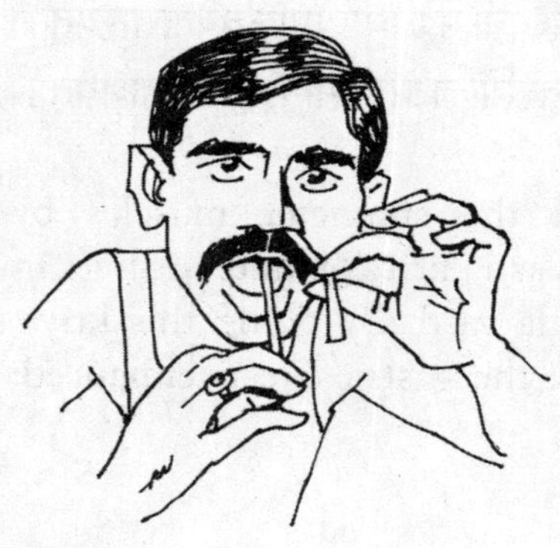

Instrument: To do this neti kriya, a one foot long cotton thread is required. Nowadays, a rubber tube called catheter is available in the medical stores, which can also be used.

Method: Apply some wax on one end of a fine thread and make it firm. Then, insert it into one nostril. It will come down to the mouth. Pull it out of the mouth using your other hand and move it to and fro 25-30 times. This should be done from both the nostrils one after the other. Be completely alert while doing this kriya.

Benefits:

- Both the neti kriyas give many benefits.
- The acharyas of *Gheranda Samhita* believe that it makes one capable of moving in the sky.
- All diseases of the phlegm are destroyed by these netis.
- Diseases of the eyes are cured and one is blessed with clairvoyance.

Note: Apart from Jala neti and Sutra neti, yogis also teach Dugdha neti, Ghrita neti, Tela neti, Dahi neti and Svamutra neti.

Lauliki Nauli (Moving the intestine)

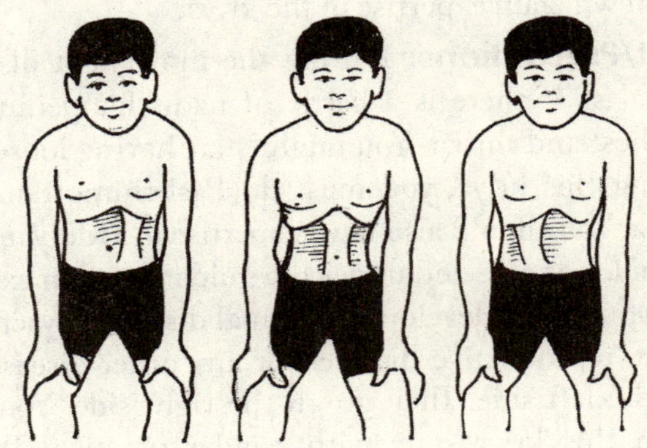

अमन्दवेगेन तुन्दं भ्रामयेदुभपार्श्वयोः ।
सर्व रोगान्निहन्तीह देहानल विवर्द्धनम ।। (Gherand Samhita 1/52)

Meaning: Move your abdomen with great speed from one side to the other. This is called Lauliki. It destroys all kinds of diseases. It increases the gastric fire and strengthens the digestive system.

Note: Please see Udara Shakti Vikasaka kriya No. 10 too.

Explanation: Do this kriya in the morning when the stomach is clear and light. Stand with a distance of one or one and a half feet between your legs. Bend forward a little and apply some pressure on your knees using your hands. Before beginning the kriya – exhale. Try to throw out all the air from the stomach and pull the stomach in so that it touches the inside of the back. Then, expand. Repeat this process so that doing nauli kriya becomes easy. Press your knees and contract the central abdominal muscles from the lower abdomen to the centre and try to expand them. This process is called Madhyama nauli.

Bend slightly to the left and increase the pressure of the left hand. The muscles of the abdomen will move to the left. This process is called Vaama nauli. When the same is done on the right, all the abdominal muscles shift to the right. This process is called Dakshina nauli.

With an even speed and a lot of willpower, do Madhyama

nauli, Vaama nauli and Dakshina nauli in sequence. With patient practice, you will gain expertise in the kriya.

Comment/Precautions: During the movement of the nauli, you will feel as if there is a battle of nadis happening in your forehead, chest and throat. You might start having loose motions. Before doing this kriya, you must do Pashchimottanasana and Mayurasana. You should also have expertise in Uddiyana bandha. Do it with a lot of care and under the guidance of an expert guru, otherwise, you might develop abdominal diseases, dysentery, pain in the waist, reproductive diseases, or any other disease. Always start with the left side. Then go on the right side. You can gain expertise in this kriya only with regular practice. Those with swelling in the stomach, disorders of bile, dysentery, chronic diarrhea, high blood pressure and heart diseases should not do this kriya.

Benefits:

- Nauli kriya is believed to be the highest of all the kriyas. *(Hatha Yoga Pradeepika)*
- It is beneficial in the disorders related to the digestive system.
- It reduces fat.
- It gives many benefits like mental peace, awakening of kundalini, improved dhyana or concentration etc.
- It cures all kinds of disorders of the wind.
- Acharyas have called this kriya a Sanjeevani booti.

Trataka (Gaze)

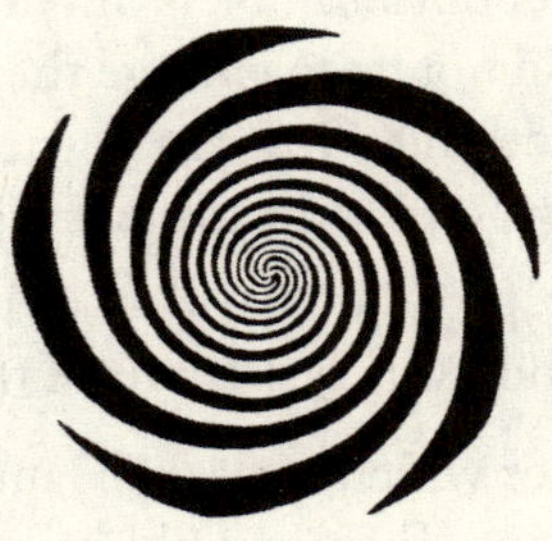

According to the author of this book, gazing continuously at a minute object or symbol for a long time without blinking is called by doing trataka. Mastery over Shambhavi mudra is obtained by doing trataka. Eye disorders are cured and one gains clairvoyance.

Trataka is considered an integral part of Hatha Yoga. Even though some practitioners do trataka without even knowing about Hatha Yoga, they get benefits from its practice. Trataka has its own significance. The other name for it is hypnotism. It is impossible to not have attractive eyes for someone who practices trataka. The fact is nowadays trataka has become a thing to be flaunted. Seminars are organised and the speakers speak about trataka for an hour and so. Neither do they explain their approach in a practical way nor is it comprehensible for a common man.

Trataka not only increases the attraction of the eyes, but also enhances the willpower of a person to such an extent that they are able to understand what is on somebody mind. By doing this kriya, the path to meditation is defined and one is able to receive a lot of spiritual energy. If one to make one's life beautiful, they must practice trataka in the right way with a lot of patience. By mastering trataka, you can not only hypnotise the person sitting in front of you, but attract a whole gathering towards yourself.

The eyes of a person who practices trataka become beautiful, large, attractive, charming, radiant and very mysterious. We have a few examples as proof in front of us: Bhagwan Rajnish (Osho), Swami Vivekananda, Swami Vishuddhananda Paramhansa (Gyanganj, Himalayas), among others are some of the few thousands who have been successful crowd-pullers by their power of attraction. The writer of this book is Surya Trataki. The objective of doing trataka should not be to enlarge the eyes. One should also aim at achieving something. One can befriend their enemies and transform deadly beasts into mild animals with the help of trataka.

There are many popular ways of doing trataka. We shall explain the main method for the benefit of the readers.

Method: Select a place which is clean, beautiful and peaceful, and has a good environment. There should be no disturbance in that place as long as you are practising.

Sit in Sukhasana at a distance of 4 feet from the object (candle) you will focus on. Light a candle and keep it at the required distance from the eyes (4 feet). The flame of the candle and the eyes should be at the same level. Keep the candle protected from three sides with a cover so that the flame doesn't move and cause distraction. Fix your gaze joyfully on the flame and do not blink. Initially, you may experience some burning sensation in the eyes. Have patience. Keep looking at the flame with full concentration and without blinking. Do not try to do this for a long time on the very first day, otherwise you will have problems on the following day. In about 5-6 months, you will start getting the benefits of this kriya. You can use a lamp or incense stick instead of a candle, but do it in a dark room.

Try to fix your gaze for as long as you can do without any discomfort, then, close your eyes and visualise the same flame. You will be able to see the flame for some time even after you close your eyes. This is called antaha trataka. Both your concentration and gaze will become stable.

There are many other ways of doing trataka, like point, circle, Sun, Moon, stars, mirror, tip of the nose, statue of your god, a shiny object, etc. Nowadays, ready-made trataka charts are also available in the market. You can use them for your practice. Some sadhakas use pranava mantra *Om* for doing trataka.

Comment: Do this kriya with a stress-free attitude. Be joyful. Observe celibacy and eat vegetarian food as far as possible. The sadhaka who does not pay any attention to the cardinal desires and takes pure vegetarian food, experiences the genesis of mystic power within himself. He gradually starts knowing the past and the future too. He is able to awaken many powers within himself, and eventually reach the pinnacle of life.

Note: If you feel a burning sensation in your eyes, do not rub them. Splash cold water or rose water on them. Those who have weak eyes should do this trataka kriya with a lot of wisdom.

This practice is not so simple and easy as it appears to be. It needs a lot of patience, self-confidence and wisdom.

To do Antarika trataka, close your eyes and try to look in between your eyebrows.

Benefits:

- One achieves clairvoyance.
- Ordinary eye disorders are cured.
- Many aspirations of life are fulfilled.
- One gets both spiritual as well as worldly happiness.
- It gives physical and mental benefits.
- It gives fame.
- It is a powerful medium to awaken the kundalini.
- The strength, aura and vitality are enhance.
- The concentration power and memory power develops.
- The spiritual power develops and one is able to work towards the betterment of this life as well as the life after.

Kapala-bhati (Frontal Brain Purification)

(To know more, please see the Kapal-bhati topic in Pranayama chapter.)

वात क्रमेण व्युत्क्रमेण शीत्क्रमेण विशेषतः।
भालभातिं त्रिधा कुर्यात्कफ़दोषं निवारयेत्।। (Gherand Samhita 1/55)

Meaning: There are three types of Kapal-bhati: Vaatkrama Kapal-bhati, Vyutkrama Kapal-bhati and Sheetkrama Kapal-bhati. By doing these, the disorders related to phlegm are destroyed.

भस्त्रावल्लौहकारस्य रेचपूरौ ससम्भ्रमौ।
कपालभातिर्विख्याता कफ़दोषविशौषणी।। (Hath Yog Pradipika 2/35)

Meaning: To do rechaka and puraka with great speed and calmness like the bellows of an ironsmith is called as Kapal-bhati by the yoga shastras. It destroys all the disorders of the phlegm.

Vatakrama Kapal-bhati (Breathing exercise)

इडया पूरयेद्वायुं रेचयेत् पिंगलां पुनः। पिंगलया पूरयित्वा पुनश्चंद्रेण रेचयेत्।।
पूरकं रेचकं कृत्वा वेगेन न तु धारयेत्। एवमभ्यास योगेन कफ़ दोषं निवारयेत्।।
(Gherand Samhita 1/56-57)

Meaning: Inhale from the left nostril (Ida nadi) and exhale from the right nostril (Pingala nadi). Then, inhale from the right nostril and exhale from the left nostril. The speed of rechaka and puraka should not be very high. This type of practice destroys the disorders of the phlegm.

Vyutkrama Kapal-bhati (Sinus cleansing kriya)

नासाभ्यां जलमाकृष्य पुनर्वक्त्रेण रेचयेत्।
पायं पायं व्युत्क्रमेण श्लेष्मा दोषं निवारयेत्।। (Gherand Samhita 1/58)

Meaning: Take in water from both the nostrils and expel it from the mouth. Then, take in water from the mouth and expel it from the nostrils. This kriya is called vyutkrama kapal-bhati. It destroys all the disorders of the phlegm.

Sheetkrama Kapal-bhati (Mucous cleansing kriya)

शीतकृत्य पीत्वा वक्त्रेण नासानालैर्विरचयेत।
एवमूभ्यास योगेन कामदेव समो भवेत्।।
न जायते वार्द्धकं च ज्वरो नैव प्रजायते।
भवेत स्वच्छंद देहश्च कफ़ दोषं निवारयेत् (Gherand Samhita 1/59-60)

Meaning: Sadhaka should drink water from the mouth with a *s....s...s...* sound and expel it from the nostrils. This is called sheetkarma kapal-bhati. By doing this kriya, the sadhaka becomes beautiful, radiant and full of vitality like the God Cupid. He does not become old; his body becomes cleansed, and all the disorders of the phlegm are destroyed.

Precautions: Those suffering from a weak heart, vomiting, acidity, lack of sleep, high fever, etc. should not do this kriya.

Benefits:

- All the Shatkarmas give a new life to the sadhaka.
- They remove wrinkles from the face and other parts of the body, making it radiant.
- Kapal-bhati removes many impurities from the body.
- Shatkarmas are very important for awakening the kundalini.
- Shatkarmas grant spirituality.
- The whole body becomes strong, firm, radiant, glowing, attractive and beautiful by doing it.

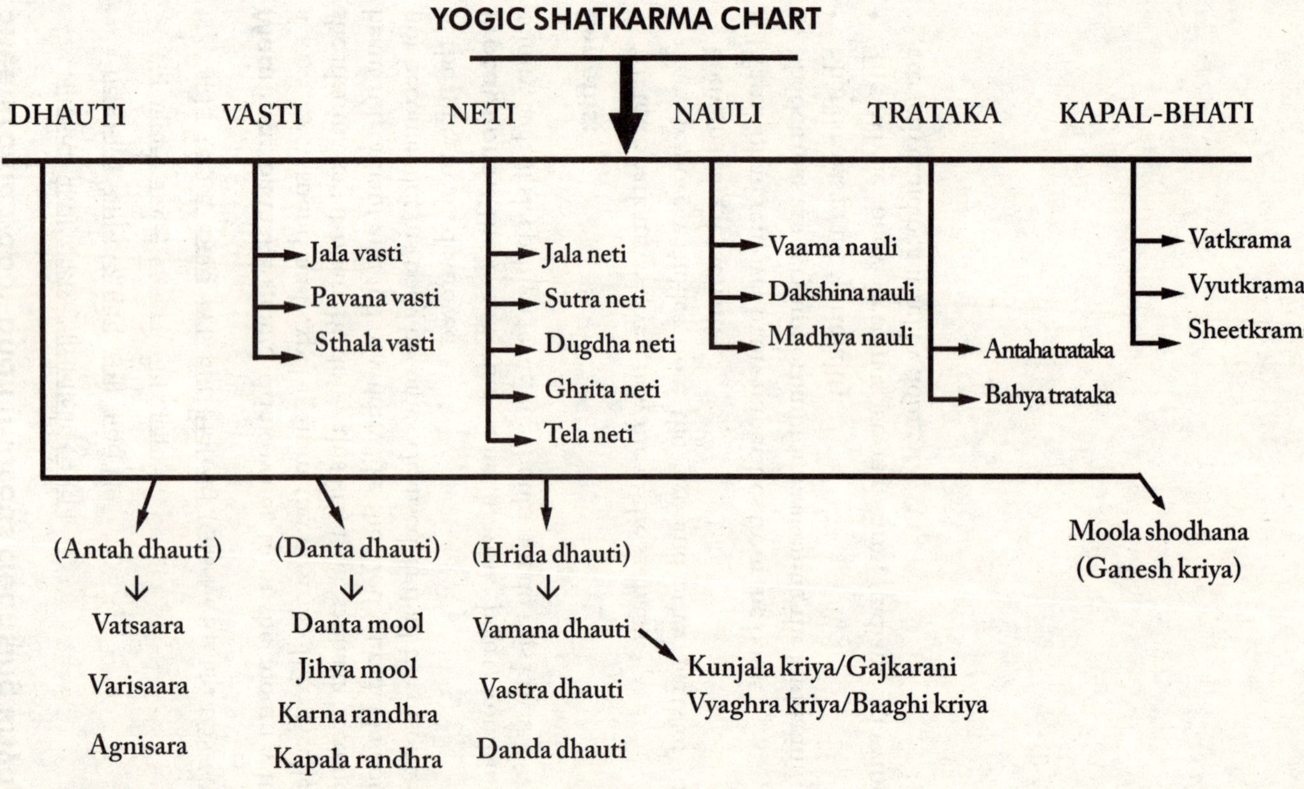
YOGIC SHATKARMA CHART
DHAUTI
VASTI
NETI
NAULI
TRATAKA
KAPAL-BHATI
Jala vasti
Pavana vasti
Sthala vasti
Jala neti
Sutra neti
Dugdha neti
Ghrita neti
Tela neti
Vaama nauli
Dakshina nauli
Madhya nauli
Antahatrataka
Bahya trataka
Vatkrama
Vyutkrama
Sheetkrama
(Antah dhauti)
Vatsaara
Varisaara
Agnisara
Bahishkrita
(Danta dhauti)
Danta mool
Jihva mool
Karna randhra
Kapala randhra
(Hrida dhauti)
Vamana dhauti
Vastra dhauti
Danda dhauti
Kunjala kriya/Gajkarani
Vyaghra kriya/Baaghi kriya
Moola shodhana
(Ganesh kriya)

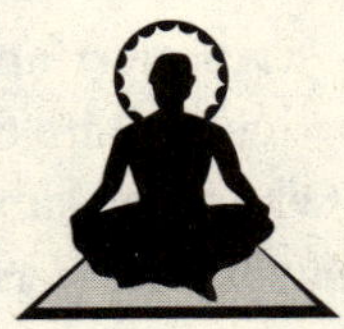

Yoga Nidra (Yogic Sleep)

A modern person's life has become disoriented owing to the changing lifestyle, atmosphere, environment and social norms. When one is disturbed and tensed, one does everything that one should not do simply to find a way out, such as taking intoxicating substances, fighting and losing temper. This is reflected everywhere – it in the family or in the neighbourhood. To avoid this situation, one must practice Yoga Nidra everyday to make the present happy and peaceful and the future ensured.

What is Yoga Nidra?

Yoga Nidra is a kriya, a kind of yogic sleep which develops our dormant willpower into a fresh and positive one immediately. In this method, one enters into the depths of one's own mind by means of autosuggestion. One activates one's subconscious mind and in a few moments, experiences freshness and new energy.

One must practice Yoga Nidra everyday in one's life. It should become a part of one's life as only 5-10 minutes of Yoga Nidra can make the entire 24 hours of the day well-organised, happy and energetic.

Yoga Nidra is an advanced method of relaxation. Often we do not feel rested or feel fatigued even after a whole night's sleep. This fatigue can be overcome only by the practice of Yoga Nidra.

In this process, a person sleeps while being awake. The body is in a state of rest, while the conscience is completely awake and alert. Yoga Nidra is to sleep with total alertness, because even in the restful state a person stays alert and awake. There are many states of the mind. This particular state of mind is the interim state between sleep and awake, where the subconscious mind is at work and the body gradually relaxes. The person gets rid of all kinds of tension, whether physical, emotional or mental. We can call this the best method to drive away depression.

There are many ways of doing Yoga Nidra. Different yoga centres teach it in distinctive ways. Here, we have only mentioned the most popular method.

Method: First ready for Yoga Nidra. Lie down on your back with ease; use a mat. Keep your body loose. Maintain some distance between your legs. Place your hands a little away from your body. Let the palms face the sky. There should not be any rigidity in the body. If you feel that any part of your body is rigid or tensed, relax it and leave your body absolutely loose from head to toe. Then, close your eyes. Do not open your eyes till you are asked to open them. Do not move any part of your body, let your body be absolutely loose and relaxed.

Take a deep breath. Take a few more deep breaths slowly. Slowly take in a deep breath; slowly let it out. Repeat once more.

Be determined mentally that you are completely ready to do Yoga Nidra, and tell yourself that you will not sleep, not sleep, not sleep. Now, carefully read the directions given here. Do not let your mind indulge in any kind of thought or imaginary ideas. Let your mind be completely free of all kinds of thoughts. You should work only at the level of hearing and being conscious. However, physically you will be unconscious. Now, let your mind move from the head to the toes.

Let your conscious mind move through the entire body. Be aware of the parts of your body and be absolutely focused.

Let your consciousness move to the various chakras and parts of the body. Mentally repeat the sequence mentioned below and accordingly concentrate on that specific part of the body.

Focus on your left hand. Take your conscious mind to your left thumb, index finger, middle finger, ring finger, little finger, left palm, wrist, elbow, arm, shoulder, armpit, the left side of the waist, thigh, left knee, left calf, ankle, heel, sole of the left foot, toes of the left foot, thumb, first finger, second finger, third finger, fourth finger, thumb of the right hand, index finger, middle finger, ring finger, little finger, palm of the right hand, wrist, elbow, arm, right shoulder, right armpit, the right side of the waist, right thigh, right knee, right calf, right ankle, toes, right thumb, first finger, second finger, third finger, fourth finger, crown of the head, forehead, right brow, left brow, centre of the brows, the eyelashes of the right eye, the right eye ball, the entire right eye, eye lashes of the left eye, left eye ball, the entire left eye, right ear, right cheek, left ear, left cheek, right side of the nose, left side of the nose, the entire nose, lower lip, upper lip, chin, the entire neck, right side of the chest, left side of the chest, the entire chest, navel, stomach and the lower abdomen.

The entire right hand, left hand, right leg, left leg, right buttock, left buttock, spine, the entire back, stomach, chest, front of the body, back of the body, the entire body. Focus on the entire body.

Experience your entire body lying on the ground in a semi-conscious state.

Focus on inhalation and exhalation. Experience the process consciously. Breathe normally.

Imagine that you are taking a stroll on a beach. The waves of the sea are splashing against your feet. You are feeling the cool water. A gentle fragrant breeze is blowing. You are feeling physically and mentally healthy. The Sun is rising in the horizon in front of you. Gradually, its gentle rays are falling on you. You are feeling energised. You are experiencing a new awareness and consciousness at the moment. The rising Sun is red in colour. Its rays are lighting up a nearby garden.

Now, you are moving towards the garden. On reaching the garden, you see numerous beautiful colourful flowers blooming. Their fragrance is reaching you. You can feel a new freshness arising inside you. You sit down in the garden. There is peace all around. Gradually and consciously come back towards your body. Become aware of your body lying loose and relaxed. Become aware of the breath coming in and going out. The breath is coming in; it is going out. Observe the breath. Now turn your entire body to the left and then to the right side. Turn left again then get up and sit up right. Chant *Om* in a long sonorous voice. Keep your eyes closed.

ॐ असतो मा सद्गमय।
तमसो मा ज्योतिर्गमय।
मृत्योर्माऽमृतंगमय।
ॐ शान्ति शान्ति शान्तिः।

Rub your palms together and place them on your eyes. Move your palms over the face and slowly open your eyes. Feel the new energy flowing in your body and start your life afresh with new enthusiasm. This way you can start a new life.

Variations: There are many more ways of doing Yoga Nidra, such as focusing on the chakras, by counting first in the ascending order and then in the descending order, among others. You can visualise the heaven, rivers, ponds, the form and formless, only the soul, the snow-clad peaks of Himalayas, religious place, holy place, etc.

Benefits:

- You become stress-free physically as well as mentally.
- You can cure the diseases of your body through Yoga Nidra. You must visualise those diseases being destroyed. The immunity of the body increases and as a result the diseases are cured by thinking this way.
- Mental powers can be enhanced. Memory power can also be improved. It can be very helpful in the mental development of children.
- A new energy is generated in the body by doing Yoga Nidra.
- You can transform the energy of all the seven chakras of your body through Yoga Nidra.

- You can make your energy flow upwards through it.
- You can progress in all the fields, whether worldly, familial, or spiritual.
- You can put an end to anger, pride, illusion, greed etc. through Yoga Nidra.
- You can become a good human being by thinking in a positive way. For example, you can think that you are honest; you are completely healthy; you are compassionate, etc. and change any situation in your life.

Precautions:

- While doing Yoga Nidra, the person should not sleep.
- He/she must listen carefully to the instructions being given.
- If someone falls asleep while doing Yoga Nidra, he/she should be woken up by gently touching his/her forehead. Touch the big toe of his/her feet to wake them up.

All the kriyas of yoga sadhana should be done
with patience, self-confidence and perseverance.
Only then can they make one experience the highest
form of spiritual bliss along with providing other
physical and mental benefits.

–RJT

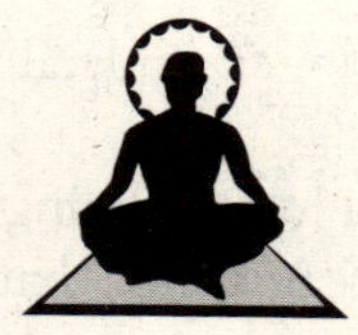

Dharana

Pancha Dharana (Five Focus)

In this section we shall mention five types of dharana. When we meditate on these dharanas, the effects of worldly passion start diminishing. The ill-effects 432of our actions can be reduced and spiritual benefits can be gained by meditating upon them. A detailed explanation on dhyana and dharana can be found in Jain literature.

Maharishi Gheranda has said that if you master the dharanas, you can automatically become capable of executing any job. The five dharanas are:

1. Parthivi dharana
2. Ambhasi dharana
3. Agneyi dharana
4. Vayaviya dharana
5. Akashi dharana

1. Parthivi Dharana (Focusing the mind on the Earth element)

यत्तत्वं हरितालदेशरचितं भौमं लकारान्वितम्।
वेदास्त्रं कमलासनेनसहितं कृत्वा हृदिस्थापितम्।।
प्राणंत्रय विलीय पंच घटिकाश्चित्तान्वितां धारयेत्।
ऐषा स्तम्भकरी सदा क्षितिजयं कुर्यादधोधारणा।।
पार्थिवीधारणामुद्रां यः करोति तु नित्यशः।
मृत्युंजयः स्वयं सोऽपि स सिद्धो विचरेभुवि।। (Gherand Samhita 3/17-18)

Meaning: The Earth element or the Prithvi tattva is yellow. Its root mantra or beeja mantra is 'Lam' (लं); its shape or form is square, and its presiding deity is Bramha. The practitioner should meditate on this tattva and hold it in his/her heart. He/she should draw the prana vayu and do kumbhaka for five ghatikas (two and half hours) while meditating on this element. This is called Parthivi dharana or the Adho-dharana. When one gains absolute mastery over this dharana, one can win over the Earth. The one who practices this Dharana continuously can conquer death, and move fearlessly on earth.

2. Ambhasi Dharana (Fixing the mind on the water element)

शंखेन्दुप्रतिमं च कुन्द् धवलं तत्वं किलालं शुभम्।
तत्पीयूषवकारबीजसहितं युक्तं सदा विष्णुना।।
प्राणं तत्र विलीय पंच घटिकाश्चित्तान्वितां धारयेत्।
एषा दुःसह ताप पापहरिणी स्यादाम्भसी धारणा।।
आम्भसीं परमां मुद्रा यो जानाति स योगवित्।।
जले च घोरे गंभीरे मरणं तस्यनो भवेत्।।
इयं तु परमा मुद्रा गोपनीया प्रयत्नतः।
प्रकाशात्सिद्धिहानिः स्यात्सत्यं वच्मि च तत्त्वतः।। (Gherand Samhita 3/19-21)

Meaning: The colour of the element water (Jala tattva) is white like that of a conch, the Moon or the jasmine (kunda). Its form is circular like the Moon and its presiding deity is Vishnu. Its beej mantra is 'Vam' (वं). With the help of yoga, meditate on the above mentioned element in your heart. Simultaneously, draw in your breath and hold it in kumbhaka for five ghatikas (two and half hours). This is Ambhasi dharana. It destroys the greatest of the sorrows and sins. The sadhaka who practices this dharana can be known as the greatest of yogis. He/she will never die in the deepest of waters because of his/her mastery over their breath.

3. Agneyi Dharana (Fixing the mind on the fire element)

यन्नाभिस्थितमिन्द्रगोपसद्रशं बीजं त्रिकोणान्वितं -
तत्वं वह्निमयं प्रदीप्त मरुणं रुदेण यत्सिद्धिदम्।
प्राणं तत्र विलीय पंचघटिकांश्चित्तान्वितं धारयत्।
एषाकालगभीर भीतिहरिणी वैश्वानरी धारणा।। (Gherand Samhita 3/22)

Meaning: The place of the fire element (Agni tattva) is the navel. Its colour is red like a ladybird. Its beeja mantra is 'Ram' (रं). Its form is triangular and its presiding deity is Rudra. It is a source of light – bright and luminous – and giver of many siddhis. Awaken this tattva in your mind and infuse it in your heart. Hold it in your heart and do kumbhaka of the prana vayu for five ghatikas (two and a half hours). This is called Agneyi dharana mudra. By regular practice of this dharana, the fear of death can be eliminated. If such a person falls into fire, he/she will come out unharmed.

4. Vayavya Dharana (Fixing the mind on the air element)

यदिभन्नांजन पुंज सन्निभमिदं धूम्रावभासं परं।
तत्त्वं सत्तवमयं यकारसहितं यत्रेश्वरो देवता।।
प्राणांस्तत्र विलीय पंच घटिकां चित्तान्वितां धारयेत्।
एषा खे गमनं करोति यामिनां स्याद्वायवी धारणा।।
इयं तु परमा मुद्रा जरामृत्यु विनाशनी।
वायुनाभ्रियते नापि खे च गतिप्रदायिनी।।
शठाय भक्ति हीनाय न देयं यस्य कस्यचित्।
दत्ते च सिद्धिहानिः स्यात्सत्यं वच्मि च चण्ड ते ।। (Gherand Samhita 3/24-26)

Meaning: The colour of the air element (Vayu tattva) is blackish, smoky grey like surma. Its beej mantra is 'Yam' (यं) and its presiding deity is Ishwar. This element is full of Sattvagun. Awaken this tattva with the power of yoga, and hold it in your heart. Hold the prana vayu in kumbhaka for five ghatikas (two and half hours). This is called Vayaviya dharana. By practicing this mudra, one can never be killed by aerial disturbances and is able to walk in the air and move in the sky. It destroys old age and death. This should not be taught to fools, wicked people or the faithless. If done, success is lost and one does not gain mastery over it.

5. Akashi Dharana (Fixing the mind on the ether element)

यत्सिन्धौ वरशुद्धवारिसदृशं व्योमाख्यमुद्भासते।
तत्वं देवसदाशिवेन सहितं बीजं हकारान्वितम्।।
प्राणांस्तत्र विलीय पंच घटिकाश्चित्तान्वितं धारयेत्।
ऐषा मोक्षकपाटभेदनकरी कुर्यान्नाभो धारणा।।
आकाशीयधारणां मुद्रां यो वेत्ति स योगवित्।
न मृत्युर्जायते तस्य प्रलये नावसीदति।। (Gherand Samhita 3/27-28)

Meaning: The colour of the sky element (Akash tattva) is blue like the water of the ocean. Its presiding deity is Sadashiva and the beeja mantra is 'Ham' (हं). Fix your mind on this tattva and hold the prana vayu in kumbhaka for five ghatikas (two and a half hours). This is called Akashi dharana. This mudra leads to nirvana and the sadhaka who masters it becomes a yogi. He/she cannot be destroyed by death and cannot perish even during pralaya.

Comment: Mentioned above are all the dharanas in their set sequence along with each of their meaning. We request the readers and sadhakas to understand them correctly. Learn them from an expert and practice them with a calm mind. Before you learn these mudras, you must inculcate all the qualities mentioned repeatedly as essential in this book. Acquire those qualities from your gurus. Immense patience and perseverance is needed to acquire these siddhis. Therefore, this is our humble request to the knowledge-seeking sadhakas that they use their wisdom to gain benefit from these dharanas.

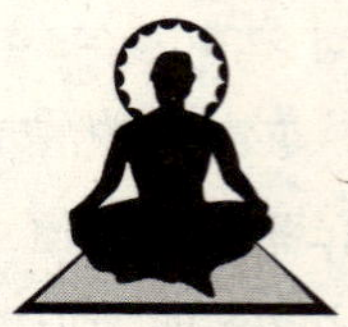

Dhyana Yoga (Meditation)

Dhyana, or meditation is a very significant practice. It is not possible to attain salvation without this sadhana. All the kriyas mentioned in the earlier chapters are related to the physical body, but dhyana is a process of the soul which takes the sadhaka to the highest knowledge, that is the Kaivalya Gyana, or the Divine Knowledge. In almost all the sacred texts of all the religions, great importance has been given to dhyana. Jainism believes that without focused meditation, one cannot expiate one's karmas. According to Hinduism, one must pray to God and do dhyana everyday. Dhyana, or meditation is as significant from religious point of view as it is from the point of view of our worldly life.

There are many ways of doing dhyana. Different ways of doing dhyana are mentioned in different texts. In *Goraksha Paddhati*, the writer states that to purify the mind as mentioned in the yoga shastra and to focus on the Supreme is called Dhyana. Depending on the saguna and nirguna type of devotion, dhyana is of two types. To think of the dark-complexioned Vishnu is saguna dhyana. To sit in a lonely place in Padmasana, Siddhasana or any posture of Sukhasana and focus on the Kundalini Chakras, or to fix one's gaze on the tip of the nose and to focus on the chakras along with the desired object is called nirguna dhyana. This is dhyana mudra, and the yogi who does this is liberated from all sins. In my opinion, there are nine places to focus on during meditation:

1. Mooladhara **2. Svadhishthana**
3. Navel (Manipuraka) **4. Anahata**
5. Vishuddhi **6. Ghantika moola**
7. Lambika sthana **8. Agya chakra**
9. Sahasrara chakra

There is ether or space above the Sahasrara. Yogis find these nine places ideal for focusing during meditation. When one focuses on these places along with the associated elements earth, water, fire, air and sky, one can attain the eight siddhis like Anima etc.

It is written in *Viveka Choodamani* that just as gold looses all its impurities on being heated and becomes pure and precious, similarly, the mind polluted by the triguna – tama, raja and sata, becomes pure by dhyana and attains self-realisation. It is further written that just as insects focus on constant movement and resultantly become restless, such as the bumble bee, similarly, the sadhaka, by focusing on the Supreme, becomes like the Supreme. Hence, the sadhaka can achieve God-like soul or divinity through meditation.

According to Yoga Sutra:

To keep the mind or the chitta stable in one place or object is dharana, and to continuously stay in this situation is dhyana. This means to focus on the desired object at length without distraction, or in a continuous flow (like pouring honey). The ultimate state of dhyana is samadhi. When dhyana is so deep that all you are aware of is the object in focus, such a state is called samadhi. When dharana, dhyana and samadhi are present simultaneously at the same place and time, such a state is called sanyama or sangama.

According to *Gheranda Samhita*:

स्थूलं ज्योतिस्थासूक्ष्मं ध्यानस्य त्रिविधं विदुः।
स्थूलं मूर्तिमयं प्रोक्तं ज्योतिस्तेजोमयं तथा।
सूक्ष्मं, विन्दुमयं ब्रह्म कुण्डली परदेवता।। (Gherand Samhita 6/1)

According to Maharishi Gheranda, dhyana is of the three kinds: Sthoola dhyana, Jyoti dhyana and Sookshma dhyana. In Sthoola dhyana, the manifested form of the desired God (saguna) is focused on. In Jyoti dhyana the self-illuminated soul (nirguna) is focused on. In Sookshma dhyana the focus is on the Bindu (Bramha kundalini).

Sthoola Dhyana (Intense meditation)

Acharyas believe that the sadhaka should visualise that he is an ocean of nectar and in the middle of this ocean is an island made of priceless jewel. The island is surrounded with sand made of precious elements. There are Neem trees laden with flowers on all the sides. This island is full of beautiful flowers such as malati, jasmine, saffron, champa, bakayan, land lotus, etc. and the air is fragrant with their intoxicating smell.

In the middle of the island is a divine wish granting tree (Kalpa Vriksha). The yogi should imagine that this Kalpa Vriksha is very beautiful and attractive. Its four branches are like the Vedas and it is eternally laden with fresh fruits and flowers. The lovely melodious sound of the cuckoo and the bumble bee is clearly heard. The sages are giving religious sermons and their voices are echoing in the air. Under the tree there is a mandapa made of diamonds and under the mandapa, a lovely throne made of diamonds and other precious stones is placed. On this throne sits his God, his focus of devotion and concentration. The sadhaka should think and pray to Him in the manner taught by his guru. How does the God look? He is adorned with jewels and ornaments. This kind of dhyana is called Sthoola dhyana by the learned.

Types of Sthoola dhyana: There is a thousand-petalled lotus called the Sahasrara on which yogis meditate. In the middle of the lotus, there is another lotus with twelve petals – is radiant and white in colour. On the twelve petals, twelve beeja mantras are written: Ha, Sa, Ksha, Ma, La, Va, Ra, Yu, Ha, Sa, Kha and Fren. In the middle of this lotus, there are three lines with the letters A, Ka, and Tha in the form of a triangle and the letters Ha, La, and Ksha are combined. Right in the middle is the pranava mantra 'Om'.

The yogi should imagine that there is a beautiful throne on which a pair of swans is seated. This pair represents the charana paduka (slippers) of the guru. Visualise a guru with two hands, three eyes, wearing pure white clothes and a garland of white flowers. His body is anointed with pale yellow paste, giving out a lovely fragrance. On his left is Shakti in red clothes. In this way, if one focuses on the guru, he can attain Sthoola dhyana.

Jyotirmaya Dhyana (Resplendent meditation)

Maharishi Gheranda asks the reader to listen to explanation of Tejodhyana after hearing about Sthoola dhyana. Mastering Tejodhyana makes the pure inner soul manifest itself.

The Kundalini Shakti is present in between the rectum and the genital, lying dormant like a sleeping snake. In it, the Supreme God is present in the form of a lamp's burning flame. Focusing on this illuminated God is called Jyotirmaya dhyana.

In between the brows and in the upper part of the heart, there exists a flame which is the manifestation of Omkara and is infused with cosmic illumination. This is the Tejomaya or the Jyotirmaya, and to meditate upon it is Tejomaya dhyana or Jyotirmaya dhyana.

Sookshma Dhyana (Micro meditation)

Maharishi Gheranda says after listening about Tejodhyana, listen to the details of Sookshma dhyana.

The sadhakas who have awakened their kundalini is indeed very fortunate. They reach a state where they can join their souls and leave their bodies through the portal of their eyes and enjoy walking on the royal road (astral walking). However, they are not visible to anyone because of their subtleness and great changeability. Then they practice Shambhavi mudra to focus on their kundalini shakti and attain stability. This is called Sookshma dhyana. This is very difficult to attain even for the devas and is very confidential.

Jyotirmaya dhyana is hundred times more fruitful than Sthoola dhyana; and Sookshma dhyana is a hundred thousand times more fruitful than Jyotirmaya dhyana, and it is also very difficult to attain.

Maharishi Gheranda says, 'I have told you about this precious dhyana by which one can have a direct perception of the self. Hence, it is the best form of dhyana.'

Significance of dhyana and its impact on the mind: The main significance of dhyana is to attain or reach God or the Supreme. By doing dhyana, not only the actions or the karmas are destroyed, but one is also able to attain God – the most difficult thing in life. It gives us extreme bliss. In this state, there is only knowledge, and having reached there, the yogi can sit in Samadhi for a long time and experience and see the Supreme about whom it is impossible to express anything in words. By dhyana, the unsteadiness of the mind is destroyed; the chitta becomes stable and unite with the unconscious mind. By doing dhyana, the sadhaka experiences profound peace and many difficult tasks become easy to perform. The disorders of the mind like cardinal desires, anger, greed, attachment, violence, falsehood, stealing, immodesty, hoarding, etc. are destroyed and one's development reaches its peak. Dhyana leads to the upliftment of the soul.

By focusing on the hundred thousand white, yellow and
red colours, which are present in our body from
head to toe and are luminous like the sun, all the
diseases are destroyed and our lifespan is improved.

– Bindu Yoga

Kundalini Science

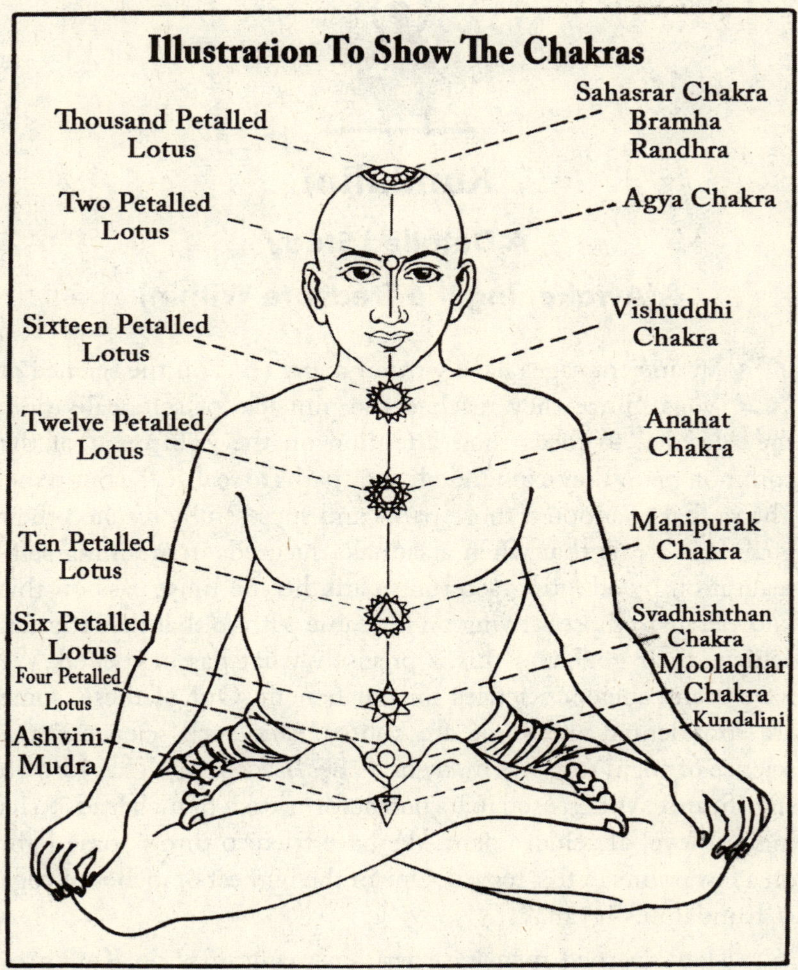

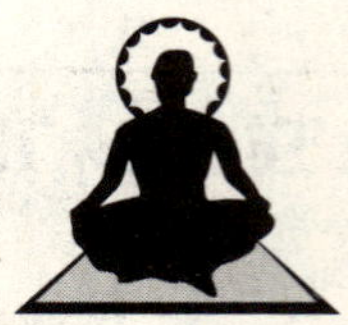

Kundalini

A Detailed Study

(Awakening the Treasure Within)

Our ancient sages have written many texts on the science of yoga. Since they reached the pinnacle of self-realisation, they decided to focus their attention on the upliftment of the common man. They expounded many paths to realise the Supreme. The sadhakas adopted those paths and successfully reached their goal. It is a rule that when a sadhaka succeeds in attaining self-realisation by adopting a certain path, he/she must pass on this knowledge to those striving on the same path so that they too can achieve their goal, and this is precisely what has happened. We have many ancient sciences for our benefit. Out of these, some are confidential and some are known. One such science is the science of yoga. Yoga has many branches. Each branch has its own significance. When used in its purest form, each branch leads to its highest level of achievement. We have tried to throw some light on a few points in this regard. One of the highest branches of yoga is 'Kundalini Vigyana'.

Many learned men have written many texts on Kundalini Vigyana and made it so simple that people from all walks of life could easily understand and put it into practice under the guidance of a guru, while enjoying its sweet benefits.

Many methods of awakening the kundalini have been developed from time to time, whether it is awakening the power by driving a wooden nail into the head or by the use of herbs.

However, the utmost development in this regard has been done by yoga. In yoga Vigyana, a persistent sadhaka, reaches his/her goal without fail. Here, we shall mention only seven chakras which are subtly present in the body. But first, let us know what's written in various text about kundalini.

According to *Shiva Samhita*:

The Shaktichalana kriya used to awaken the dormant kundalini shakti by prana vayu is the most powerful kriya. The yogi who does Shaktichalana kriya everyday to acquire siddhis, his kundalini power automatically awakens and starts flowing upwards. One attains various siddhi by persistent practice.

It is further written in *Shiva Samhita* that by the forceful strokes of the prana vayu, all the presiding deities of the various chakras awaken and the kundalini moves up and unites with Shiva who resides in Kailasha.

The power of the Moon which flows in the left nadi is in the form of Shakti and the power of Sun which flows in the right nadi is in the form of Shiva. The sadhaka who practices Shaktichalini mudra everyday gain a long life and disease-free life.

It is written in *Shandilya Upanishada* that the Kundalini Devi resides below the navel. It has eight characteristics and eight kundals. It rectifies the Prana vayu and brings it back to its original form. It balances the food and water in the body, illuminates the fire of the face and the Brahmarandhra.

According to *Yoga Kundalinyopanishada*:

While practising Moola bandha, let the downward flowing Apana vayu be forcefully pushed upward. By doing this, it gets enkindled and moves upward along with the fire.

It is further written in the same Upanishada that wise people should give direction to their Kundalini Shakti. When the energy wave rises from the Mooladhara and reaches the place in between the brows (Agya) and one is able to hear the cosmic sounds, then one must understand that one has successfully awakened their kundalini.

According to *Gheranda Samhita*:

The wind can be mastered by practising the Moola bandha. In other words, through Moola bandha one is able to control the air in their body. Observe silence while doing it.

Aitareya Aranyaka

Prana is the protector of all the senses. It can never be destroyed. It comes and goes through different nadis. Every moment it enters and exists our body through the mouth and the nose. In its spiritual form, prana is present in the body in the form of air, however, it is the Sun God in the form of our own deity.

Tantrasara

The Kundalini Shakti moves around riding on swans (self) in (the field of the) soul.

According to *Dhyanbindu Upanishada*:

With its mouth, the Kundalini Shakti covers the gate of the road through one can reach the Bramhasthana, lying sleep in the body. It can only be awakened by the combined efforts of fire, mind and well-directed prana vayu. Just as a thread follows the needle, the kundalini follows the prana vayu along the path of Sushumna and moves up. Just as a locked door is opened with a key, the yogi can open the door to salvation with the Kundalini Shakti.

There are many other texts which have expounded the kundalini in detail and many wise and learned men who have said a lot on this topic.

Pandit Gopinath Kaviraj explains that 'Bindu' is another name for Kundalini Shakti. It is called Chidakasha. It is the Mahamaya Shakti of the Supreme. There are two kinds of power of the Parameshwara or Parama Shiva: Chidroopa and Achidroopa.

Similarly, various religions have perceived it in different ways.

Now, we shall explain the seven chakras briefly. They are:

1. **Mooladhara chakra**
2. **Svadhishthana chakra**
3. **Manipuraka chakra**
4. **Anahata chakra**
5. **Vishuddhi chakra**
6. **Agya chakra**
7. **Sahasrara chakra**

1. Mooladhara Chakra (The root chakra)

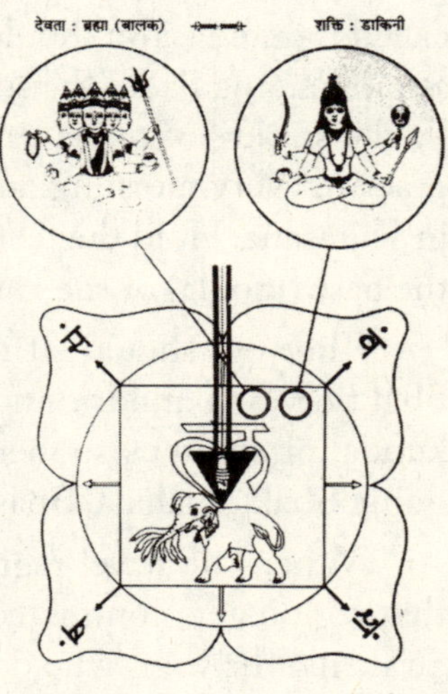

This chakra is two finger spans above the anus and two finger spans below the genitals. In other words, this chakra extends up to four finger spans and is situated in the perineum. In many texts, this place is called the kanda, where the snake power, the kundalini, sits with its body coiled in three and a half wraps. It is written in *Shatchakra Niroopana* that there is a Bhoo-ling inside the triangle of the Mooladhara on which the super subtle Kundalini Shakti, bright like the full moon, lies asleep covering the gate of the Bhoo-ling is like the stalk of lotus.

In the golden Mooladhara, there is a red lotus with four petals. Its main presiding diety is the four armed Bramha and goddess is Dakini. On each of its petals the mantraksharas 'Vam' (वं), 'Sham' (शं), 'Shham' (षं), and 'Sam' (सं) are written respectively. At the centre of this lotus is the Earth element, square in shape, golden yellow in colour and has the shining Asthashoola in it. The beeja mantra of this square is 'Lam' (लं) which is mounted on the Airavat elephant. In the middle of this lotus is a soft, beautiful and bright triangle called Kamroopa. This triangle points downwards. The goddess residing inside this triangle is Tripura Sundari and the triangle itself is called Shakti peetha or the seat of power. There is Svayambhoo Linga inside this triangle which is dark like smoke; the snake power kundalini is coiled around it.

According to *Hatha Yoga*, just as a person opens the door with the help of a key, a yogi, with regular practice of *Hatha Yoga*, opens the path to Sushumna and attains salvation. The Paramatma or the Supreme, is situated at the uppermost end of the Sushumna. The kundalini covers the opening path of the Sushumna and lies asleep. This kundalini is a bondage for the ignorant and the path to salvation for the yogis.

The Sushumna nadi in between the Ida and Pingala nadis is called Balranda. You should use it with the help of Hatha Yoga and attain Parama Pada. The sutrakara says that the kundalini awakens by the strokes of prana vayu's control. To master this, one should practice every morning and evening for one and a half hours. Sit in Vajrasana. Hold the feet above the heels and press them against the base (moola) or the anus.

The yogi should sit in a stable posture in Vajrasana and do Shaktichalana mudra and Bhastra Kumbhaka Pranayama. The kundalini awakens sooner by this method. It is a rule that after doing Shaktichalana, Bhastra should be done only in Vajrasana.

When the navel region is contracted, the Sun or the fire of that region gets contracted too. Resultantly, the Kundalini Shakti awakens. The yogis who do this kriya have no fear of death.

The sadhakas who observe celibacy and eat sparingly can attain siddhi in the first instant or very quickly. The yogi who moves the kundalini and does the Bhastra Kumbhaka in the special way, does not even fear the Yama. He can give up his body at his will.

The middle nadi called the Sushumna becomes easier to open for the sadhaka with the practice of asanas, pranayama and mudras or in other words, it can be easily mastered.

In this way, the sadhaka should regularly practice the above mentioned method patiently under the guidance of a guru to awaken the kundalini. The sadhaka achieves success and siddhi along with attaining knowledge. He becomes famous and is revered by all.

If one focuses on the Mooladhara in an ordinary way, one can get many benefits like enhancing the glow, aura and vitality of the body, curing of blood disorders, sexual disorders, skin disorders, eye disorders, urinary disorders, etc. When the chakras are not well-developed, many diseases emerge in the body. Therefore, the sadhaka should focus on the chakras.

2. Svadhishthana Chakra (The sacral chakra)

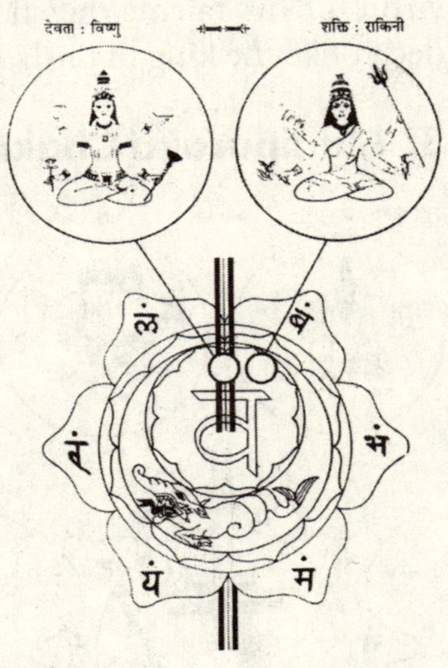

This second chakra is situated about two fingers above the Mooladhara and a little below the navel. The lotus of this chakra is orange coloured and has six petals. The mantras written on these petals are 'Bam' (वं), 'Bham' (भं), 'Mam' (मं), 'Yam' (यं), 'Ram' (रं), and 'Lam' (लं). At the centre of this lotus is a half moon which is white in colour. Inside this moon is the Varun Beej 'Vam' (वं), mounted on an alligator. Its element is the blue water. On the Bindu (anusvara) of the beeja mantra is Lord Vishnu seated on Garuda, holding the conch, disc, mace and lotus in his four hands respectively. His clothes are yellow. The goddess of this chakra is Devi Shakini who is dark-complexioned. Blood continues to flow from one of her pierced nostrils. This chakra is related to the reproductive organs, emotions, both the legs and the will to expand one's family. If this chakra is disturbed, all the above mentioned parts will be affected.

It is written in Gorakha method that if one focuses on the tip of their nose and meditate on the sagun or nirgun form of Svadhihthana chakra, one can reach a state of bliss.

There are many other benefits of meditating on this chakra: The body becomes disease free. One becomes fearless. The mind becomes calm. Jealousy, attachment and hatred are destroyed. The body starts glowing and our speech becomes powerful and polished. The reproductive organs become well-developed and function efficiently.

Conclusively, one must meditate on the Swadhishthana chakra. It is written in *Saundarya Lahri* that a person who worships the kundalini spreads the light of his/her success everywhere. His/her personality becomes pure and clean like the snow clad Himalayas and he/she becomes generous and prosperous. By the virtue of his talents, he/she succeeds in defeating the snake of deceit like the king of birds, Garuda.

3. Manipuraka Chakra (The solar plexus chakra)

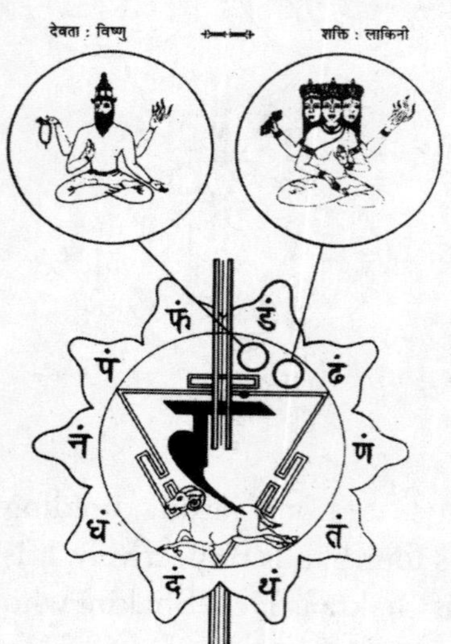

The Manipuraka chakra is situated at the root of the navel. Its element is fire and it has a lotus with ten petals. The golden-coloured petals have the mantras 'Dam' (डं), 'Dham' (ढं), 'Nnam' (णं), 'Tam' (तं), 'Tham' (यं), 'Dam' (दं), 'Dham' (धं), 'Nam' (नं), 'Pam' (पं), and 'Pham' (फं) written on them respectively. At the centre of the lotus is a red-coloured inverted triangle with the beeja mantra 'Ram' (रं). Its vehicle is the sheep. Its presiding deity is Rudra and the goddess is Devi Lakini.

This chakra is bright and radiant like a jewel. It is the centre of fire. It is the life centre of the spiritual and materialistic body. It is illuminated by awareness as well as power and is the residing place of Rudra Granthi. It is the centre of the Sun (heat). It protects a person's life.

The life of people between the ages 14-21 is affected by the Manipuraka chakra. The person impacted by the Manipuraka chakra is always ready to gain name, fame and popularity.

Since this is the centre of Sun, it manages the efficient working of the parts of the abdomen. In case of any imbalance in this chakra, the digestive system gets affected. The person suffers from disorders of blood, heart and mind. The body becomes lazy, lethargic and full of disappointment. Hence, one can get rid of the above mentioned diseases by meditating on the Manipuraka chakra. One can also gain many other benefits. One stays away from diabetes; the digestive system, diaphragm, large intestine, small intestine and the entire abdominal region receives its benefits. Spiritually, one acquires good qualities such as non-violence, truth, celibacy, forgiveness, etc. and one progresses continuously in life.

4. Anahata Chakra (Heart chakra)

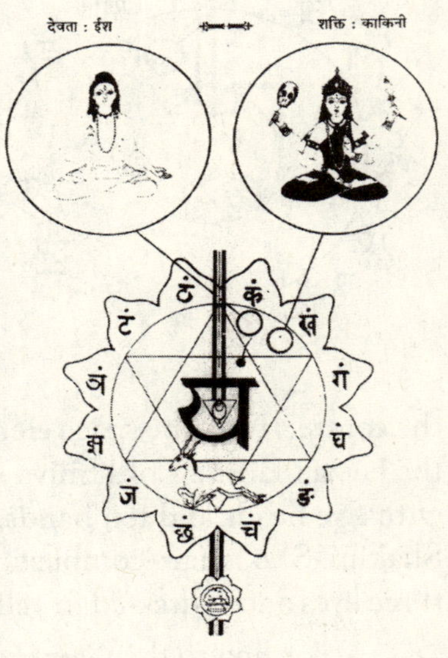

This chakra is also called the Hridaya chakra. It is situated near the heart. It has a shining lotus with twelve petals. On each of the petals, the mantras 'Kam' (कं), 'Kham' (खं), 'Gam' (गं), 'Gham' (घं), 'Na' (ङं.), 'Cham' (चं), 'Chham' (छं), 'Jam' (जं), 'Jham' (झं), 'Na' (ञा), 'Tam' (टं), 'Ttham' (ठं) are written respectively. At the centre of the lotus, there is a hexagonal form (two triangles placed one upon the other in the opposite directions). Its atmosphere is smoky and its beeja mantra is 'Yam' (यं) which denotes the air element. It is mounted on a black stag. On the bindu of the beej vayu, the presiding deity Three-Eyed Isha is seated like a swan. Both her hands are raised in Abhaya mudra. The goddess is Devi Kakini who is golden hued and has four arms. In the middle of these triangles is the Bana Ling with a half moon and a dot on it. Under it, the soul is situated like the flame of a lamp.

This chakra is related to the chest, heart, blood vessels and respiratory system. If there's is an imbalance in the chakra, diseases of the heart, respiratory problems (asthma) and mental disorders can occur. When this chakra is awakened, one can get rid of the related diseases. Pity, compassion, forgiveness, wisdom and happiness comprise the spiritual benefits of this chakra.

5. Vishuddhi Chakra (The throat chakra)

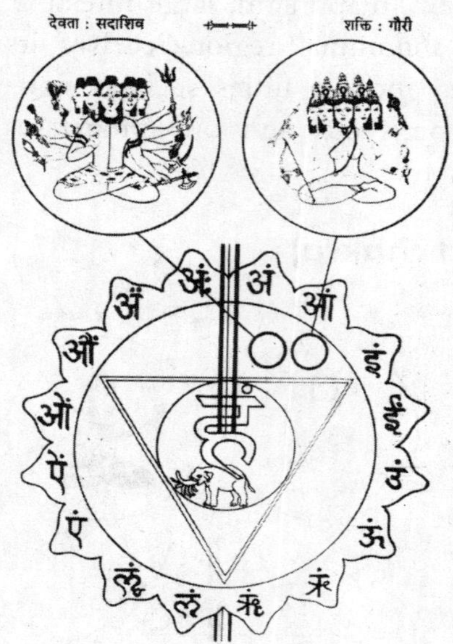

This chakra is situated in the throat region. It is a lotus with sixteen petals. It is smoky purple in colour and has sixteen mantras on its petals: 'Am' (अं), 'Aam' (आं), 'Im' (इं), 'Iim' (ईं), 'Um' (उं), 'Uum' (ऊं), 'Rim'(ऋं), 'Rrim'(ऋं), 'Lrim'(लृं), 'Lrrim' (लॄं), 'Em' (एं), 'Aim' (ऐं), 'Om' (ओं), 'Aum' (औं), 'An' (अं), 'Ah' (अः) respectively, which are bright red in colour. Inside, there is a triangle within a white circle. Inside the triangle is a full Moon with a white bejewelled elephant at the centre. It has the space element, beej mantra 'Ham' (हं) on it. In the beeja mantra, Lord Shiva sits in his Ardha Nareeshwara form with five heads and ten hands. The goddess of this chakra is Devi Shakini. She is fair-complexioned and has four arms, five heads, three eyes and is dressed in yellow clothes.

According to the *Gorakha Samhita*, if a yogi meditates on the saguna, nirguna or the flame (illuminated) form of the soul in this bright and radiant Vishuddhi chakra, situated in the throat, by focusing on the tip of the nose, he can become immortal.

By meditating on the Vishuddhi chakra, the sadhaka can stay for days at a time without feeling hungry or thirsty. One becomes reflective, thoughtful and a philosophical. One's speech becomes clear. One can savour the nectar which drips in the throat, become radiant and gain many spiritual benefits.

But when there is an imbalance in this chakra, many throat disorders occur. One's memory power becomes weak and many mental disorders also emerge.

6. Agya Chakra (The third eye chakra)

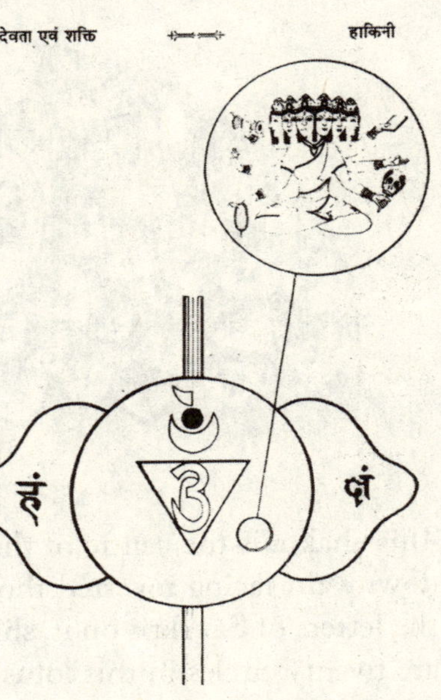

This chakra is situated in between the two brows and is called the two-petalled lotus. It is also called the third eye. The colour of the petals is bright white. The two mantras 'Ham' (हं) and 'Ksham' (क्षं) shine on these two petals. In the state of meditation, the sadhaka can have supernatural experiences. Inside this lotus is the fair Shiva illuminated in the form of a linga. The beeja mantra 'Om' (ॐ) is also illuminated here. The Bramha nadi becomes visible in this light. The triangle is situated in this lotus as a symbol of absolute power. The presiding deity is Lord Shiva and the goddess is Devi Hakini who is fair-complexioned. Her six faces are red in colour, with each face having three eyes. She has six arms and is seated on a white lotus.

This chakra is of great significance to sadhakas because it has great utility in many states of meditation. By awakening this chakra, the sadhaka becomes powerful enough to have clairvoyance, divine knowledge, power to understand the thoughts of other people, see the future, past and transmit thoughts. This Agya chakra is considered as the gateway to the upliftment of the atma.

This chakra is also called the sangama or confluence, because the Ganga (Ida), Yamuna (Pingala) and Saraswati (Sushumna) flow separately from the Mooladhara and unite in the Agya chakra. If this chakra is disturbed, there is always a danger of being prone to mental disorders. Therefore, the sadhaka should carefully meditate on this chakra under the guidance of a guru and make his life worthwhile.

7. Sahasrara Chakra (Crown chakra)

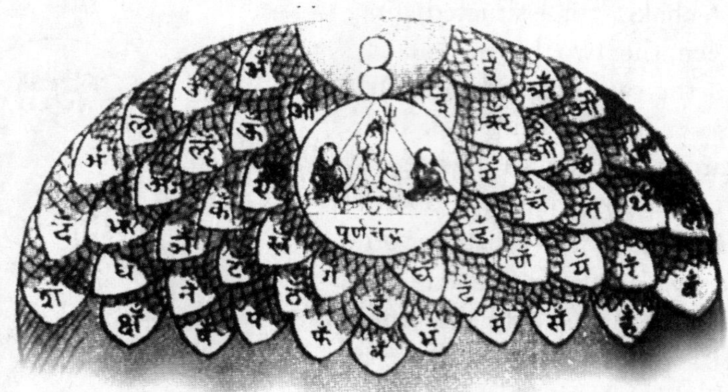

This chakra is the centre of the highest form of awareness. It is a downward facing inverted thousand-petalled lotus which has all the letters of Sanskrit on it, shining brilliantly like the Sun. There are twenty circles in this lotus and each circle has fifty petals. At the top of the crown is the visarga 'Ah' (हं). This is the centre point of all the power. At the centre of this lotus is the Shiva Linga which is luminous and a symbol of spiritual energy. He sits with his Mahashakti. The element of this chakra is Tatvateeta. Its beeja mantra is Visarga 'Ah' (हं) and the Tatvabeeja gati is Bindu. The yantra of this chakra is white full Moon.

By mastering this divine Sahasrara, one can attain the state of Asampragyata Samadhi. At this this state, the negative tendencies of the mind of the sadhaka disappear. There is only absoluteness in this state. Therefore, the sadhaka automatically enters into the state of Samadhi. It is here that the sadhaka experiences that divine state from where endless knowledge, endless happiness, and limitless power begins.

When there is an imbalance in this chakra, a person loses his/her sense of their physical and mental condition. Therefore, the sadhaka should carefully understand the chakras and meditate on them with patience under the guidance of a guru and move ahead on his chosen path.

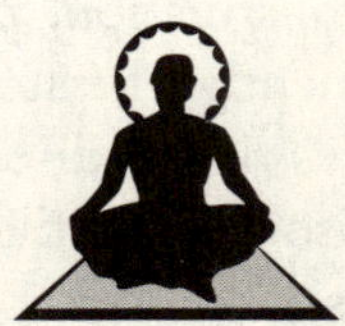

Nabhi Vigyana Parikshana

The navel is the centre point of our body. It plays an important role in poviding good health to the human body.

According to the Ayurvedacharyas, if the navel is displaced from its centre, it can lead to many diseases. When the navel is displaced, all the parts related to the Manipuraka chakra suffer from various ailments. Therefore, in order to keep the entire body healthy, it is important to keep the navel in its place.

The Main Reasons for Navel Displacement

Many people suffer from navel displacement, or do not even realise that their navel chakra is displaced. They continue to suffer and worry about the diseases which arise from navel displacement throughout their life. There are many reasons for navel displacement such as lifting very heavy objects, losing balance while walking, jumping, running, getting up suddenly from sleep, lifting too much weight with one hand, holding in the pressure of motion and urine, rubbing the abdomen without correct knowledge, some chronic disease of the abdomen, tolerating hunger and thirst for a long time, irregularity in the time of sleeping and waking up, mental disorders like fear, too much worry, anger, etc., intaking impure food or food that causes harmful gas, too much food, blocking sneeze or yawn, blocking the apana vayu, not doing the yoga kriyas in the correct manner, among other things.

Diseases Caused Due to Navel Displacement

Due to navel displacement many symptoms and diseases emerge. A person suffers from constipation, passes very less stool, or passes less stool very frequently; the stool gets stuck to the walls of the intestine which gives rise to disorders of the wind; several disorders arise, such as disorders of the eye, hair fall, premature graying of hair, weight loss, reproductive disorders, foul smell of the mouth, disorders of blood and heart, etc.

Yogasanas to Cure Navel Displacement

The following asanas are useful and beneficial in curing navel displacement: Supta Vajrasana, Pashchimottanasana, Ushtrasana, Chakrasana, Dhanurasana, Naukasana, Halasana and Uttanpadasana.

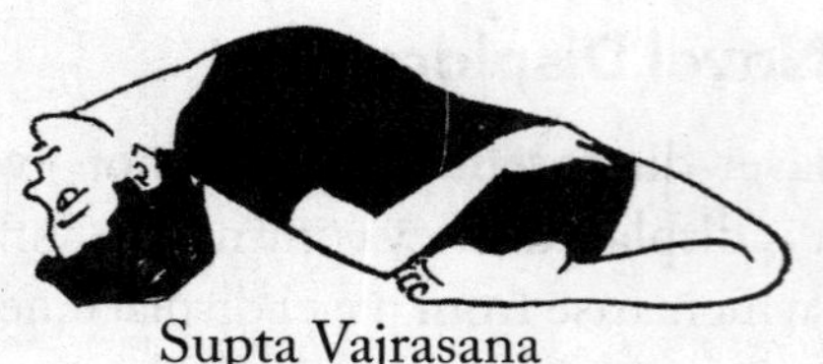

Supta Vajrasana

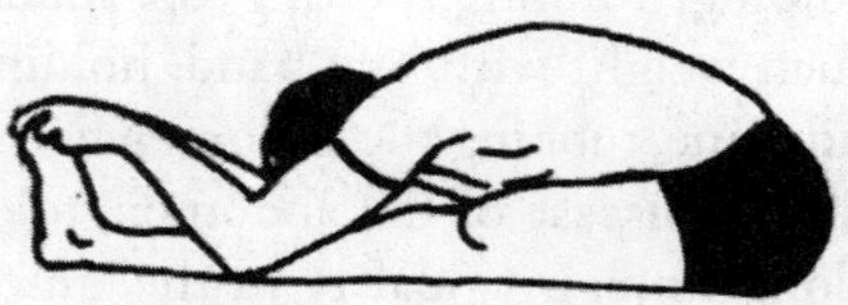

Pashchimottanasana

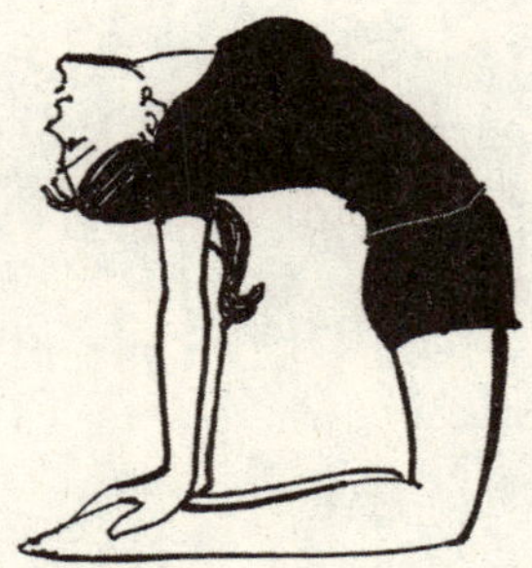

Ushtrasana

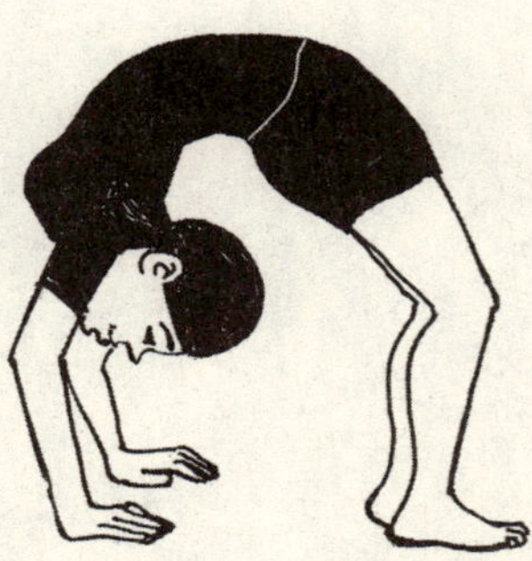

Chakrasana

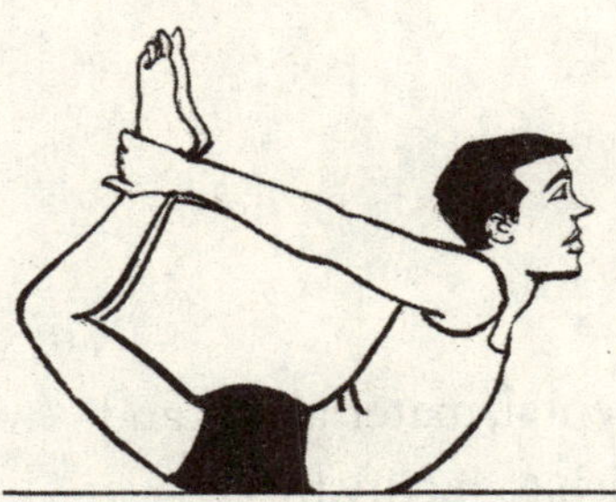

Dhanurasana

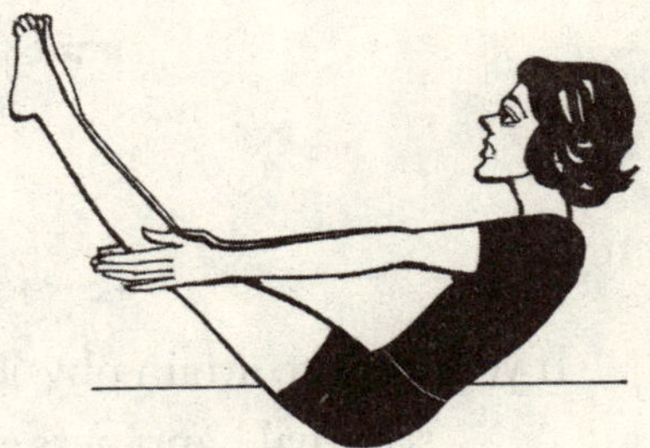

Naukasana

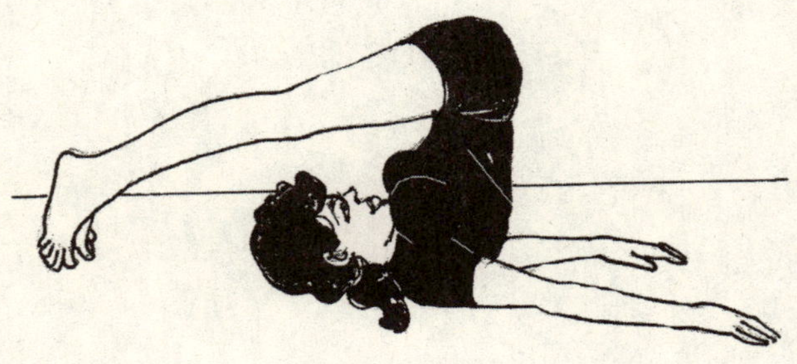

Halasana

If you want to experience heavenly pleasures,
you must do unconditional dhyana.

–RJT

If you want to attain physical, mental, materialistic and
spiritual happiness and wish to rectify this
life as well as the next, you must study
Ashtanga Yoga in depth.

–RJT

According to Ayurveda: Many kinds of herbal treatments are used in Ayurveda to cure navel displacement.

1. Take 10 grams of fennel seeds and 10 grams of jaggery; chew them well (till you become healthy again) every morning on an empty stomach. The navel will come back to its original position.
2. Tying Vitex Negundi leaf (Nirgundi) on the stomach proves beneficial for the navel.
3. Apply some castor oil on the ripe leaves of Calotropis (Aak) and heat it over the flame, give hot fomentation with this on the stomach and then, tie it on the stomach. This helps in bringing the displaced navel back to its place and reduces the inflammation and swelling in the internal parts of the abdomen.
4. For severe dysentery, filling up the navel with the milk of a banyan tree is very beneficial.
5. Cut a tomato into half and remove its seeds. Fill the hollows with 9 ratti dry roasted borax powder (suhaga)and heat it over direct flame. Sucking this tomato slowly helps in bringing the displaced navel back to its position.
6. Make a decoction from the flesh of Beach Almond fruit (baheda) and drink it once every hour. This cures the displaced navel as well as severe dysentery.

The significance of the navel has been explained in Vedas and Puranas and our other ancient texts. Nowadays, due to the lack of complete knowledge, we do not get the right treatment and suffer from various diseases. Hence, we must focus on this aspect also in order to gain more benefit. This topic is very vast. Due to the lack of space, we shall stop at this juncture.

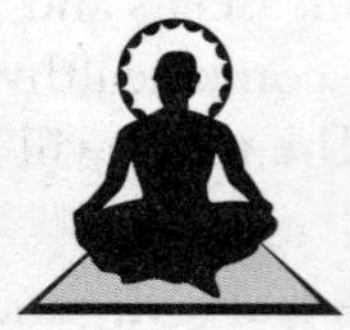

Ideal Diet: A View

There is a very old saying: 'As you eat so shall you be, and as the kind of water you drink, so shall be your voice.' We eat our food for the sake of our body. So, have we set any parameters for it? Or have we considered questions such as: What kind of food will be beneficial for us and to what extent? How much should we eat? What kind of food is ideal for us? When should we eat? What should be the quality of food?

Whether we consider view of the shastras, or listen to modern doctors, we will find one thing in common: Both are of the opinion that pure vegetarian food is the best for us. Vegetarian food provides us with many kinds of proteins, vitamins, minerals and salts. Food plays a significant role in our life. It also leaves a great impact on our mentality, and this is the reason that wise men have stressed on sattvik food.

It is written in *Hatha Yoga*:

सुस्निग्धमधुराहारश्चतुर्थांशविवर्जितः ।
भुज्यते शिवसंप्रीत्यै मिताहारः स उच्यते ।। (Hath Yog Pradipika 1/58)

Meaning: The sadhaka should eat sparingly. His food should be completely smooth and sweet. He should fill half of his stomach with food, one fourth with water and leave the other one fourth for prana vayu.

Food to be Avoided/Unsuitable Food

The writer says that sadhakas should not eat the following types of food: Bitter, sour (tamarind, etc.), tangy (chilly, spices etc.), food with too much salt, too warm like jiggery, some typical green leaves, sesame, alcohol, fish etc. and non-vegetarian food, yoghurt, butter milk, asafoetida, garlic, onion, turnip, black gram, intoxicating drinks etc.

It is further mentioned in *Hatha Yoga* that one should not eat food which is reheated over fire (pulses, rice, etc.) and dry food without ghee. One should avoid food which has too much salt. We should not talk too much while eating. It is written in *Skanda Purana* that one should give up bitter and sour food, and always drink a lot of milk. It is further written that non-vegetarian, tangy and pungent food like chilly should be avoided, or not eaten at all. Stale food and food with a foul smell should not be eaten.

Sadhakas should give up excessive indulgence in intimacy, bad people, eating too much fruits, observing too much fast, lifting heavy load, doing Surya Namaskara too many times, etc. In other words, it is mentioned in this sutra that too much of anything should be avoided. For example, if you do not observe celibacy or do too much fast, your body will become weak and you will not be able do the required sadhana. Therefore you must use your wisdom.

Suitable Diet (Food worth taking)

Acharya Maharaj says that in order to keep their bodies healthy and the mind happy, sadhakas should take complete vegetarian food which is beneficial for them. Wheat, cereal, milk, ghee, mishree, butter, dry ginger, parval, etc., five kinds of leafy vegetables, green moong and pure water (clean filtered water) – all these are beneficial for the body. It is further clarified that to make the body healthy, we should take milk with sugar and ghee (cow's milk is best), nutritious laddoos and pancakes, and all those ideal vegetarian food items which will benefit the body and are as per the norms of the shastras.

The sadhaka should keep all the above mentioned facts in

mind and prepare his/her diet schedule. He/she should take pure and fresh food everyday. He/she should have dinner in the evening or during dusk so that the food is properly digested. If you go to sleep immediately after having your meal, the food remains in your stomach all night and makes you feel lazy. There may be chances of having constipation and the muscles of the abdomen would be unable to absorb the vitamins and proteins from the food. As a result, possible diseases would emerge in the body. Therefore, if you want to make your body beautiful, well-built, strong, disease free and full of vitality, you must take care of your diet.

The Benefits of a Suitable Diet

Such items which, when eaten, generate energy and build up the fibres while repairing the damaged ones, assist in the various functions of the body. This is nothing else than food.

The amount of food a person consumes when he/she feels hungry is called appetite. Every person has a different appetite. Appetite depends on age, season, body built, and social milieu.

Balanced Diet

Our food should be rich in vitamins, carbohydrates, fats, proteins, and mineral salts. In order to maintain the balance of the body, we need food which has 75 percentage of salty and 25 percentage of acidic elements. We should not take the same type of food in excess, rather take food which has various qualities and many nourishing elements.

Based on the Trigun theory, there are three types of food:

1. Sattvika **2. Rajasi** **3. Tamasika**

1. Sattvika food: Such food items which give life, health and happiness, and are acquired from nature in a simple manner enhance our lifespan and intellect. These foods pacify our mind and make our intellect sharper and our conduct balanced. Such foods nourish the annamaya, pranmaya, manomaya and vigyanmaya kosha equally and keep them all balanced.

Pulses, rice, cow's milk, ghee, sweet fruits etc. as well as milk products, plant-based products and ghee are categorised under sattvika food.

All those foods which enhance our lifespan, intelligence, strength, health, happiness and compassion, and which are smooth, juicy and stable are called sattvika food.

2. Rajasi food: Food which are pungent, acidic, salty, very hot, and prepared using in various inflammatory spices, oil and ghee to make them taste better are called rajasi food. Garam masalas, tea, coffee, tobacco, black pepper, etc. come under the category of rajasi food. Such food speed up the processes of the body and as a result, the prana starts flowing with great speed, which is not right for our body. It becomes the cause of imbalance in the panchkosha. According to *Gita*, food which are bitter, sour and too salty give rise to sorrow and pain. Rich diets such as halwa, puries or deep fried food also come under the category of rajasi food.

3. Tamasika food: Food which is stale, outdated (beyond the date of expiry) or which is fermented is called tamasika food. Meat, fish, eggs, stale food, or food taken in excess quantity, and alcohol come under the category of tamasika food as they give rise to tamasika behaviour. Polluted, canned and packaged food also come under the category of tamasika food. According to *Gita*, food which has been cooked long time back, dry food, food with foul smell and impure food are all tamasika; onion and garlic are also tamasika food.

Impact of Different Kinds of Food On the Mind

It is said that what a person eats decide his thoughts and actions. The type and quality of food has its impact on the body as well as on the mind of the person.

1. Sattvika food: When we take sattvika food, the thought and actions related to sattvaguna are generated in our day-to-day life. It results in positive sattvika qualities like truth, knowledge, sharp intellect, peace, stability and profundity of mind, purity of the heart, simplicity of the heart, bliss, happiness etc. One develops self-control and tolerance. The body becomes healthy and free of disorders. The mind too becomes pure.

2. Rajasi food: Rajasi food result in unstable mind, jealousy, hatred and quarrel, harshness in speech, stress, tension and sorrow. This kind of food give rise to anger, provocation or excitement, and cardinal desires. The mind always remains unstable; body seems to become heavy; mind becomes unfocussed and the nervous system is always tensed.

3. Tamasika food: Tamasika food results in laziness, ignorance, attachment, pride, anger and heaviness. It results in harshness, cruelty and violence in the behaviour. One becomes selfish, quarrelsome and intolerant by nature. One's behaviour becomes very harsh and inhuman, resulting in problems and sufferings.

Impacts and Ill-effects of Unsuitable Food

When we eat unnatural or unsuitable food many thoughts accumulate in our mind. We become prone to many diseases. Body's strength starts depleting. Most of the diseases of the modern age are a result of incorrect food habits. Diabetes, high blood pressure, and various diseases of the intestine and liver are a result of wrong food habits.

Ill-effects of Non-vegetarian Food

- Most of the animals drink dirty and toxic/impure water. As a result, many kinds of chemical elements enter their body and make their flesh toxic, poisonous and infected. When the animals are killed, adrenal and other hormones related to fear, anger, depression, etc. are released which become a part of their flesh, and reach our body when we eat that infected flesh and generate negativity in us.
- The teeth structure of carnivorous animals is designed to tear and chew flesh. Their teeth are sharp and pointed and nails are huge and hard, whereas, the teeth structure of herbivorous animals is designed to chew and pound the food.
- Non-vegetarianism is against the nature of man.
- Humans are designed as vegetarian machines. The intestine is six times longer in ratio to the body, whereas

the intestine of a carnivorous animal is in exact proportion to their body.

- More acidic elements are discharged from the intestines of carnivorous animals, helping them easily digest the meat they consume. Conversely, the intestines of human beings discharge less acidic elements which is unable to fully digest the non-vegetarian food.
- The jaws of carnivorous animals move up and down while chewing, while the jaws of herbivorous animals move freely in all directions. Keeping all these things in mind, we can say that vegetarian food is the most ideal food for humans.
- Non-vegetarian food lead to mental tension and physical imbalance, whereas vegetarian food give mental peace and physical balance.
- When we eat meat, many parasites like Ascaris, Taenia Solium, etc. enter our body and give rise to many diseases. The meat of some animals, when eaten, lead to diseases like fits and mad cow disease.

According to World Health Organization, about 160 types of diseases are caused by non-vegetarian food. Non-vegetarians have greater chances of developing diseases like indigestion, constipation, acidity, hernia, problems of the pancreas, piles etc.

According to scientific study, vegetarians are 50 percent less prone to breast cancer, cancer of the large intestine, cancer of the prostate, etc. as compared to non-vegetarians, because vegetarian food has elements which protect the body from cancer and increase immunity.

Baldness, ulcers, diabetes, fits, high blood pressure, etc. are found less in those who take vegetarian food.

WHAT TO EAT AND WHAT NOT TO EAT IN WHICH ILLNESS

Illness	What to eat, drink and do	What not to eat, drink and do
Diabetes	**Grains:** Roti made of multi grain atta (wheat, barley, gram), rotis made of flour with wheat husk, sprouted grains and easily digestible food Vegetables, salad, sour fruits, lemon, fenugreek, bitter gourd, palak, snake gourd, turnip, gourd, tinda, parval, French beans, chaulai, radish, radish leaves and tomato **Fruits:** Jamun, amla, orange, cucumber, sweet lemon **Dry fruits:** Coconut, peanuts, walnuts, cashewnuts, etc. **Spices:** Ginger, dry ginger, turmeric, garlic, coriander, cinnamon, ajmod, etc. **Others:** One should take soyabean, curd, buttermilk, fenugreek seeds and always keep one's stomach clear by avoiding constipation	Rice, meat, fish, egg, milk powder, singhada, ghee, butter, sugar, jaggery, honey, glucose, jam, sweets, jelly, toffee, chocolate, ice cream, mango, banana, cold drinks, tea, coffee, rabdi, sesame, potato chips, arbi, beet root, black gram, puries, parathas, samosa, kachori, alcohol, ice, cold water, food items made using wheat flour, spices, heavy food, stay away from fear, worry, and disturbance
High blood pressure	**Grains:** Kabuli chana and other grams, sprouted grains, roti made from a mix of wheat and gram (chew well and while eating) **Vegetables:** Parwal, arbi, potato, tinda, snake gourd, mint, gourd, palak, pumpkin, cabbage, chaulai, boiled green vegetables, garlic, grapes, apple, orange, pears; do apan vayu mudra and yoga nidra	Spices, deep-fried stuff, salty stuff, stale food, meat, fish, eggs, tea, coffee, alcohol, tobacco, full-cream milk, butter, pickles, chutney, tangy food should be totally given up. Do not intake too much salt and give up heavy and intoxicating food items.

Illness	What to eat, drink and do	What not to eat, drink and do
Low blood pressure	Light, easily digestible, nourishing food, food items made from soya bean **Fats:** Milk, raisins, almonds, munakka, cashew nuts, pistachio, chhuhara, ghee, oil, etc. **Fruits:** Grapes, sweet fruits and their juice, carrots, apple juice **Vegetables:** All vegetables, salad, raita Soak 32 raisins in water overnight and eat them in the morning everyday. Tea, coffee	Heavy greasy food, food which is not nutritious, deep-fried stuff, cold drinks, alcohol, tobacco. In case of low blood pressure, if the left nostril is functional, immediately start breathing from your right nostril and sleep on your left-hand side.
Heart diseases	**Grains:** Rotis made from atta, porridge, soya bean and soya bean chunks, green moong daal, sprouted grains, black chana **Vegetables:** gourd raita, palak, garlic, carrots, radish, bathua, tomato, bitter gourd, ginger, coriander, chaulai, arbi, gourd, snake gourd, tinda, parval, mint, etc. **Fruits:** Pine apple, pomegranate, grapes, jamun, amla, apple, leechi, guava, lemon, sweet lime, orange, papaya, banana, coconut water **Fats:** Sunflower oil, soya bean oil, mustard filter oil, fresh sweet curd, cow's milk, jaggery, almonds, pistachio, buttermilk, food items rich in calcium, sodium and vitamin B-1	Rich food, spicy food, pickles, papad, chutney, ghee, butter, vanaspati ghee, coconut oil, cream, mava, rabdi, kheer, ice cream, cake, chocolate, biscuit, cheese, mutton, fish, eggs, alcohol, strong tea, coffee, tobacco, cold drinks

Illness	What to eat, drink and do	What not to eat, drink and do
Constipation	**Grains:** Sprouted grains, wheat sprout juice, mixed atta rotis, porridge, rotis made of atta with fibre (chew well while eating) **Dal:** Green moong dal, tuwar dal, mixed dal **Green vegetables:** Fenugreek, palak, cucumber **Fruits:** Banana, apple, guava, papaya, pomegranate, carrot, mango, water melon, musk melon, lemon, and coconut water. Try to keep some cloves or jaggery in mouth and suck slowly like a toffee. Take fruit juice in large quantity, trifala powder or fenugreek seeds before going to bed.	Pure wheat atta rotis; stale, cold, rich spicy food; sweets, spices, masoor dal, chana dal, urad dal, arbi, ladies' finger, brinjal, onion, radish, meat, fish, eggs. Do not eat to the full capacity of the stomach and do not take too much tea or coffee
Jaundice	Light, easily digestible and fresh food **Grains:** Rice, porridge, khichadi, millets, barley, rotis made of atta with fibre, sabudana kheer or semolina kheer **Dal:** Moong masoor, tuwar **Vegetables:** Radish, gourd, bitter gourd, cucumber, onion, mint, cauliflower, palak, coriander, fenugreek, parval, carrot, garlic, cabbage, tomato **Fruits:** Papaya, watermelon, amla, sapota/cheeku, dates, grapes, pomegranate, sweet lime, apple, orange, musk melon **Drinks:** Skimmed milk, cane juice, boiled water, lemon juice and coconut water. Drink as much water as possible	Rich food, spices, salt, sour stuff, pickles, food made from maida, oil, ghee, meat, fish, eggs, besan, milk, sweets, heeng, arbi, urad dal, sugar, jaggery, tea, coffee, tobacco, alcohol, packaged and canned food

Illness	What to eat, drink and do	What not to eat, drink and do
Diarrhea	ORS, curd, rice, khichadi, water of cooked rice, water of cooked moong dal, arrowroot, makhana, sabudana kheer, buttermilk, lauki raita, lassi, banana, lemon, sweet lime, orange, pomegranate juice, cane juice, papaya, apple	Stale, deep-fried, rich, spicy stuff, eatables made of wheat, milk, alcohol, tea, coffee, potato, brinjal, arbi, cauliflower, pickles
Malaria	Eat sattvik and easily digestible food. After the fever has subsided, take sabudana kheer, water of cooked rice, grapes, rice, semolina kheer, light milk, unripe banana, parwal, curry made of banana flowers. Drink water in which lemon and sugar has been added In the season of malaria, if you grind four leaves of tulsi and four black pepper corns together and consume them in the form of small balls, you will not catch malaria	Rich spicy food, meat, fish, eggs, alcohol, and all such stuff which are cool in nature
Typhoid (internal fever)	In the initial stages of fever, take barley, sabudana, arrowroot, water of curdled milk and biscuits. Add 8-10 cloves to one litre of water and boil it. Sieve it and let cool. Drink this water. Take tea and coffee in less quantity. ½ or 1 gram of cinnamon powder taken with sugar syrup twice a day can keep typhoid away.	Heavy spicy food, food that cause gas, open, contaminated food and contaminated water

Illness	What to eat, drink and do	What not to eat, drink and do
Night fall	Eat only easily digestible food. Take safed moosali with milk in the night. Eat dry fruits, banana, jamun, and naturally sweet food items.	Do not let constipation occur. Do not eat food items that cause excitement or intoxication, avoid wrong mentality, do not stay awake till late in the night. Give up oil, spices, chillies and non-vegetarian food.
Stone in the kidney and other diseases of the kidney	Eat rotis made of atta from which the fibre has been removed. Eat barley chapattis, sattu, sahijan beans, fresh fruit juice, bitter gourd, fresh green peas, turnip, beet root, old pumpkin, ginger, mango, apple, musk melon, water melon, papaya, grapes, cucumber, coconut water, pears, carrots, etc. it is beneficial to chew cardamom and sugar cane. Drink water many times in small quantity.	Supari, all types of gutkha, rich foods which take long time to digest like chutney, savouries, papad, pickles, tea, coffee, alcohol, beer, soda, cold drink, meat, fish, palak, brinjal, tomato, radish, zameenkand, onion, ladies' finger, beetroot, rice, raisins, munakka, dry fruits, milk and milk products, curd, paneer, butter, chocolate, food stuff with high sodium, bread, cake, pastry, etc.
Migraine	Eat light and easily digestible food. Mix curd, rice and mishri and eat it every morning and evening with meals. Put two drops of fresh ghee made from cow's milk for relief. Put 7 to 8 drops of mustard oil in the nostril on the side which hurts to get relief. Before sunrise, eat jalebis made in pure ghee with milk, or eat rabdi, lemon juice, drink neembu shikanji (with sugar) after meals. In the morning and evening, before meals, take one cup grape juice. Take heeng, dry ginger, mustard oil, tulsi, etc. and observe celibacy.	Do not eat non-vegetarian food. Give up food that take a long time to digest. Do not hold in your urine or sneeze. Do not sleep or stay awake, for long hours. Do not eat too much of food which is sour, chilly, etc. Do not drink tea or coffee frequently. Give up tuwar dal, garam masala and all such stuff which cause heat. Sweets, savouries, maida, oil, rice, curd, eggs, milk, butter milk, ghee, mango powder, tamarind, stale food, alcohol, cold drinks, ice, ice cream, urad dal, almonds, coconut, yeast, cold water, heavy and rich food, radish, banana, tobacco. Stay away from dust and smoke. Do not eat anything which causes phlegm. Rich food, deep-fried and spicy food, alcohol, tobacco, gutkha, tea, coffee, cold drinks, salt, meat, fish, eggs, etc.

Illness	What to eat, drink and do	What not to eat, drink and do
Asthma	**Grains:** Simple easy to digest food, rotis made with atta with fibre, porridge, cake, biscuits, moong dal **Vegetables:** Boiled vegetables, palak, parval, fenugreek, turnip, bitter gourd, onion, coriander, mint tinda, chaulai, sahijan beans, ginger, garlic, potato **Fruits:** Papaya, musk melon, cheeku, anar, mulberry, carrot, banana, water melon, jiggery, grapes, raisin, dates **Others:** Turmeric, rock salt, green cardamom, chana, cloves, coffee; grind together suhaga flower and mulethi and take it with warm water	Sweets, savouries, maida, oil, rice, curd, eggs, milk, buttermilk, ghee, dried mango powder, tamarind, stale food, alcohol, cold drinks, ice, ice cream, urad daal, almonds, coconut, yeast, cold water, heavy and spicy food, radish, banana, tobacco. Stay away from dust and smoke. Do not eat anything that causes phlegm
Anemia	Wheat, chana, moth, sprouted moon with lemon juice for breakfast, take peanuts with jaggery in the morning and evening, take milk and dates. **Vegetables:** Palak, mustard, bathua, fenugreek, turnip, beet root, green coriander, mint, tomato, papaya, grapes, pomegranate, banana, guava, apple, cheeku, lemon, grains, dals, munakka, raisin, dried goose berries, carrots, dates, radish leaves, orange, amla, etc.	Heavy, spicy deep-fried food, alcohol, tobacco, gutkha, tea, coffee, cold drinks, salt, non-vegetarian food

Irregular Menstrual Cycle – What to Eat, Drink and Do?

There are two main problems related to irregularity in menstrual cycle:

1. Very scanty bleeding or blockage of some kind.
2. Too much bleeding

For problems related to menstrual cycle, the following things can be taken:

Coconut

Helps remove blockages and lets the flow become normal

Peas

Removes the blockages of periods

Tulsi

Grind dried (in shade) tulsi roots to make a fine powder. Wrap it in a beetle leaf and chew it. This will help stop the excess flow or bleeding. Take a balanced diet. Include lemon, sweet lime, hot tea, coffee, carrots, mustard, fennel, etc. in your diet

To reduce the flow

Grind pomegranate peel to make a fine powder. Sieve the powder and take one teaspoon with chilled water. It will help stop the excessive flow

Taking a little heeng is also helpful

What not to eat, drink, or do

Oil, rich and very spicy food, pickles, sweets, polished rice, meat, etc.

To get rid of obesity

Take two glasses of water everyday to which half a lemon has been squeezed (Keep the water overnight in a copper vessel and use it in the morning.). Porridge, bottle gourd, snake gourd, beans, palak, horse gram, and salad should be eaten in more quantity. Take tomato soup, bottle gourd soup and buttermilk everyday. Always eat simple, balanced and easily digestible food. Go for a walk every morning. Do light exercise, yogabhyas and pranayama regularly. Take precaution for disease such as thyroid which result in obesity. Give up laziness. Do as much work as possible depending on your capacity.

What not to eat, what not to do

Do not eat food deep fried or cooked in ghee and oil, rich food, sweets, rice, potato, banana, eggs, meat, fish, alcohol, beer, tea, cold drinks, etc. Totally give up resting in the day, going to bed immediately after dinner, getting up late in the morning, laziness, etc.

Note: The above mentioned facts regarding what to eat and what not to eat in which illness are generalised instructions. You should use your wisdom and follow the instructions as per your body condition and consult a nutrition and diet expert. For more information and help, you can contact the author as well.

Mudras gradually lead a person towards the upliftment of the soul as well as towards purity.

–RJT

Thousands of diseases are caused due to the imbalance of air, bile and phlegm. Please keep these below mentioned facts in mind in your day-to-day routine.

Imbalance of	What to eat, drink and do	What not to eat, drink or do
Air	Cow's milk, ghee made from cow's milk, mishri, ginger, parwal, bottle gourd, bathua, chaulai, grapes, papaya, roti made from wheat flour, urad, mustard, matured rice, hot food, sweet, sour and salty eatables, fenugreek seeds, cardamom, harad	Bitter food, tangy food, stale food, packaged and canned food, cold drinks, chana dal, deep-fried stuff, chana leaves, masoor dal, peas, cauliflower, tea, coffee, alcohol, non-vegetarian food, intoxicating items, etc.
Bile	Sweet, cold food items, sattu, moong, masoor, cow's milk, ghee made from cow's milk, sweet lassi, parwal, tinda, cucumber, green coriander, mint, lemon, sweet lemon water, water melon, apple, pomegranate, amla, baheda, gulkand, petha	Urad dal and stuff made from urad dal, sour and sweet food which generate heat, meat, alcohol, coffee, hot environment. Do not do very laborious work.
Phlegm	Atta made from matured wheat, moong, chana, masoor, barley rotis, goat's milk, carrots, apple, water melon, dry fruits, saunth, amla, black pepper, turmeric, cloves, basil, lukewarm water	Sour, sweet, salty and heavy food, stale food, fresh wheat, fresh rice, ghee, butter, buffalo's milk, sugar cane, potato, brinjal, banana, guava, meat, fish, eggs, alcohol etc.

Note: Apart from all these things, remember one thing – avoid eating out as much as possible.

What to eat in which month?

An old saying	Month	What to eat/do
चैत चना, बैशाखे बेल,	1. March-April	Gram (Chick peas)
जेठे शयन, आषाढ़े खेल,	2. April-May	Bel (Aegle marmelos)
सावन हर्रे, भादों तिल।	3. May-June	Sleep
कुवार मास गुड़ सेवै नित,	4. June-July	Play
कार्तिक मूली अगहन तेल,	5. July-August	Harad (Myrobalan)
पूस करे दूध से मेल।	6. Aug-Sept	Sesame
माघ मास घी-खिचड़ खाय,	7. Sept-Oct	Jaggery
फागुन उठ नित प्रात नहाय।	8. Oct-Nov	Radish
	9. Nov-Dec	Oil
	10. Dec-Jan	Milk
	11. Jan-Feb	Ghee-khichadi (Ghee-Jumble)
	12. Feb-Mar	Early morning bath

What not to eat in which month?

An old saying	Month	What to eat/do
चैते गुड़ बैशाखे तेल,	1. March-April	Jaggery
जेठ के पंथ, अषाढ़े बेल।	2. April-May	Oil
सावन साग, न भादों मही,	3. May-June	Going out
क्वार करेला, कातिक दही।	4. June-July	Bel (Aegle marmelos)
अगहन जीरा, पूसै धना,	5. July-Aug	Green veggies, Sattu
माघै मिसरी, फागुन चना।	6. Aug-Sept	Buttermilk
जो कोई इतने परिहरै,	7. Sept-Oct	Bitter gourd
ता घर बैद पैर नहिं धरै।	8. Oct-Nov	Curd
	9. Nov-Dec	Jeera (Cumin)
	10. Dec-Jan	Coriander
	11. Jan-Feb	Mishri (Sugar dandy)
	12. Feb-March	Chana (Chick peas)

The above mentioned explanation has been done on the basis of old sayings, hence, apply them as per the region, time and physical condition.

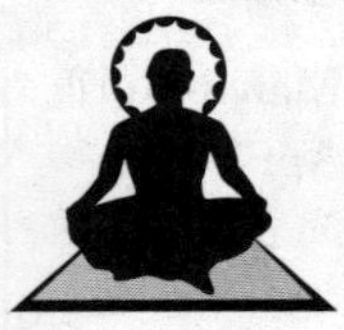

The Science of Human Anatomy and Bodily Functions

The human body is a wonderful creation and a gift of God. In this chapter, we shall explain human anatomy and the related functions which will help you associate them with various yogasanas.

It has been observed that the first impact of the yagasanas is on the muscles, glands and spine. This chapter is written with the special intention of understanding this wonderful form called the human body.

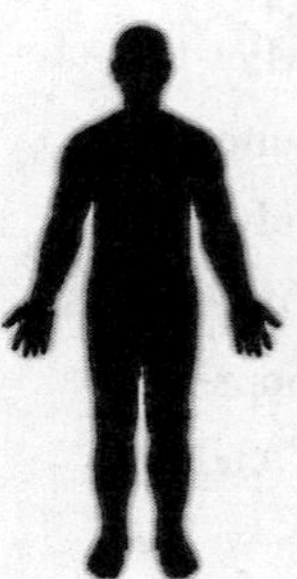

Anatomy

The human body is made up of numerous minute cells. These cells combine to make tissues, and tissues make the muscles. Similarly, various muscles combine to make other glands and organs.

In order to study the human body, let us divide it into six parts: Head, neck, upper limbs, lower limbs, abdomen and thorax.

Head

The bony structure of the head is called the skull. It is made up of many bones. There are two major bones in the skull – the cranium and the mandible. The hollow inside the cranium, called the brain box, is where the brain is encased.

Neck

The neck joins our body with the head. It has many parts such as the thyroid gland, parathyroid gland, thymus gland, arteries, veins, nerves, trachea, oesophagus, etc.

Upper Limbs (Hands)

The structure of our upper limbs are as follows:

1. Shoulders
2. Upper arms
3. Forearms
4. Palms

The shoulder is divided into three parts:

(1) Pectoral region (2) Axillary region (3) Scapula

Lower Limbs (Legs)

Usually all animals use all the four limbs to walk. However, human beings use only the lower limbs, or the legs, to walk.

The structure of the lower limbs is as follows:

1. Pelvic girdle – Hip bone + Sacrum + Coccyx
2. Femur
3. Tibia and Fibula
4. Foot-tarsals and Metatarsals

Abdomen

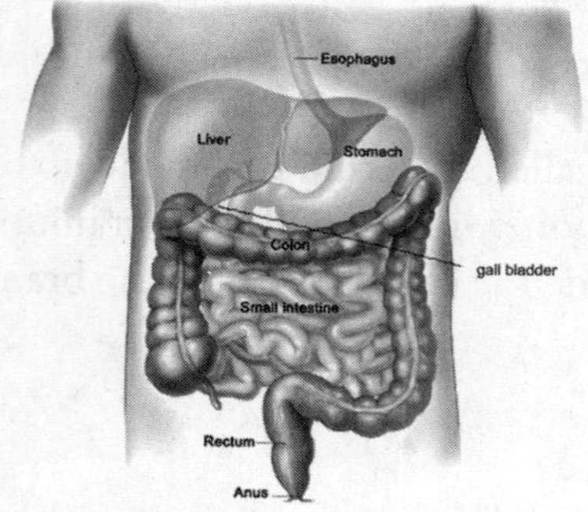

The abdomen is a very large and significant part of the human body. It consists:

Liver, pancreas, stomach, intestine (small and large), spleen, uterus and ovaries in women and testis in men.

Thorax

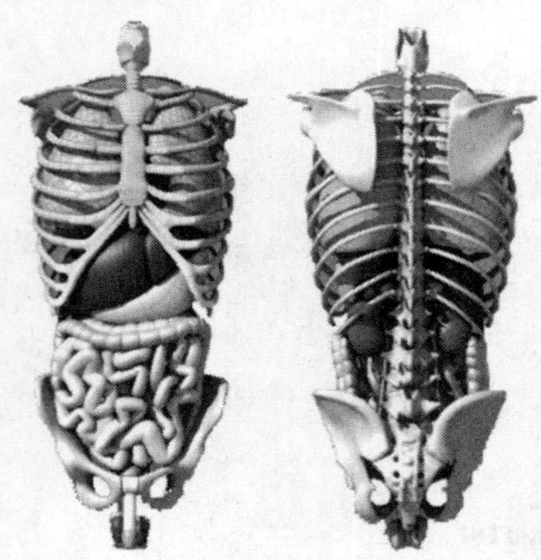

This part is below the neck region and extends up to the xiphoid process of the sternum. There is a skeletal structure in the thorax which is made of ribs and is connected to the sternum in the front and to the vertebral column at the back. The heart and lungs are enclosed in this rib cage and they control the respiratory and circulatory processes of the body.

The Air Sinuses of the Skull

Some cavities in the skull which are filled with air. They are called air sinuses.

They are generally found in the frontal, sphenoid, ethmoidal and maxillary parts of the skull. They produce sound and help in reduce the weight of the face and the forehead.

Sinusitis

The infection of the nose reaches the sinus which in turn becomes infected and inflammatory. When such an inflammation occurs, it is called sinusitis. In this disease, that particular part of the head starts aching where the sinus problem has occurred, making one suffer from persistent cold. When this cold is prolonged, one nostril constantly flows, and might give out foul smell at times. This is called chronic sinusitis.

Articular System

The place or spot where two or more bones join is called as joint. The study of bone joints is called arthrology. These joints are made up of bones, cartilages, ligaments, fibrous tissues and synovial membranes. The joints can be divided into three categories:

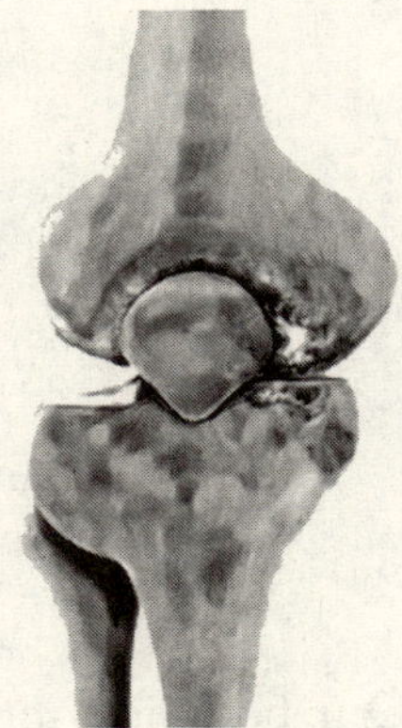

1. Fibrous joints
2. Cartilaginous joints
3. Synovial joints

Gout

In this disease, the amount of uric acid in the blood increases and particles of sodium urate accumulate in the joints, resulting in inflammation.

Generally this inflammation begins from the toes and thumbs of the feet. The feet swell and one suffers from fever, pain in the hands and legs, along with excessive sweating.

Functions of the Body (Physiology)

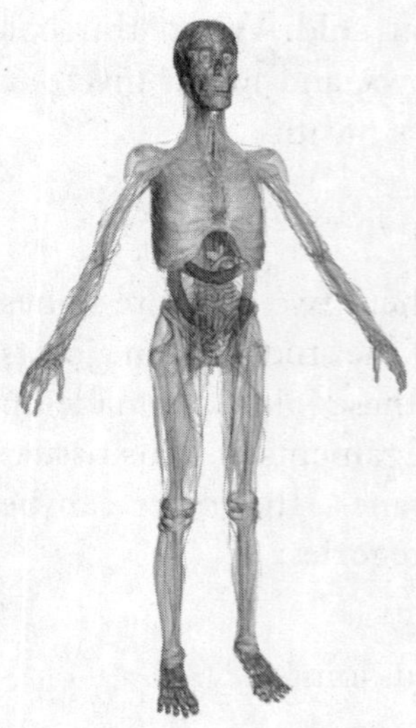

Our body is controlled and directed by various systems, that is functions are carried out by different systems. The circulatory system circulate blood in our body. Similarly, other systems too carry out their respective functions.

All the functions of our body are carried out by the following systems:

1. Circulatory system
2. Lymphatic system
3. R E system
4. Digestive system
5. Respiratory system
6. Endocrine system
7. Urinary system
8. Reproductive system
9. Nervous system

Circulatory System

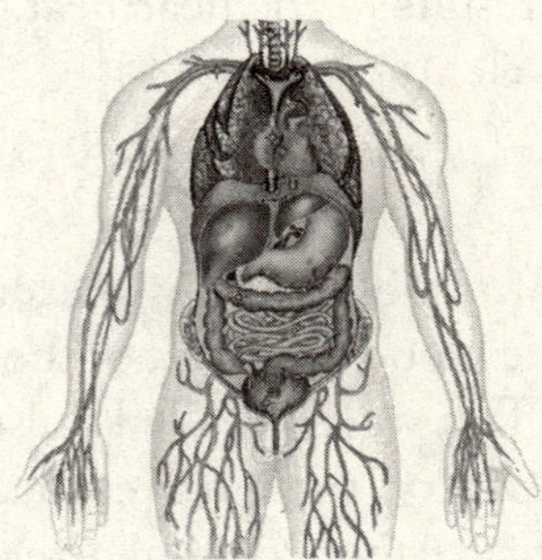

The main functional organ of the circulatory system is the heart. The blood vessels, spread in the entire body, are connected to the heart. They circulate the blood in the body.

There are two kinds of blood vessels in our body:

1. Arteries 2. Veins

The position of the heart

The heart is located in the middle of the chest in the Medeasteneum behind the sternum. Its larger side is on the left.

The Cardiac Cycle

The heart is like a pump. All the processes related to the circulation of blood in the body are done by the heart, and these processes are collectively called the cardiac cycle. The process of the heart begins from the sinus arterium node and after being circulated in the entire body, ends up in the ventricles, causing the ventricles to contract. The process of the atrium and the ventricles can be divided in two: Systole and diastole. In systole, the heart contracts and in diastole, the heart expands.

Heart's Sounds

Due to the contraction of the ventricles, the arterial ventricular valves close and cease to work for a short while. While closing, the sound created is called the first heart sound. We hear it as 'Lubb'. As soon as the contraction is over, the aortic valve close and the second heart sound is created. We hear it as 'Dubb'. The complete working of the heart results in the heartbeat. It indicates that the heart is functioning well.

What is Pulse?

When the pressure of the blood flow is exerted on the arteries, and simultaneously the blood flows out of the heart, a wave passes through the arteries. This wave is called pulse. We see this pulse mostly in the radial artery, though we check the pulse in the brachial artery, popliteal artery, femoral artery and dorsalis pedis artery as well. The ideal reading of the pulse should be 72/minute in a grown-up person and 140/minute in an infant.

The amount of blood in the body is approximately 5 litres.

Blood Pressure

The lateral pressure exerted by the blood on the walls of the arteries and veins during its circulation is called the blood pressure. The instrument used to measure blood pressure is called the Sphignomeno metre. The increase in blood pressure is called hypertension and the decrease in blood pressure is called hypotension. The Sixth Joint National Committee adopted the following criteria to categorise hypertension:

JNC VI Criteria for Classification of Blood Pressure

Category	Systolic mm HG	Diastolic mm HG
Optimal	<120	<80
Normal	<130	<85
High Normal	130-139	85-89
Stage – 1 Hypertension	140-159	90-99
Stage – 2 Hypertension	160-179	100-109
Stage – 3 Hypertension	>180	>110

Digestive System

The following parts of the body combine to make the digestive system:

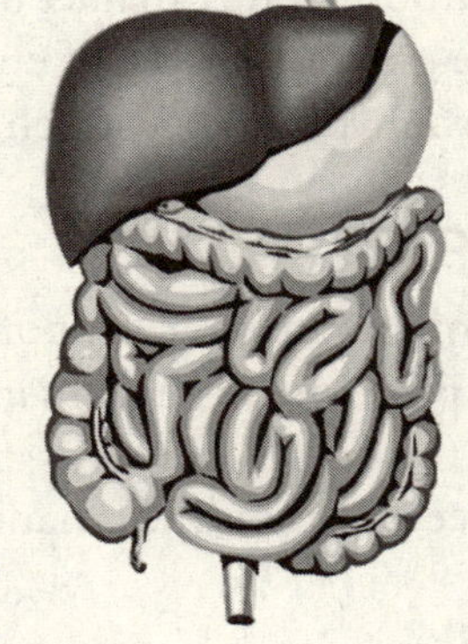

1. Mouth
2. Pharynx
3. Oesophagus
4. Stomach
5. Small intestine
6. Large intestine
7. Rectum
8. Anus
9. Liver

All these parts together form the elementary canal. The digestive process starts from the mouth and ends at the anus. There are a few other central parts which help in the digestive process: Glands, salivary glands, pancreas, gall bladder, etc.

The Digestive Process

Whenever a morsel of food is put into the mouth, the salivary glands become active and start secreting saliva. This saliva mixes with the food that we chew. After being chewed, the food goes into the oesophagus. From there it goes into the stomach. Here, it goes through a few chemical and mechanical processes, mixing with endocrine juices. In this way, the food takes the digested form.

The food then goes into the small intestine where its absorption takes place. It moves to the large intestine by the contraction and dilation movement of the small intestine. Here the undigested food is converted into waste matter and moved into the rectum under the large intestine. Then, it moves out of the anus.

The important elements of the body:

1. Carbohydrates
2. Proteins
3. Fat
4. Vitamins
5. Mineral salts
6. Water

Carbohydrates

Carbohydrates makes up for a large part of our food. It is also the greatest source of energy for the body. The main categories of carbohydrates are starch and sugar.

Protein

Proteins are a very important part of our diet. The main constituent of proteins is the element nitrogen. It helps build the protoplasm of the cells and the tissues. It is found in soya bean, pulses, milk, cheese, groundnut, channa, moong dal etc.

Fat

Just like carbohydrates, fats too have carbon, hydrogen and oxygen elements, but their ratio is different. It is found in butter, ghee, vanaspati ghee, etc.

Mineral Salts

Mineral salts are important for all the organic processes that take place in our body. We receive these mineral salts through our food. They are present in our body too. The main minerals are: Calcium, phosphorus, iron, sodium, potassium, magnesium, and iodine.

Calcium

Calcium is mostly found in the bones and the teeth and is important in building them. It makes the bones strong and hard. The normal requirement of calcium in an adult is 1 gram per day. Pregnant women need 1 ½ grams per day. Calcium is found in milk, curd, cottage cheese, almonds, and the leaves of radish, cauliflower, fenugreek, carrots and pulses, etc.

Phosphorus

Phosphorus is found in practically every cell of the body. It helps in building the bones and teeth. It keeps the nervous system healthy. Pregnant women and children need it more. Phosphorus is found in cabbage, apples, radish, soya bean, carrots, corn and potato.

Iron

It is very helpful in the increasing haemoglobin present in the red blood corpuscles. Ordinarily, a person needs 20-30 grams of iron every day. Iron is found in apple, spinach, peas, jaggery, carrots, cucumber, onion, tomato, grapes, potato, etc.

Sodium

We generally use sodium in our daily food in the form of salt. It combines with chlorine in salt to form sodium chloride. We need about 2-5 grams of salt every day.

Potassium

Potassium is most needed by the intercellular fluids. It is important for the chemical processes that take place in the cells. It is also necessary for the transmission of emotions in the nerves.

A person generally needs about 4 grams of potassium every day. It is found in all those food which are rich in protein.

Magnesium

It is found in our bones and teeth. 50 percent of the magnesium in the human body is in the bones. A person needs about 200-300mg of magnesium every day. It is found in fruits and vegetables.

Iodine

Thyroid gland is present in our throat. Iodine is needed for the proper functioning of this gland. It helps the thyroid gland in manufacturing hormones like thyroxin and triodothyromin. Iodine is found in onion in abundance. It is also found in sea products and salt. Its deficiency causes goitre.

Vitamins

Vitamins are chemicals which are present in minute quantities in almost all food items. Vitamins are of two types: Fat soluble and water soluble.

Fat soluble – A, D, E, K

Water soluble – B and C

Vitamin A

Vitamin A is found in plants and also in the form of carotene. It is converted into pro-vitamin retinol in the intestine. Vitamin A enhances our eyesight. It helps in manufacturing the retinal pigmentation which in turn helps us see even in dim light as well as protects us from infection. This vitamin helps in maintaining the reproductive power and controls the development of other cells. It is generally found in green vegetables, butter, and milk. Its deficiency causes diseases like night blindness and xerophthalmia.

Vitamin D

Vitamin D is of two types.
Vitamin D – D2 Calcifer of Cholecalciferol D3
Vitamin D helps our body absorb calcium. This vitamin assists in the development of bones. It helps in manufacturing phosphorus in the kidneys. The most vitamin D that we receive is from the sun rays. Its deficiency causes diseases like rickets in children and osteomalacia in adults.

Vitamin E

This vitamin dissolves in the skin. It is also known as tokopherol. It is mainly found in vanaspati oil, cotton seeds, sunflower seeds, butter, etc. We need about 0.8 mg of this vitamin every day. It prevents unnecessary oxidation in the body due to its anti-oxidant qualities. It also prevents sterility and is very helpful in the development of the womb.

Vitamin K

We know it as the vitamin which stops the flow of blood. In other words it helps in blood clotting. It is found in green vegetables and fruits. It is found in large quantity in cow's milk.

Water soluble Vitamins B and C

There are many kinds of Vitamin B:

Vitamin B1 Complex

Vitamin B2 Riboflavin

Vitamin B6 Pyridoxin

Vitamin B3 Pantotheric acid

Vitamin B12 Cyanocobalamin

Vitamin C (Ascorbic Acid)

We know this vitamin as ascorbic acid. It is soluble in water and destroyed by heat. It is generally found in fresh fruits, specially fruits which have citrus acid such as orange, lemon, amla, tomato, papaya, grapes, beetroot, sweet lime, etc. It helps in the manufacture of insulin. Its deficiency causes scurvy.

Endocrine System

The glands of our body are divided into two types: One which secretes the hormones directly into the blood stream because they do not have any ducts. These are called endocrine glands. The others are those which have ducts. They are called exocrine glands.

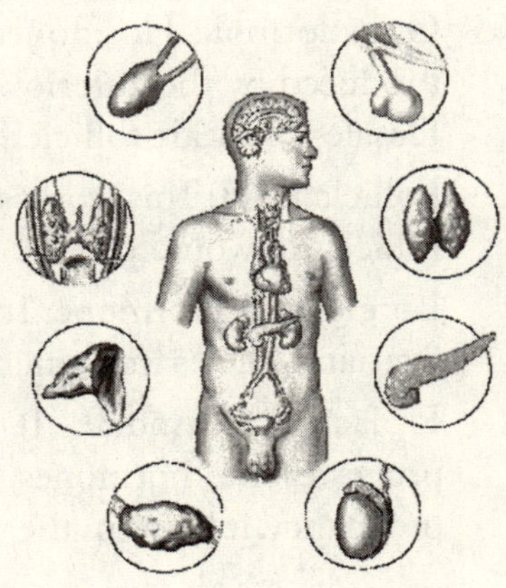

Hormones

Some glands in our body secrete certain juices which mix in the blood and gets circulated in the body. The functional elements of these secretions are called hormones.

Endocrine Glands

1. Pituitary gland
2. Thyroid gland
3. Parathyroid gland
4. Thymus gland

5. Adrenal gland
6. Islets of the Langerhans of the Pancreas
7. Pineal gland
8. Sexual gland

Pituitary Gland

This gland is situated inside our head. There are anterior lobe, posterior lobe and the pars intermedia in this gland. This gland is reddish-brown in colour. The hormones secreted by the anterior lobe are as follows:

1. Growth Hormone: Its function is to promote the growth of the body.
2. Adrenocorticotropic Hormone (ACTH): It is necessary for the development of the cortex of the adrenal gland.
3. Thyroid Stimulating Hormone (TSH): It works to develop and enhance the capacity of the thyroid gland.
4. Gonadotropic Hormones: Two reproductive hormones are produced by the anterior pituitary glands in both males and females. They are follicle FSH and luteining hormones.
5. Follicle FSH: This works to help in the growth of the ovarian follicles in women.
6. Luteinizing Hormone: It helps in the full maturation of the ovarian follicles in women.
7. Prolactin Hormone: It works with the oestrogen and progesterone hormones to develop the breasts. During pregnancy, it helps in the secretion of milk.

Hormones Secreted by the Posterior Lobe:

1. Anti-diuretic Hormone: This hormone increases the permeability of the kidneys and helps them absorb more water.
2. Oxytocin Hormone: The main function of this hormone is to contract the myoepithelial cells in the breasts of a woman and help in the secretion of milk.

(I) Thyroid hormone

It is secreted by the thyroid gland. The hormones thyroxine T4 and triodothyronine T3 are secreted from the thyroid. It controls the growth and development of the tissues. Its deficiency or excess gives rise to many diseases like hypothyroidism and hyperthyroidism.

(II) Thymus gland

This gland is situated in the middle of the chest. It has two parts. It becomes active infancy. Its function is to maintain the antibodies and the immune system.

(III) Adrenal gland

This gland is situated above the kidneys. Many hormones are secreted from this gland, such as gluco cartecoid, mineralocartecoid, steroids etc.

Islets of the Langerhans in the Pancreas

This gland has ducts. Its tissues secrete digestive juices which help in digestion. These bunches in the pancreas are called islets of langerhans which are endocrine glands. They can be divided into two categories: The ones in which the cells secrete glocogen hormone and the other in which the cells secrete insulin hormone.

Pineal gland

This is a 10 cm long reddish-brown coloured gland situated near the corpus calossum, behind the third ventricle below the brain.

Sexual gland

It refers to that arrangement in the body parts of men and women which produces sperms and eggs.

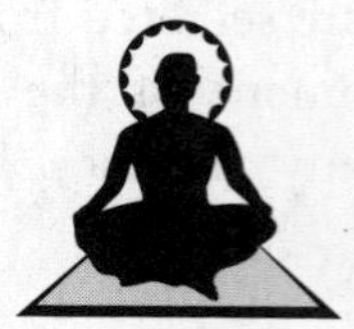

Acupressure

India is the only country in the world where various skills and talents have been born. Due to certain reasons, some of this precious knowledge was lost. But if we make proper use of the knowledge which is still with us, we can live a healthy life till our last breath. One such knowledge is the science of acupressure, which means 'to apply pressure'. Since ancient times, acupressure has been used as treatment in some form or the other in India. In this approach, a calculated degree of pressure is applied on specific parts of our body to cure related diseases.

Our body is made up of five elements and is directed by an energy which we know as the soul, conscience or life force. This energy is present in our entire body. 7,200 nerves terminate in our palms and soles. The mounts in these parts of the body are the main pressure points. The switch board of the life energy flowing in our body is situated in them. If we go by the theory of acupressure then, due to our imbalanced lifestyle, many foreign elements enter our body and get accumulated inside parts. In whichever part of the body they get accumulated, diseases related to that part start emerging. These foreign elements also get accumulated in the related acupressure points in the palms and soles and the diseases start spreading quickly. In order to remove these foreign matters from the body, necessary pressure is applied on the related acupressure points (reflex points). With regular treatment, the disease gradually vanishes from the body.

According to Dr F M Gheiston (acupressure specialist), live energy is present in our body. When it leaks out of the palms and soles, the parts of the body related to that particular point become prone to diseases. When we apply pressure on these points, the leakage of energy is blocked and the impact of the flow of energy in that part of the body is normalised. Hence, the disease starts healing.

This approach is simple, less time consuming, less expensive and purely non violent. It calms the body and mind as well as increase our energy. Due to the lack of space, we have given only the basic introduction of this approach here. Those who wish to use this method of treatment should contact the experts in this field to gain benefits. We have provided an illustration with details of the pressure points and the corresponding parts of the body.

You can balance vata (wind), pitta (fire) and
kapha (water) in your body through determination.

To get rid of Vata, give up tension.

To get rid of Pitta, work on your fitness.

To get rid of Kapha, balance your temper.

–RJT

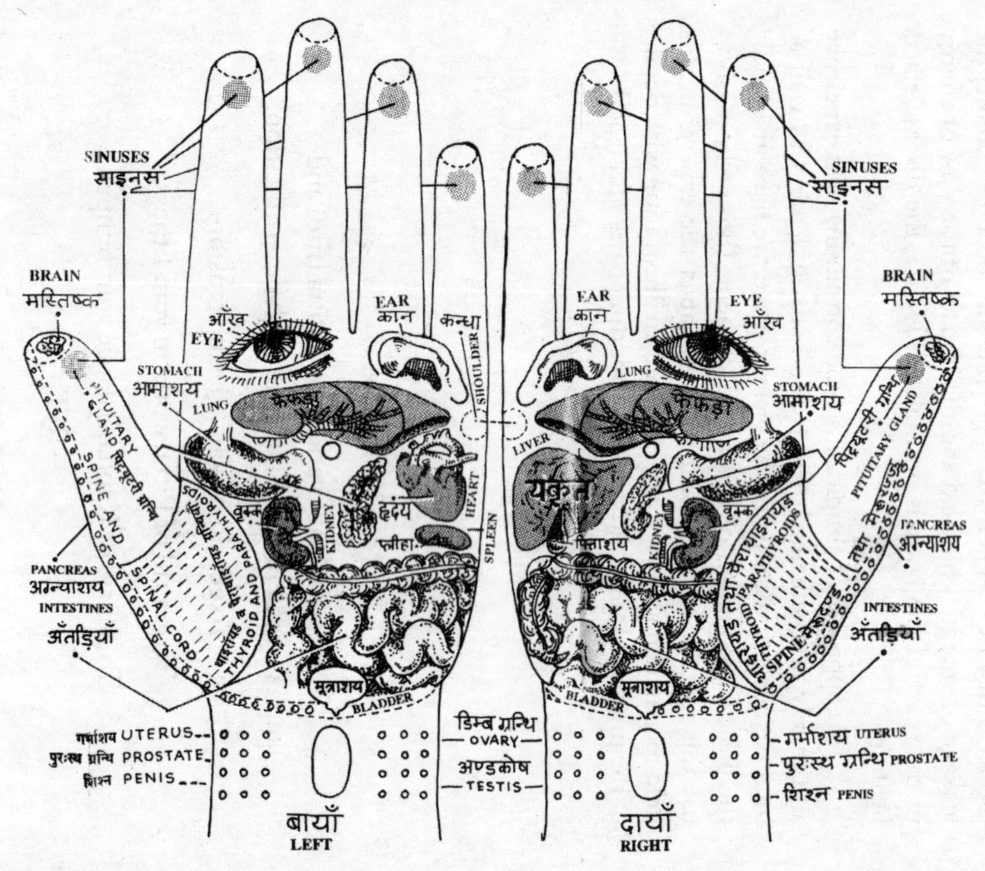

SINUSES
साइनस
BRAIN
मस्तिष्क
EYE
आँख
EAR
कान
कन्धा
SHOULDER
STOMACH
आमाशय
LUNG
फेफड़ा
PITUITARY GLAND
पिट्यूटरी ग्रन्थि
SPINE AND SPINAL CORD
THYROID AND PARATHYROIDS
KIDNEY
वृक्क
हृदय
HEART
प्लीहा
SPLEEN
LIVER
यकृत
पित्ताशय
PANCREAS
अग्न्याशय
INTESTINES
अँतड़ियाँ
मूत्राशय
BLADDER
गर्भाशय UTERUS
पुरःस्थ ग्रन्थि PROSTATE
शिश्न PENIS
डिम्ब ग्रन्थि
OVARY
अण्डकोष
TESTIS
बायाँ
LEFT
दायाँ
RIGHT

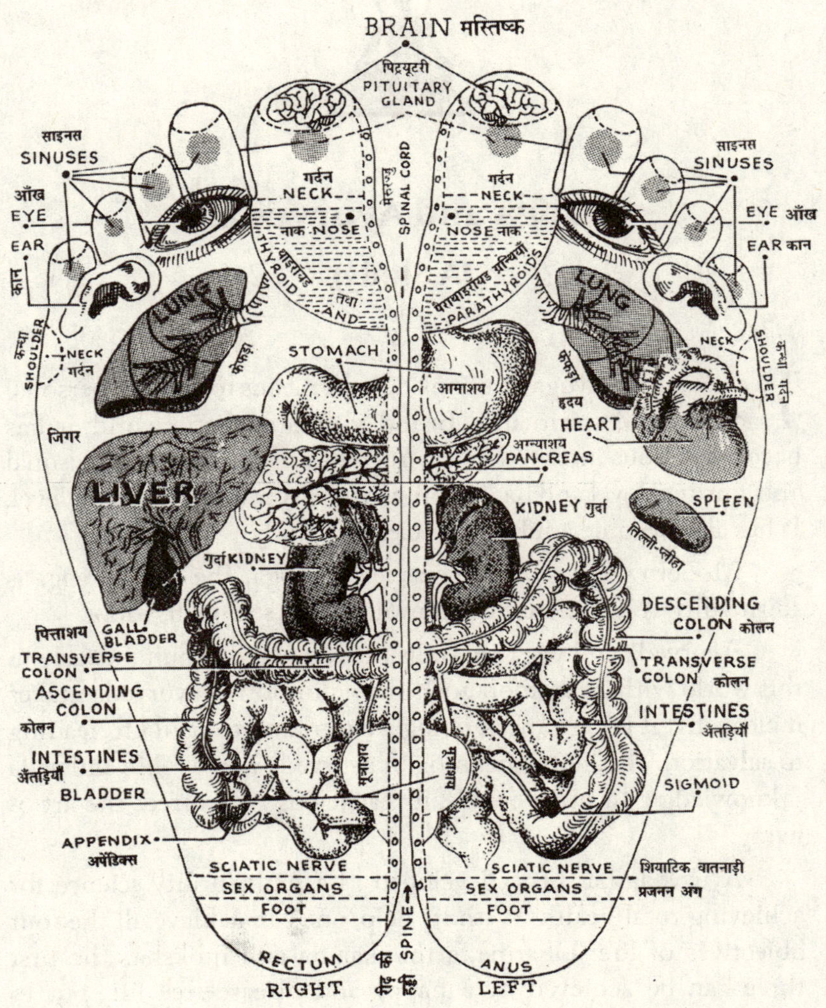

BRAIN मस्तिष्क
पिट्यूटरी
PITUITARY GLAND
साइनस
SINUSES
आँख
EYE
EAR
कान
गर्दन
NECK
नाक NOSE
मेरुरज्जु
SPINAL CORD
THYROID
तथा
AND
PARATHYROIDS
LUNG
फेफड़ा
SHOULDER
NECK
गर्दन
STOMACH
आमाशय
जिगर
LIVER
पित्ताशय
GALL. BLADDER
गुर्दा KIDNEY
TRANSVERSE COLON
ASCENDING COLON
कोलन
INTESTINES
अंतड़ियाँ
BLADDER
APPENDIX
अपेंडिक्स
साइनस
SINUSES
EYE आँख
EAR कान
गर्दन
NECK
NOSE नाक
SHOULDER
NECK
हृदय
HEART
अग्न्याशय
PANCREAS
KIDNEY गुर्दा
SPLEEN
DESCENDING COLON कोलन
TRANSVERSE COLON कोलन
INTESTINES
अंतड़ियाँ
SIGMOID
SCIATIC NERVE
SEX ORGANS
FOOT
SCIATIC NERVE शियाटिक वातनाड़ी
SEX ORGANS प्रजनन अंग
FOOT
SPINE
RECTUM
ANUS
RIGHT
LEFT

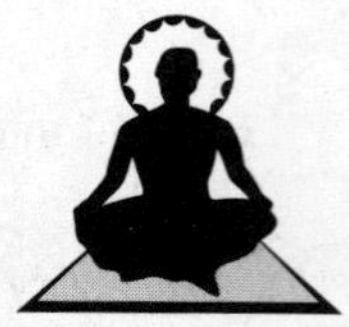

Yoga and Ayurveda

(A Study)

In earlier times, yoga was considered a means to achieve personal sadhana and spirituality. In today's materialistic world, it has become famous internationally. Yoga has risen above the personal and spiritual level and has become extensively useful at social level. It has also become a subject of scientific study.

Modern yoga is only one aspect of yoga. The base of yoga is spirituality. It is a science of knowledge and self-realisation.

Ayurveda and yoga are skills that emerged simultaneously in this world with a common goal. The definition of ayurveda makes it clear that it is a means of living a happy and fruitful life, leading to salvation. The literal meaning of ayurveda is ayu = life and veda = knowledge. In other words, it teaches us the correct the art of living.

Ayurveda has been developed as a multi-utility science for achieving total health. With its help, one can achieve all the four objectives of life: Dharma, artha, kaama and moksha. The first three can be achieved by a happy and disease-free life, but to achieve the fourth, ayurveda recommends yoga along with herbal medicines.

While ayurveda gives us physical health, yoga is a science of consciousness which leads us towards self-awareness along with helping us get rid of our inner sorrows and taking us towards salvation. Both yoga and ayurveda are related to the mind and conscience, physical and mental health respectively. In spite of these specialisations, yoga is a part of ayurveda. Possibly, the detailed knowledge of the treatment of the mind and conscience in ayurveda became an off-shoot and emerged in the form of yoga.

Many learned and wise men are of the opinion that it is the same acharya who created ayurveda for the body, yoga for the mind and grammar for the voice/speech. This great acharya is none other than Maharishi Patanjali who expounded the science of yoga. In the first shloka of *Charaka Samhita*, the writer says:

पतञ्जलमहाभाष्यचरक प्रति संस्कृतेः।
मनोवाक्कायदोषाणं हर्सेऽहियतये नमः।।

In the first text of ayurveda, *Charaka Samhita*, all the theories of yoga are already present in a precise and summarised form. There is a description of yoga and pure intellect in the Gyana and Tatva Anubhuti Moola chapter of Naishthika Chikitsa in *Charaka Samhita*. This summarised version of yoga vidya has been explained in detail in the *Yoga Sutra* written by Patanjali.

According to Shri Atrideva Vidyalankara, people of Yayavara clan, who were the followers of the charaka branch of the Krishna Yajurveda, were very adept in ayurveda and yoga. They were nomads by nature, that is why they were called charaka.

The basic principles and the cleansing theories of ayurveda and yoga are very similar and closely related. The main cleansing kriya of ayurveda is the Pancha Karma in which the acharya has included vamana, virechana, anuvasana, asthapana and shirovirechana. In the *Yoga Sutra*, Maharishi has explained the Shatkarma for the cleansing of the body, which are dhauti, vasti, neti, nauli, trataka and kapal-bhati. There is a lot of similarity in these and the Pancha Karma mentioned in ayurveda. Shatkarma is present subtly but in its totality in ayurveda. They were developed in Ayurveda and later included in Hatha Yoga.

The main objective of yoga is to lead people towards salvation, whereas this is merely one aspect of the science of life or ayurveda. Ayurveda is the guiding text for the entire life and its ultimate goal is related to spiritual development. Apart from spiritual development, ayurveda also preaches about physical and mental development.

Ayurveda is the science which provides remedies to the physical, mental, spiritual, and materialistic problems. It is this total health which leads a person to the attainment of the four goals of life, namely, dharma, artha, kaama and moksha. Whereas yoga is a means to get relief from the spiritual problems and achieve moksha.

As mentioned earlier, three different texts were written for the purification of mind, speech and body by the same person. Patanjali's *Yoga Sutra* was written for the purification of the mind, *Mahabhaashya* for speech and *Charaka Samhita* for the purification of the body. It is on this basis that the eight parts of ayurveda and the eight parts of *Yoga Sutra* appear to be so similar.

The first section of *Yoga Sutra* is Yama, under which non-violence, truth, non-stealing, celibacy and non-hoarding are explained. In ayurveda, they are explained in detail under svastha vritta, aachaara, rasaayana, paapa karma, tri-upstambha and hitayu respectively. Under the second section of *Yoga Sutra* fall shaucha, santosha, tapa, svadhyaya and ishvara pranidhana. These are also explained in a very organised and simple way as the main parts of svasthya vritt and dincharya. Similarly a detailed, clear and comprehensive explanation of asana, pranayama, pratyahara, dharana, dhyana and samadhi can also be found in ayurveda. Out of these, dharana, dhyana and samadhi have been mentioned by the acharyas as the main technique in treating mental disorders. The explanation of Pragya and Yoga Purusha in ayurveda is similar to the Ritambhara, Pragya and the Yoga Purush of *Bhagvada Gita* mentioned in *Yoga Sutra*.

In this way we see that yoga is a mere part of ayurveda. When we see the theories and principles of ayurveda, we find that it has been created by keeping in mind the happiness of a person in this life and in the next one. It is a guide to attain money, a good life and the next life along with the four goals – dharma, artha, kaama and moksha. While this is the means to achieve happiness in this life through medicine, food and habits, yoga aims to build the next life through spirituality, divine knowledge and experience. Even though yoga is an aspect of ayurveda, they are also complementary to each other. While ayurveda leads to salvation through physical, mental and spiritual cleansing, yoga leads to salvation through physical, mental and spiritual cleansing via various kriyas. Though yoga is only a means of attaining nirvana, one cannot attain nirvana till one is healthy and normal. That is why ayurveda is considered the main means of attaining salvation after having lead a happy and healthy life, while yoga is considered as a mere assistant to it.

Yoga exercise was as much needed by humankind
yesterday as it is needed today, and
will be needed tomorrow as well.

–RJT

Tips for Total Good Health

- Get up in the morning before sunrise.
- Fill a copper vessel with water at night and drink at least two glasses of this water next morning.
- Use one teaspoon triphala.
- Take pure food for breakfast (do not take packed or tinned food).
- Give up intoxicating substances.
- Take vegetarian food, salad, fruits, juice, etc. in your diet.
- Try to take your first meal before noon and dinner four hours before going to bed. Sleep early at night.
- Sattvika and pure food not only builds up the aura and vitality. It also generates positive emotions such as happiness and love.
- Do not hold in your cough, sneeze, yawn, vomit, urine and motion. Trying to hold them gives rise to many diseases.
- Stop eating the whole day. When you chew bubblegum, chewing gum, gutkha, tobacco, paan-beedi, cigarette, etc. you actually chew our own precious life. Therefore, never indulge in these things.
- You must wash your hands, feet and face before going to bed. By doing this, one sleeps well and maintains good health.
- Stomach ailments, constipation, indigestion, disorders of the wind, bile and phlegm can be controlled by observing fast.
- Eat to live, do not live to eat.
- When our food is pure, our conscience too is purified. A pure conscience leads to pure intellect and good memory, and good memory results in opening up all kinds of physical and mental blockages.

- Wind, bile and phlegm lead to good health as well as ill-health depending on their balance or imbalance. Keeping these things in mind decide your food habits, behaviour, exercise, daily routine and other things.
- Balance the air, bile and phlegm using your willpower. To calm the air, give up worry; to calm the bile, enhance your capabilities; and to calm the phlegm, bring stability in your behaviour.
- Soak two almonds in water overnight and the next morning, peel and eat them along with milk. This will enhance your memory and sharpen your intellect.
- Do surya namaskara with light exercises and light asanas.
- For good health, do yogasanas regularly.
- Do meditation.
- The kriyas related to yogasanas do not merely give us good health but also give us mental fitness.
- Adopt celibacy, and make your life strong and firm.
- Nowadays, yoga is the only alternative which can make the spine flexible. It also gives good health and peace to the body, mind and intellect. It has been aptly said: A healthy mind resides in a healthy body.
- It is written in Upanishada that he who has trained his body in the fire of yogabhyasa is not troubled either by disease or by old age. Even death does not go near him.
- Have a positive attitude.
- Thinking big really works. Imply it.
- Read good literature; become energetic.
- Be humble; you will become powerful.
- Even if you are busy the whole day, be alert towards your body.
- Give your family members a lot of affection without expecting anything from them.

- Be aware of these ten things and follow them in your life – kshama, maardan, aarjava, shaucha, satya, sanyama, tapa, tyaga, akinchanatva and bramhacharya.
- Give up four things: Anger, pride, illusion and greed.
- Keep five things in mind which are not worth adopting: Violence, falsehood, stealing, immodesty, and hoarding.
- Do not worry about what you are in the eyes of other people. Rather, consider what you are in your own eyes.
- Start making life beautiful for others. The troubles of your life will automatically convert into benefits.
- It is not important how many languages you know. What is more important is how cultured you are.
- Massage your head with pure oil. Avoid scented oils available in the market. Use pure coconut, mustard or almond oil. They cool your head and freshen it up.
- Develop a habit of reading good literature every day. Knowledge is never wasted.
- When the clouds of sattvika rasa pour down your body, the river of your life span increases and swell day-by-day.
- Always remember that if you think you can be beaten, you are beaten, and if you think that you can win, then you have already won.
- Those who have a strong willpower are supported even by gods.
- Always remember that just as the picture quality will not be good if any part of the television does not function well. The screen will have lines and the picture will be blurred. Similarly, if any part of your body does not function well, your life will be like the spoilt image on the screen. If you take care of your health, you will always present a good picture of yourself.
- Our body is a collection of many minute atoms. It is made up of numerous atoms and molecules. They have innumerable

secrets of the universe hidden in them. Try to know yourself. You can never know when or which secret would grant you a mysterious power.

- If you use fraudulent material in building your house, your house will collapse and perish. Similarly, the food that you eat builds you up. So, it is up to you how you wish to build this house called YOUR BODY.

Always remember, if you are doing anything against nature, you are reducing the cosmic sound of the universe. Live in tune with the it and in a natural way.

–RJT

The highest form of prayer is the one which has compassion for all the living creatures.

–RJT

The Role of Yoga in Stress Management

Stress, like other necessities of life, is significant for our progress, but when it goes out of control, it becomes fatal. Yoga, through its perspective and philosophy of life and its treatment, keeps stress under control. Positive stress brings mobility and progress in life, but in excess, it fills our life with distress.

Modern life and gadgets have taken people away from humanistic values. A lot of stress has spread all over the world like an epidemic, giving rise to many mental and physical diseases. Yoga teaches us to follow the yama, niyama, asana, pranayama, pratyahara, dharana, dhyana and samadhi. It asks us to stay away from cardinal desires, anger, greed, attachment, jealousy, hatred, etc. on the one hand, while drawing our attention towards the higher goals of life on the other. Most of us simply while away our life in stress and tension without realising that there is a higher state of life and that one can live a higher life.

Positive tension brings positive results like competitive spirit and gives us the necessary energy and ability to work till we achieve its highest quality. It plays an important role in helping be careful and move towards victory. Yoga plays a role in helping us use stress in a positive way.

The negative effects of stress give rise to many diseases such as high blood pressure, diabetes, constipation, unhealthy digestive system, ulcer, poor eyesight, loss of the working capacity of various parts of the body, breathlessness, excessive secretion from the adrenal glands, insomnia, irritation, excitement, worry, fear, unwillingness to work, heart problems, heart attack, depression, arthritis, etc.

The practice of non-violence, truth, non-stealing, non-hoarding and celibacy under Yama creates a healthy and protective environment in the society. If all of us individually follow these qualities, many reasons of stress and tension will automatically vanish due to a secure and healthy environment.

Under Niyama: Shaucha, santosha, tapa, svadhyaya and

ishwara pranidhana teach us to live a contented life. By following the practice of tapa, svadhyaya and ishwara pranidhana, you can automatically feel a sense of dissatisfaction, discontentment, incorrect logics and negative thinking vanish from your life. If these feelings persist, life becomes an experience of aimless wanderings.

While doing the asanas, the mind combines with the body to make it strong, tolerant, calm and stress-free, and enhances the capacity which is called siddhi in the yogic jargon. The maximum therapeutic impact of the asanas has been seen on the mental and physical diseases.

By doing pranayama, the mind becomes unmindful, your emotional balance increases and the mind becomes one with the soul. The inherent qualities of a person are developed and their chances of blooming into a fully wonderful human being become 100 percent. The endocrine secretions like the adrenal can be made ineffective and then, stress can be used as a motivating force.

In pratyahara, the senses are directed inwards and are trained to receive their subject at the inner shrine. This reduces the distraction of the mind. Its wanderings stop and it becomes stress-free.

By practicing dharana, dhyana and samadhi, alpha rays are emitted from the brain, which make the mind calm and creative. Sleep, laughter, play and seclusion have also been observed to give healthy results but they are very limited when compared to dhyana.

Yoga also motivates you to take a sattvika and balanced diet. Today, modern science has accepted the impact of food on psychological disorders. The mind which was earlier looking for taste and excitement has now started looking for nutrition and health in food.

Yoga and Mental Health

Personality – Definition and Factors

When we look at the Indian and the world philosophies, it comes into light that while at one hand philosophers have been intrigued by the external atmosphere of humans, on the other they have sufficiently tried to understand their humanistic qualities. People have many ideologies related to personality. A lot of efforts have been made globally to do a scientific and detailed study of personality. But even today, a common acceptable definition of personality is yet to be established. In the initial stages, some psychologists stressed on the mental, animate, chemical and physical aspects of human beings, while the others stressed on the external behaviour.

The following experts and learned men have defined personality from time to time. Out of these, the definition given by Allport is considered satisfactory:

1. Morton Prince, 1924
2. John B Watson, 1924
3. Edwin Ray Gathrie, 1948
4. Murray, 1948
5. J P Guilford, 1956
6. Warren, 1930
7. Boring, 1950
8. Pervin, 1971
9. Gordon W Allport, 1961

Professor Gordon W Allport has defines personality in his book, *Personality: A Psychological Interpretation* published in 1937 as: The dynamic organisation – within an individual – of those psycho-physical systems that determine his/her characteristic behaviour and thought.

This definition given by Allport covers all the theoretical ideologies. Most of the psychologists consider it satisfactory, directly or indirectly. This definition can be analysed under three points:

1. Psychophysical systems
2. Dynamic organisation
3. Characteristic behaviour and thought

In this way, it is clear that the concept of 'personality' is very wide. It includes all the characteristics of a person in a coordinated manner.

Personality Determinants

There are many determinants of personality which control and direct the behaviour of a person. The main determinants are:

1. General activities/general openness
2. Neuroticism
3. Emotional instability
4. Authority/submissiveness
5. Depression
6. Sociability
7. Ego power

Factors Which Influence the Personality

Personality is a dynamic organisation of the external and internal characteristics of a person. The biological, cultural, social and psychological factors play a special role in the development of a person's personality. When a child is born, they acquires certain hereditary traits from their parents. Apart from these, family, school, social milieu, etc. contribute significantly to build a child's personality.

The factors that affect a person's personality have been divided into four categories:

1. Biological 2. Cultural 3. Social 4. Psychological

1. Biological Factors

These are called internal factors because a person does not have any control over them. The main factors under this category are hereditary or biogenic processes like the endocrine glands, physique, chemical composition of the body and the nervous system. Heredity and environment, both are significant factors which influence personality.

Heredity: With the help of study of the reproductive system, efforts have been made to locate heredity among the biological factors affecting a person's personality. According to Mendel's theory, there are three laws of reproduction:

1. The law of segregation
2. The law of dominant and recessive genes (Or the law of dominance)
3. The law of independent assortment

It has been discovered that the effect of heredity is passed from one generation to the other through genes. After the birth of a child, four biological factors play a special role in deciding its personality:

1. Endocrine glands
2. Physique
3. Body chemistry
4. Nervous system

2. Cultural Determinants of Personality

Every society has a different and unique culture. It has a deep impact on the food habits, behaviour and personality of a person. Rituals, habits, traditions dressing styles, food habits etc. are some of the main traits of culture.

Many experimental and anthropological proofs have been presented through various studies with regard to the cultural impact on personality.

Culture is of two types:

1. Material culture
2. Non-material culture

3. Social Determinants of Personality

After a child's birth, the environment around him/her has a clear impact on his/her personality. According to Herlock, 1974, the social situations decide the learning process according to the age. By doing this, the 'I' or the 'ego' of a person develops and the feeling of social responsibility increases. The social determinants of personality are responsible for the total transformation of the original matter. Out of these, the factors related to the family and the school are central.

4. Psychological Determinants of Personality

1. Intellect
2. Motivation
3. Interest
4. Attitude
5. Worry
6. Frustration
7. Values
8. Momentum
9. Lifestyle

Factors Related to Family

The relationship between the parents and the child according to the studies of Harlow, 1966, Michael,1958 and Green Stein, 1966

- Very alert parents
- Very harsh/strict parents
- Insulting parents
- Parents who are partial
- Mutual relationship between the parents
- Size of the family
- Sequence of birth and personality – first, middle and the last child

Socio-economic Condition

The urban or rural environment of the family plays an important role in deciding one's personality. Like social situation, the economic condition of a family also influences one's personality. Too rich or too poor, both kinds of environment act as hurdles in the proper development of a child's personality.

Groups' Influence

The type of group to which a person belongs influences his/her personality. The group may be primary or secondary. Its membership may be compulsory or optional. Similarly, the personality of a leader and a member are clearly different.

Impact/Influence of School

1. Curriculum
2. Teacher
3. The general discipline of the school
4. Friends in the school
5. The age of going to school

The Role of Yoga in Determining One's Personality

With regular practice of yoga, the Intelligence Quotient of a person increases. Frustration, loneliness and inferiority complex vanish from his/her personality. His/her interests are developed and defined. His/her values are socially accepted. Moreover, his/her lifestyle is modern yet yogic. To sum up, there is a positive development of his/her personality.

Yoga's Influence on Personality Development

Personality is best understood in terms of internal and external influences. At every moment our genes, experiences, environment and free will determine our personality. Every person has a speciality in terms of certain characteristics such as feelings, behaviour, capabilities, ideals, etc. One's personality is understood by what one thinks and how one acts.

According to modern psychology, the various personality theories fall into five major perspectives:

1. The **Psychoanalytic perspective** defines personality in terms of the dynamics that underline behaviour.
2. The **Trait perspective** defines personality in terms of behaviour.
3. The **Humanistic perspective** pays attention to the potential of growth in people.
4. The **Social Cognitive perspective** emphasises the ways in which our personalities are influenced by our environment.
5. The **Evolutionary perspective** asserts that the patterns of behaviour seen in a species is a product of evolution.

According to modern psychology, the following factors of personality can be balanced and developed through yoga:

1. Intelligence Quotient: By doing asana and pranayama along with trataka and meditation, the Intelligence Quotient increases.

2. Motivation: The sadhaka is always filled with a positive energy due to which he/she is able to win over many obstacles and always feels motivated and enthusiastic.

3. Interest: The sadhaka becomes introvert or extrovert according to his interests. He/she gets both worldly and spiritual achievements. When he/she is extrovert, he/she gets the worldly gains, and when he/she is an introvert, he/she gets the spiritual gains. Both the directions are necessary to lead a life of excellence in this world.

4. Attitude: Yoga teaches how to develop qualities such as service, love, sacrifice, etc. That is why a person who practices yoga always has a positive attitude in life.

5. Worry and Frustration: Yoga sadhana reduces the feelings of loneliness and inferiority. By practicing yoga, unity and integrity infuse in one's personality and one experience a feeling of completeness in oneself.

6. Values (Six types of expounded values):

1. Values based on knowledge through which a person is always in pursuit of truth and knowledge; for example, The philosophers and scientists.
2. Values based on beauty which create various interests towards life; their goal is talent and beauty. For example, painters, poets, singers, dancers, etc.
3. Values based on money which make a person look at life from the monetary and utilitarian perspective. For example, industrialists, businessmen.
4. Values based on politics direct a person towards politics. For example, politicians and leaders.
5. Values based on religion – the religious gurus and sages who have interest in religious activities come under this category.
6. Values based on social norms – people involved in various social activities and reforms come under this category. For example, social reformers, social workers, etc.

7. Momentum or Force of Desires: By doing yoga, one gains control over their momentum, otherwise a person may fall under the influence of this force and take impulsive decisions which may be wrong or unwanted, and later he/she might regrets them.

8. Lifestyle: The sadhaka's is modern while being yogic. He/she gives more importance to inner bliss as compared to the sensual pleasures. He/she is more involved in self-realisation than in running after materialistic goals.

According to Indian perspective, the essence of human personality is the Self. Self-realisation is the goal of human life, according to Indian psychology. Self-realisation brings about a transformation in the thinking and behaviour of a person. The human personality is made up of the three gunas and the pancha koshas. Their development and balance leads to the development of the personality. The control and direction of our behaviour, thinking and reflection leads to the balance of the three gunas, namely, sattvika, rajasika and tamasika. The following are the five koshas of the human body:

1. Annamaya kosha
2. Pranmaya kosha
3. Manomaya kosha
4. Vigyanmaya kosha
5. Anandmaya kosha

Development of these koshas through yoga and sadhana leads to the development of our personality.

Shatkarm (Cleansing processes)

The annamaya kosha or the physical body is cleansed and developed by the practice of neti, dhauti, vasti, nauli, trataka, kapal-bhati and asanas. The pranmaya kosha is developed by the practice of pranayama. By developing the life force and the immunity system, the quantity of prana increases in our body. The manomaya kosha is developed through pratyahara and dharana; vigyanmaya kosha is developed through dhyana and anandmaya kosha is developed through samadhi.

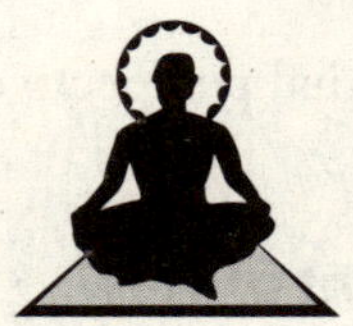

Prayer

The literal meaning of prayer is, 'a solemn request to God or true humility'.

Prayer is the total surrender of the self to God, with absolute devotion and faith. True prayer is one where we merge our lesser self in the flow of the greater self. We spread the light of our soul in the world, merging it with the light of the universe, while forgetting our megre individuality in the divine experience of the endless eternal power. When this happens, our little ego is destroyed while we gain the knowledge about our true self.

Prayer can be verbal as well mental. Prayer can also be triggered by situations. It has many forms and levels such as prayer of the lower level and higher level. The former is one where a person prays for the destruction or death of his enemy or prays for any kind of harm for others. The highest level of prayer is devoid of all selfish intentions. It is totally selfless. It does not involve any kind of pleasure for the self.

The effect of prayer is destroyed when the mind is diverted towards materialistic objects. It is very important that the mind should stay stable and absolutely focused on the deity or the object of devotion.

A true prayer should be short because in cases of long prayers, there are chances of the mind going helter-skelter. The best form of prayer takes one to that highest level of experience, where prayer is not required anymore as the devotee unites with the Supreme.

Types of Prayers

From the social and spiritual perspective, there are three kinds of prayers:

1. From the social point of view:

a) Personal prayer
b) Collective prayer
c) Universal prayer

2. From the spiritual point of view:

a) Prayer for the self
b) Selfless prayer
c) Destructive prayer

Explanation of prayers from a social point of view:

a) Personal prayer

Personal prayer is one where the person himself surrenders to God. In this kind of prayer, the divine qualities of God and the wish to receive God's grace is expressed in the form of prayer. For example,

त्वमेव माता च पिता त्वमेव, त्वमेव बन्धुश्च सखा त्वमेव।
त्वमेव विद्या द्रविड़म् त्वमेव, त्वमेव सर्वम् मम देव-देव।।

b) Collective prayer

A prayer which is done in a group or between the guru and disciple for the welfare of the group is called a collective prayer. A good example is found in the Vedas and Upanishads.

Example: The following prayer said by a guru and his disciple in the *Atharva Veda* is a beautiful example of a collective prayer.

सहनाभवतु, सहनौ भुनक्तु, सहवीर्यम् करवावहै।
तेजस्विनावधीतमस्तु मा विद्विषावहै, ॐ शांति शांति शांतिः।।

c) Universal prayer

This is a prayer which is done for the welfare of the entire world. In this prayer, there are no personal aspirations or expectations in the heart of the person who is praying. He/she prays selflessly for the welfare of the world.

Example,

सर्वेभवन्तु सुखिनः सर्वे सन्तु निरामयाः।
सर्वे भद्राणि पश्यन्तु, मा कश्चित् दुःखभागभवेत्।।

From the spiritual perspective, there are three types of prayers.

a) Selfish prayer or prayer for the self

Selfish prayer is a prayer done with the intention of happiness, health, money, and victory for the self and the near and dear ones. A prayer with the motive of improving someone is done in the following manner:

सुधरे वह सुशील बन, पालन कर आचार।
कर्म धर्म में रत रहे, सब कुव्यसन निवार।।

b) Selfless prayer

Selfless prayer is done to awaken one's consciousness, cleansing the mind, purify the heart and expiate the sins, and for the well being, health, happiness and upgradation of others without any selfish intention. Though the above mentioned intensions are a kind of wish, they are worldly desires. The one who is praying has no personal benefit in mind. Therefore, it is a selfless prayer. A prayer which is done for the well-being of others and for self-development helps a person achieve higher goals of self-realisation. Such prayers can also be done for the progress and welfare of the country.

Example: The following prayer can be said for the welfare of the self:

जगे चेतना विमलतम, हो सत्य सुप्रकाश।
शांति सर्व आनंद हो, पाप ताप का नाश।।

बुद्धि वृद्धि, विवेक, बल, आत्म बल बढ़ जाए।
सदिच्छा मानस बल बढ़े, धृति धर्म को पाए।।

In the same way, a selfless prayer can be said for the progress of the nation in the following way:

सदाचार सत्कर्म का, करें पालन सब लोग।
मेल एकता साध के, हरे देश के रोग।।

c) Destructive prayer

A prayer which is directed towards the destruction of the enemy or to harm someone is called a destructive prayer. Such a prayer is done under the influence of selfish actions like cardinal desires, anger, pride, greed, attachment, etc. Such prayers are of a low category because they do not benefit anyone; rather it lowers the spiritual status of the person.

To pray in order to harm someone or to cause someone harm, to physically harm someone, to pray for somebody's monetary loss, to pray for injustice towards someone, to pray to free a criminal etc. are considered as prayers of low category and hence, banned by the learned men and sages.

The Utility and Significance of Prayer in Daily Life

Prayers have great significance in the life of a person. The various situations of prayer not only give us support but also liberate us from fear. Prayers provide us with the base to live our life, and additionally influence our entire personality.

1. Means To Attain Total Good Health

There are three aspects of a person's total health. The first is physical health which is bulky; the second is mental health which is subtle, and the third is spiritual health which is related to the soul. There is a deep traditional relationship and coordination between these three. In the absence of prayer, the spiritual aspect is constantly neglected. Resultantly, the soul is filled with sorrow and then the mind becomes restless, unstable and sorrowful. If this situation persists for a long time, many psychological diseases such as worry, fear, mental depression etc. emerge. These diseases give rise to high blood pressure, diabetes, heart diseases, hysteria, diseases of the stomach like disorders of wind, etc.

Prayers give strength and power to the soul which help us face tension, confusion as well as unfavourable circumstances and turn them in our favour. With regular and constant prayer, we gain the strength to fight against our diseases and eventually, the ill-effects of the diseases decrease. This helps us cure the diseases quickly. Hence, it is clear that regular prayer strengthens all the three aspects of a person's health and leads him/her to total good health.

2. Means of Knowing the Self

One of the main objectives of prayer is the progress of the conscience. First the sadhaka does penance to expiate his/her sins, and then resolves to never indulge in sinful acts again. Prayer is like a dutiful guard in the life of a sadhaka who prohibits thieves and anti-social elements to come near the house. Repeated prayers give the sadhaka a chance to do repeated self-evaluation. This helps him know where he/she went wrong in between the two successive prayers. When the sadhaka sits in meditation in this manner, he/she regrets his/her wrong deeds and resolves to never indulge in those sins. Just as bathing and taking medicines cleanse and treat our bodies and internal systems, prayers treat and cure the soul or the conscience.

3. Means To Attain Spiritual Capabilities

Prayer not only works as a treatment, but also grants us spiritual capabilities. Regular prayer puts an end to the restlessness of the mind and helps it reach a state of stability. The sadhaka gains control over the tendencies of the mind. The level of mental concentration also increases gradually and the ego is destroyed. Thus, prayer takes the sadhaka to great heights where he/she can experience the omnipresence of God and is able to establish contact with the Supreme.

4. Means To Attain Salvation

By regular and continuous prayer, we gains control over the tendencies of our mind. Along with the control over the mind and the heart, prayer provides such a divine protection to the sadhaka that it fills him/her with a feeling of pride when the materialistic distractions unsuccessfully try to lure him/her during dhyana and other practices of the higher order. In such a situation, our pride and ego can be ceased through prayer.

There are many examples of great people who have exhibited great coordination and balance even in the most dire and sorrowful circumstances of their life. Jesus, while being crucified, prayed for forgiveness of those who were killing him, thereby proving the omnipresence of God and being liberated from his physical agonies. Mahatma Gandhi played a significant role in India's freedom struggle, through non-violence and truth, on the basis of the power of prayer.

If we seriously consider the utility of prayer, we will find that in the modern world prayer is used as a medicine to treat many serious diseases. Researches on *Om* have proved that through prayer (chanting *Om*), illnesses like high blood pressure and low blood pressure can be cured and the person can be brought back to his/her normal condition.

Stress, Confusion and Despair

In modern times, the main reasons for most of the mental illnesses are stress, confusion and despair. When we wish to make a permanent position for ourselves in the society, try to live upto the expectations and values of our family as well as the society's. Resultantly, we fail to fulfill our own desires and such situations give rise to stress.

Meaning of Stress

In psychology, the word stress is used in context of reason and impact.

Stimuli as the Reason for Mental Stress

Stress is related to stimuli. An event or factor which generates or creates stress is called a stimulus. These stimuli are physical, social and psychological. Fatigue, pain, illness etc. are physical stimuli. The social factors leading to mental disorders are categorised as social stimuli, such as poverty, unemployment, untouchability, etc. The psychological stimuli are events which create mental disturbance, such as losing a job, death of a dear one, marital disturbances, etc.

Stimulus as an Impact of Mental Stress

Stress is related to the mental situation or psychology. It means that stress is the impact of an event or its result but not the reason. Various scientists have defined stress in different ways. The definitions given by Reiths and Nevid, 1991, Rebar, 1995, and Davidson and Neil, 1996 are more acceptable and popular.

Types of Stress

On the basis of intensity:	1. Low
	2. High
On the basis of duration:	1. Short term
	2. Long term
On the basis of consciousness:	1. Conscious stress
	2. Unconscious stress
On the basis of direction:	1. Directed towards work
	2. Directed towards the self/ego

Reasons for Stress in Modern Life

In today's competitive social environment, a person experiences stress due to various reasons. He/she feels tired and bored after a busy day, an irregular schedule and by his/her failed attempt to establish coordination between various demands of daily life. He/she feels that life is no longer enjoyable and normal. He/she is not able to solve the problems related to family, neighbours and work place. As a result, he/she gets more tensed. Some of the main reasons for stress are:

1. The day-to-day problems

(a) Family problems, (b) Problems related to health, (c) Problems of the pressure of time, (d) Internal problems, (e) Environmental problems, (f) Problems related to monetary responsibilities, (g) Professional problems, (h) Problems related to a secure future

2. Change in life

A sudden, unwanted change in life is also one of the main reasons for stress.

3. Pain and troubles

Physical problems or diseases

4. Frustration and confusion

When one is unable to fulfill one's own necessities or those of the family, one starts feeling frustrated which later becomes stress. Confusion might also lead to stress.

5. Natural and technological calamities

This is one of the major reasons for stress in modern life. Storms, flood, blasts, epidemics, etc. are some of the examples of natural calamities which have a direct impact on life. People are affected by them and therefore, become prone to stress.

The calamities generated by technology also create great problems, such as Bhopal gas tragedy, fire in the Jaipur Petrol Depot, atomic explosion, etc. affect people living many kilometers away from the spot of the tragedy, and hence, create stress in their lives.

Confusion or Struggle

1. Advent (Advent struggle): This happens when a person faces two strong goals and is not able to decide which one to achieve first , such as whether to eat first or to go to sleep. The solution to such dilemma is easy. The person should first eat food and then go to sleep.

2. Avoidance (Avoidance struggle): This kind of dilemma offers two choices. For example, if there is a lion on one side and a cliff on the other, which should the person choose? Most people try to choose a third alternative.

3. Advent (Avoidance struggle): In this situation, a person is stuck between the positive and negative goals and it becomes difficult to choose between the two. For example, a person you consider your enemy has invited you to dinner. In such a case, if you refuse to go, you will be called unsocial and uncultured and if you accept the invitation, you will hurt your ego.

The Sources of Struggle

1. Broken families
2. Faulty tendencies of the parents
3. Faulty education system
4. Incorrect professional planning
5. Social prohibitions/taboos
6. Contradictory cultural values
7. Contradictory form of Id and super ego

The word 'frustration' is derived from a Latin word meaning 'waste'.

Factors of Frustration

External factors	Internal factors
1. Worldly factors 2. Social factors 3. Economic factors	1. Physical problems 2. Mental problems 3. Contradictory desires or objectives/goals 4. Very high level of aspiration 5. Weak ego 6. Wrong mental attitude 7. Lack of honesty and firmness

Reactions to Despair

Depending on the degree, factors and types of despair, a person expresses his/her reaction towards frustration. These reactions are of two types:

Ordinary reaction

1. Increase in effort
2. Compromise with the situation
3. Make fun of the situation
4. Humility
5. Change the goal

Quick or impulsive response

1. Internal violence: The person can go to the extent of committing suicide.

2. External violence: The person starts scolding or beating other people.

Ways to Get Rid of Frustration and Dilemma

Mental struggles are of two types: Conscious struggles and unconscious struggles. In conscious struggle the person is aware of the struggle and is also aware of the form and result of the struggle. Unconscious struggle happens on the unconscious level and the person is not even aware of it. It is comparatively easier to face and find a solution to conscious struggles, whereas unconscious struggles are very complicated and their solutions are also very difficult to arrive at.

Solutions to conscious struggles

1. The state of debate
2. The state of decision
3. The state of determination
4. Apparent behaviour

Solution to unconscious struggles

This is a mental process by which a person faces the frustrations unconsciously. These are also called defense mechanisms. Through this process, a person finds the solution to his/her mental frustration caused due to the contradictory tendencies of the Id and the Super ego. The Ego tries to save itself from worry and stress. Therefore, they are called as ego defenses.

Types of defense mechanisms

1. Repression
2. Transformation
3. Sublimation
4. Rationalisation
5. Regression
6. Reaction formation

Lower defense mechanisms

1. Displacement
2. Projection
3. Identification
4. Internal projection
5. Compensation
6. Denial and taboo

The Impact of Meditation on the Mind

The main objective of meditation is to bring stability to the mind which is generally unstable and unfocussed. An unstable mind is not suitable for taking any decision. In fact, it increases the intensity of the problem and one gets entangled in a tough situation. A disturbed mind can rarely gain benefit from a given situation. It is generally unsuccessful.

Everyone wants peace. However, it is not possible to find it as long as we have desires in our heart. These endless desires are the cause of all the turmoil within us. While interacting with the society, the mind is always distracted and restless. If a person wants peace while being in the society, he/she must take refuge in meditation otherwise, he/she must run away from the given situation.

According to Indian sages, soul or conscience is the main source of knowledge. This knowledge flows freely from our heart when the mind experiences absolute peace and is directed inwards. The instability of the mind closes many doors of knowledge, whereas a calm and introvert mind opens many new paths towards knowledge. In other words, in order to gain knowledge a certain state of mind is required, which is stable, calm, concentrated and directed inwards. Otherwise, the mind would be diverted towards other fantasies. The only way to empty the mind of all fantasies and imagination is meditation. It makes the mind tolerant, calm, subtle and light. By doing meditation regularly, peace is established in the mind. It awakens qualities such as grace, humility, courage and patience. The relaxation that is attained from meditation frees the mind of all the stress and tension. A distressed mind is filled with hope. In short, one can say that meditation gives a fresh new life to the mind.

The mind attains both worldly as well as spiritual benefits from meditation. When it is extrovert, it gains worldly benefits, and when it is introvert, it gains spiritual benefits. In order to lead a life of excellence in this world, both the types of achievements are important. When we concentrate our mind on a particular subject every day, our abilities and potential in that subject are enhanced. It is this science of meditation which is used to enhance the capabilities of the mind. It has been seen that the capabilities of the minds of writers, artists, musicians, painters, singers and scientists are enhanced through this method of focusing. Consciously or unconsciously, everyone's mind is focused all the time, but it is not focused on one subject or topic to enhance the inherent potential pertaining to it. People, who do physical labour as well as those who do intellectual labour, both achieve power and peace through meditation.

When we do meditation, alpha rays are emitted from the brain which generates peace and creativity in the mind. Those who do not use meditation as a tool are often seen to resort to drugs to fall sleep or for peace of mind, but it has its own side effects. By meditation, the working of the right and left sides of the brain is balanced. The metabolic activities of the brain function efficiently. It has been observed that by doing meditation, the perception of the sense organs and the understanding capacity of the brain develop amazingly. The memory, emotional sympathy and the quality of sleep are enhanced, and there is a decrease in unnecessary worry and harmful addictions. Meditation proves to be very helpful in changing our habits and forming new habits.

Why is there so much adversity in spirituality regarding the mind and the thoughts? Because it is the mind which is the main cause of attachment and liberation, sorrow and happiness. In its absence, there is neither binding, nor liberation, neither happiness, nor sorrow. Through meditation, one can attain a state where the mind is at peace and is in total surrender to God.

Misconceptions Related to Yoga

There are many misconceptions in this society regarding yoga. Generally, it is popularly believed that yoga is related only to some special people or some yogis or sanyasis. This knowledge or skill is very difficult and is meant only for certain people. Ordinary people cannot use it or know about it. This is a completely incorrect interpretation. Quite contrary to this, yoga is an easy and simple path to follow. Yoga plays a special role in keeping our body and mind beautiful, clean and healthy.

Yoga has been scientifically developed as an art of living which can be understood clearly from the following table:

1. Is yoga not meant for the common man?

S. No.	Misconception	Fact
1.	Yoga is meant only for sages and recluses.	Yoga can be adopted by everyone from sages to the common man.
2.	It is necessary to observe celibacy in order to practice yoga.	Married people too can do yoga.
3.	One has to leave his/her family and live in seclusion to practice yoga.	One can practice yoga while having a family too.
4.	Yoga is related only to the Hindu religion.	Yoga is an experimental and practical skill. It cannot be related to any caste, religion or community. Hence, everyone can use yoga for one's personal progress.

2. Only asanas and pranayama are yoga

There is another misconception regarding yoga that only asanas and pranayama are yoga. Most people believe that only asana and pranayama are yoga and practice only these two aspects of it, whereas yoga is a very wide subject. Its goal is salvation, which is the pinnacle of the development of any person. Maharishi Patanjali framed the practice of yoga expanding it from Yama till Samadhi in the form of Ashtanga Yoga, out of which Yama and Niyama are only two parts. Hence, only asanas and pranayama are not yoga. Yoga takes us much beyond these aspects and makes us achieve much greater heights.

3. Yoga is a miracle

There is another misconception about yoga that it is a miracle or that to achieve it is miraculous. This is nothing but a proof of our misguided thinking because yoga is not at all related to any miracle. On the contrary, yoga considers miracle as an obstacle in moving ahead on the path of sadhana. The siddhis which are mentioned in yoga are actually a warning for the sadhaka, and not as a miracle. Hence, we can say that yoga is not a miracle.

4. Yoga is a method of treatment/medical science

Since ancient times, various meanings and uses of yoga have been propagated by man. Out of these, one is that yoga is a method of treatment or a medical science. Whereas the truth is that just as an insects gets grinded with the grain automatically; similarly, in order to achieve the ultimate goal of yoga, i.e. salvation, various aspects of yoga are used. This leads to the treatment of various diseases and total physical health. However, it does not mean that yoga is a medical science.

5. Yoga is only a philosophy

Since yoga is the topic of discussion amongst many scientists and philosophers, and its facts are put to use by them, there is a general opinion amongst common people that yoga is a subject of philosophy in which one discusses God, soul, salvation, etc. On the contrary, yoga discusses these topics merely to enlighten our path so that the path we are moving on is clear to us and we have it knowledge. Since it is also an experimental and practical subject, we can say it is not merely a philosophy.

6. Yoga is a method of doing exercise

This is a general opinion of people that yoga is a method of doing exercise which is used to gain physical health. This is an absolutely wrong notion, because the objective of yoga is not to merely gain physical health but to gain mental and spiritual health as well. Yoga works on all these aspects of health. Body is the basic foundation of life which helps us reach the ultimate goal of Kaivalya. Therefore, it is very important to keep it healthy. That is why physical kriyas are added, but this doesn't mean that yoga is a method of exercise. The goal of yoga is much higher than that.

Conclusion

Conclusively, we can see that yoga is a simple and easy skill which can be adopted by anyone to gain benefits, irrespective of religion, caste or creed, whether he is a recluse or a family man or a bramhachari. Therefore, in the light of all the above mentioned misconceptions and the related facts, we can easily give up misguided notions and adopt a new and positive perspective of yoga.

Impact of the Misconceptions on Our Mind

The misconceptions in the minds of people are reflected in their influences, it further makes yoga and the yogi infamous. The impact of such misconceptions can be understood by the following points:

1. Passiveness or disinterest towards yoga
2. Fear of the yogic kriyas and their other aspects
3. Confusion about the final goal of yoga
4. To look down upon yoga and yogi with contempt
5. Disinterest towards yogic text

The Sources of Misconceptions

1. Imagination or hearsay

To make an impression about yoga on the basis of mere imagination, or creating a misconception after hearing something from someone, or to talk nonsense about yoga is one of the reasons for these misconceptions.

2. Show off or dressing sense

Generally, we form an opinion regarding the outer appearance of a yogi and view anything related to yoga or a yogi from that perspective.

For example: A yogi has a beard and long flowing hair.

A yogi wears white or saffron clothes.

3. Differences in tradition and narrow view point

Right from the time of Maharishi Patanjali, yoga has been understood and taught by various people using different methods. As a result, there has been confusion. People become overconfident about their own methods, giving rise to a narrow point of view.

4. Partial understanding of the subject

Various discourses undertaken by those who have no practical or textual knowledge of yoga give rise to a partial understanding of the subject.

5. Difference in schools of thought

Due to a difference in the theories of different schools of thought or cults, the disciples of those schools grasp the subject according to their capacity and belief, and further propagate the same. This gives rise to difference and confusion.

6. Immature intellect

Adapting incomplete knowledge and following it continuously results in a person becoming headstrong and gives rise to an immature intellect.

7. Narrow definitions

Yoga is a complete science. But due to our rigidity or the tendency to prove ourselves as right, our definition of yoga brings to light only such facts which we deem true or significant. Such definitions come under the category of narrow definitions.

8. Disbelief in the goal and the means of yoga

Most people have no idea about what yoga is, or what can be

gained from yoga. Due to incomplete knowledge about these aspects, when we form our own means and goals of yoga, we give rise to a serious lack of understanding regarding the goals and means of yoga.

9. Difficulty in understanding the significance of the various aspects of yoga

Most people do not know what are the aspects of yoga, even after learning and doing yoga for many years. They have no idea about their significance or the reason behind their sequence. Therefore, when they speak about yoga in a confusing manner, it gives rise to misconceptions.

Solutions

The ways to solve the problem of misconception related to yoga are as follows:

1. Propagate a positive view point about yoga.
2. Motivate and inspire society to read yogic text.
3. Propagate the correct information and knowledge pertaining to yoga.
4. Show and exhibit the asanas and kriyas of yoga along with their benefits.
5. Translate the text on yoga in simple and easy languages to popularise them in the society.
6. Teach not to use the attainable aspect of yoga for monetary benefits.

Hasya Yoga Chikitsa

(Yoga Therapy through Laughter)

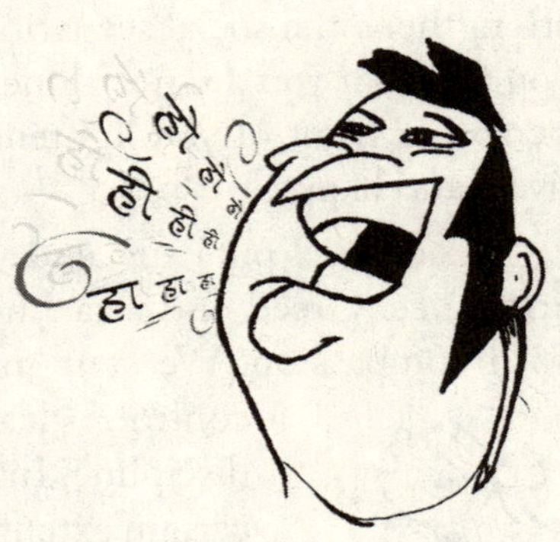

We must simply laugh and make others laugh: Ha – ha – ha . . . hi – hi – hi . . . ho – ho – ho . . .

Nowadays, people seem to have forgotten how to laugh. However, laughter is as important for our body and health as food. Gradually, man is forgetting many natural things and as a result is becoming prey to various disorders. Some people are of the opinion that if they laugh, people might form an impression that they are comedians or that they are not serious. So, they do not laugh at all. Seniors in the office often think that if they sit and laugh with their junior employees, the juniors would think that they have no class. All these things are baseless and meaningless. When we laugh, many things are triggered simultaneously. The entire environment transforms; the atmosphere becomes light and fragrant with the purity of our heart. Every face lights up with a smile. The whole body experiences tremors which affect the abdominal region as well as the digestive system and makes it function efficiently. Our breath becomes regulated, which is beneficial for those suffering from both low and high blood pressure. The force of air clears up the lungs and increases the circulation of blood. The heart too starts functioning efficiently. All the 72,000 nerves open up. This alone gives us the benefits of many exercises. Laughter is contagious. When we laugh, the person in front of us also laughs. When we smile, the other person smiles too. However angry a person may be, when we give them a lovely smile, they become happy. Many difficult jobs become easier to perform with a happy disposition. So, laugh aloud; laugh to your heart's content. It will help you get rid of many problems and tensions. You would feel a new energy being generated in your body. Laughter is a natural treatment which drives all the negativity and ill feelings out of your being. Perhaps this is the only process where the give and take is done without any monetary exchange. In this process, the more you give, the more it multiplies. It also strengthens the social scenario because when you laugh together, you feel that you are not alone. When you have a happy face, the person in front of you lightens up and the atmosphere becomes lively and happy.

Laughter puts an end to anger. It destroys pride and arrogance. Greed and attachment vanish and our heart is filled with compassion. We start moving on the path of forgiveness, control, cleanliness, penance, humility and discipline. In this way, we become spiritual to a certain extent.

So, let us all make laughter an integral part of our lives. Let us laugh and make others laugh. Let us fill not only our body, mind and soul, but also our neighbourhood, society, country and the entire world with bliss, happiness and purity.

Come on, let us laugh aloud: Ha – ha – ha . . . hi – hi – hi . . . ho – ho – ho . . .

शांति पाठ

ॐ असतो मा सद्गमय,
तमसो मा ज्योतिर्गमय, मृत्योर्माऽमृतंगमय।
लोका: समस्ता: सुखिनो भवन्तु।
ॐ त्रयम्बकं यजामहे सुगन्धिम् पुष्टिवर्धनम्।
उर्वारुकमिव बन्धनात्मृत्योर्मुक्षीयमाऽमृतात।।
ॐ शान्ति:शान्ति:शान्ति:

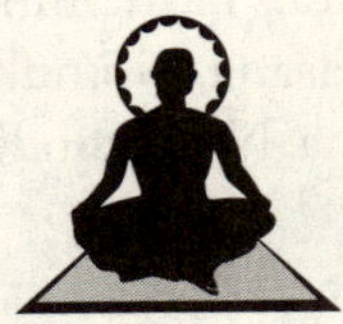

Which Asanas Should be Done for Which Disease

Asthma

Asana of the Sheershasana group, Sarvangasana, Bhujangasana, Shalabhasana, Dhanurasana, Veerasana, Ushtrasana, Paryankasana, Pashchimottanasana, Supta Veerasana, Nadi-shodhana Pranayama, Uddiyana bandha, Yoga Nidra

High Blood Pressure

Padmasana, Pashchimottanasana, Siddhasana, Pavanmuktasana, Nadi-shodhana Pranayama (do not do kumbhaka), Sheetkari, Ujjayi, Yoga Nidra

Meditate on God with a calm mind; eat vegetarian food without oil and spices

Low Blood Pressure

Salamba Sheershasana, Sarvangasana, Halasana, Karna Peedasana, Veerasana, Surya Namaskara, Shashankasana, Nadi-shodhana Pranayama, Bhastrika, Kapal-bhati, Surya Bhedana Pranayama, Shavasana

Diabetes

Sheershasana and asanas of this group, Surya Namaskara, Sarvangasana, Mahamudra, Pashchimottanasana, Ushtrasanas, Supta Vajrasana, Bhujangasana, Gomukhasana, Halasana, Ardha Matsyendrasana, Shavasana, Nadi-shodhana Pranayama (without antahkumbhaka)

Headache

Padmasana, Sheershasana, Halasana, Sarvangasana, Pavanmuktasana, Pashchimottanasana, Vajrasana, Marjari Asana, Nadi-shodhana Pranayama (without kumbhaka), Yoga Nidra

Fits

Halasana, Mahamudra, Pashchimottanasana, Shashankasana, Bhujangasana, Nadi-shodhana (without kumbhaka), Ujjayi with antahkumbhaka, Sheetali Pranayama, Yoga Nidra; eat vegetarian food and do meditation

Migraine

Sheershasana, Sarvangasana, Pashchimottanasana, meditation in Padmasana or Siddhasana, Veerasana, Shavasana, Nadi-shodhana Pranayama (without kumbhaka), Yoga Nidra

Diseases of the chest

Surya Namaskara, Sheershasana, Sarvangasana, Bhujangasana, Dhanurasana, Padmasana, Akarna Dhanurasana, Pashchimottanasana, Ardha Matsyendrasana, Bakasana, Baddhakonasana, Chakrasana, Kapotasana, Natarajasana, Asanas done by bending backwards, Ujjayi and Nadi-shodhana Pranayama, Yoga Nidra

Pain in the waist

Asanas done in the standing position and by bending backwards, Supta Vajrasana, Dhanurasana, Bhujangasana, Ardha Matsyendrasana, Parvatasana, Sarvangasana, Sheershasana, Chakrasana, Nadi-shodhana Pranayama

For the development of the brain and memory

Sheershasana and asanas of this group, Sarvangasana, Pashchimottanasana, Uttanasana, Yoga Mudrasana, Pada Hastasana, meditation in Padmasana or Siddhasana, ordinary Trataka, Shavasana, Nadi-shodhana Pranayama, Surya Bhedana and Bhastrika Pranayama, Yoga Nidra

Stomach ache

Sheershasana, Sarvangasana, Halasana, Uttanasana, Veerasana, Supta Veerasana, Vajrasana, Naukasana (In case of navel displacement, do the asanas meant for curing it.)

Kidney

Surya Namaskara, Sarvangasana, Sheershasana and asanas of this group, Halasana, Pashchimottanasana, Ushtrasana, Shalabhasana, Dhanurasana, Ardha Naukasana, Matsyendrasana, Bhujangasana, Hanumanasana, Kapotasana

To cure impotency and maintain vitality

Sheershasana and asanas of this group, Sarvangasana, Uttanasana, Pashchimottanasana, Mahamudrasana, Ardha Matsyendrasana, Hanumanasana, Kapal-bhati, Anuloma-viloma, Nadi-shodhana Pranayama (with antahkumbhaka), Uddiyana bandha, Vajroli mudra and Vipareetkarni mudra

Laziness/Lethargy

Sheershasana, Sarvangasana, Pashchimottanasana, Uttanasana, Nadi-shodhana Pranayama (without kumbhaka)

Loose motion

Sheershasana and asanas of this group, Sarvangasana, Janusheershasana, Nadi-shodhana Pranayama (without kumbhaka); check the position of the navel

Ulcers of the intestine

Sheershasana and asanas of this group, Sarvangasana, Pashchimottanasana, Yoga Nidra, Ardha Matsyendrasana, Ujjayi and Nadi-shodhana Pranayama, Uddiyana bandha with antahkumbhaka

Ulcers of the stomach

Vajrasana, Dhanurasana, Chakrasana, Mayurasana, Naukasana, Padhastasana, Uttanasana, Padangushthasana, Shalabhasana

Hernia

Sheershasana and asanas of this group, Sarvangasana, Akarna Dhanurasana

For the testicles

Sheershasana and asanas of this group, Sarvangasana, Hanumanasana, Samkonasana, Pashchimottanasana, Baddhakonasana, Yoga Mudrasana, Bramhacharyasana, Vatayanasana, Vajrasana, Garudasana

Pain/disorders of the heart

Shavasana, Ujjayi Pranayama (without kumbhaka), Yoga Nidra, Dhyana in Shavasana or Sukhasana, Nadi-shodhana Pranayama (without kumbhaka)

Diseases of the stomach such as constipation, gas, indigestion, difficulty in motions, acidity and disorders of the wind; bad breath

Sheershasana and asanas of this group, Sarvangasana, Naukasana, Pashchimottanasana, Matsyendrasana, Dhanurasana, Bhujangasana, Mayurasana, Yoga Mudrasana, Uttanasana, Padmasana, all asanas done in standing position, Vajrasana, Pavanmuktasana and related asanas, Trikonasana, Mahamudra, Shalabhasana, Matsyasana, Ardha Chandrasana, Shashankasana, Padangushthasana, and Shankha-prakshalana asanas; check for naval displacement

Joint disorders, pain in the joints/spine/shoulders/arthritis

Sheershasana and asanas of this group, Sarvangasana, Padmasana, Siddhasana, Veerasana, Paryankasana, Gomukhasana, Uttanasana, Pashchimottanasana, kriyas of the Pavanmuktasana group

Teeth/gums/pyorrhea/baldness/freshness of the face/wrinkles/ordinary eye disorders

Sheershasana and asanas of this group, Sarvangasana, Halasana, Vipareetkarani mudra, Pashchimottanasana, Shalabhasana, Vajrasana, all the asanas done by balancing on the head, Bhujangasana, Surya Namaskara, Simhasana, a series of eye exercises

Obesity

Specific exercises which provide energy, Surya Namaskara, Sheershasana and asanas of this group, Sarvangasana, Halasana, kriyas of the Pavanmuktasana group, Vipareetkarani mudra and all the asanas meant for indigestion and other stomach disorders. Be very particular about the diet

Lungs

Sheershasana and asanas of this group, Sarvangasana, Padmasana, Surya Namaskara, Lolasana, Veerasana, asanas done in the standing position, Chakrasana, Dhanurasana, all pranayamas with antahkumbhaka

Slip disc/sciatica/pain in the waist, spine and cervical/spondylitis

Asanas done in the standing position and by bending backwards such as Bhujangasana, Shalabhasana, Dhanurasana, Uttanpadasana, Vajrasana, Supta Vajrasana, Gomukhasana, Tadasana, Utkatasana, Makarasana

For increasing height

Tadasana, Surya Namaskara, Dhanurasana, Halasana, Sarvangasana, Pashchimottanasana

Paralysis/polio

Shalabhasana, Dhanurasana, Makarasana, Bhujangasana, Padmasana, Siddhasana, Kandhasana, Halasana, Sarvangasana, Shavasana, Ujjayi and Nadi-shodhana Pranayama.

It is best if the patient visits a doctor and after consultation, does the relevant yogasanas. Generally, polio is acquired at birth and paralysis after infancy. Ayurvedic medicines and yoga will be beneficial depending on how old the disease is.

Anemia

Sheershasana and asanas of this group, Sarvangasana, Pashchimottanasana, Surya Namaskara, Ujjayi Pranayama, Nadi-shodhana Pranayama, Kapal-bhati Pranayama

Piles

If you have constipation, get that treated first. Then, do Sheershasana and asanas of this group, Sarvangasana, Halasana, Vipareetkarani mudra, Matsyasana, Simhasana, Shalabhasana, Dhanurasana, Ujjayi without kumbhaka, and Nadi-shodhana Pranayama

Cough

Sheershasana and asanas of this group, Sarvangasana, Uttanasana, if suffering from cold, do Surya Namaskara, Pashchimottanasana, Ardha Matsyendrasana, along with these, see the asanas for asthma

Insomnia/worry/excitement/depression/ mental weakness

Surya Namaskara and asanas of this group, Sarvangasana, Koormasana, Pashchimottasana, Shashankasana, Yoga Mudrasana, Uttanasana, Bhastrika without kumbhaka, Nadi-shodhana and Surya Bhedhana Pranayama along with Bhramari, Moorchchha Sheetali and Sheetakari Pranayama, Yoga Nidra. You must read *Art of living through Yoga* and do specific exercises and kriyas that give energy

Irregular menstrual flow and diseases related to the overies

Sheershasana, Sarvangasana, Bhujangasana, Veerasana, Vajrasana, Shashankasana, Marjari Asana, Yoga Nidra, Nadi-shodhana Pranayama, Moola bandha, Uddiyana bandha, Vipareetkarani, Vajroli mudra, Yoni mudra and Yogmudrasana

Testis, urinary disorders

Sheershasana and asanas of this group, Sarvangasana, Halasana, Shalabhasana, Dhanurasana, Uttanasana, Naulasana, Supta Vajrasana, Baddha Konasana, Uddiyana bandha, Nadi-shodhana and Ujjayi Pranayama

Night fall

Sheershasana and asanas of this group, Sarvangasana, Pashchimottanasana, Baddha Konasana, Moola bandha, Vajroli mudra, Yoni mudra, Nadi-shodhana Pranayama (think positive). Wash your hands and feet with fresh water before going to bed at night and meditate on God

Disorders of the reproductive organs

Surya Namaskara, Vajrasana, Shashankasana, Ushtrasana, Tadasana, Uttanasana, Trikonasana, Yoga Mudrasana, Chakrasana, Tolangulasana, Dhanurasana, Makarasana, Veerasana, Dhanurakarshana Asana, Bramhacharya Asana, Mayurasana, and Kapal-bhati Pranayama

Pregnancy

Light exercises (yogic sookshma vyayama), Pavanmuktasana and related asanas, Pranayama without kumbhaka, do all the asanas under the guidance of a good trainer

Infertility

Sheershasana, Sarvangasana, Halasasana, Pashchimottanasana, Padmasana/Siddhasana, Chakrasana, Garudasana, Vatayanasana, all mudras (Vajroli Mudra, Yoni Mudra), Nadi-shodhana Pranayama, Kapal-bhati Pranayama

For women

For excessive menstrual flow: Baddha Konasana, Veerasana, Janusheershasana, Pashchimottanasana, Uttanasana and all the kriyas of the Pavanmuktasana group. Women should read the chapter on related diseases

For weak people

Pray everyday (with a heartfelt feeling) and adopt the prayer practically in your life, Pranayama, Anuloma-viloma (for a minimum of 10-15 minutes every morning), meditation during sunrise, light exercises (as per the disease), Padmasana and asanas of the medium level, see tips on total health, follow the chart on what to eat in which month, use wheat sprout in your diet

Asanas to enhance beauty

Tadasana, Vajrasana, Padmasana, Surya Namaskara, Matsyasana, Trikonasana, Marjari Asana, Uttanasana, Koormasana, Bhujangasana, Chakrasana, Dhanurasana, Pashchimottanasana, Gomukhasana, Tiryaka Bhujangasana, Meru Vakrasana, Sarvangasana, Halasana, Naukasana, Pavanmuktasana, Markatasana, Anuloma-viloma Pranayama, Kapala-bhati Pranayama, Bhastrika Pranayama, Yoga Nidra, Meditation

For total good health

Follow the rules given in this book, asanas of the Pavanmuktasana group, Sheershasana and related asanas, Sarvangasana, Halasana, Vipareetkarani mudra, Pashchimottasana, Dhanurasan, Tiryak Bhujangasana, Tiryaka Tadasana, Shalabhasana, Marjari Asana, Markatasana, Vyaghrasana (first variation), Padmasana, Yoga mudra, Moola bandha, Nadi-shodhana Pranayama, Vajroli, Yoni mudra, Mahamudrasana, Kapala-bhati and Bhastrika Pranayama

Note: The number of yogasanas is too much and therefore, it becomes very difficult to decide which asana to do and which not to do. We have given the list of asanas as per all the diseases/ categories. Do yogabhyasa under the guidance of an expert yoga guru, according to your flexibility, disease, season and convenience. Keep all these things in mind and get rid of all the diseases. Do not forget to read the benefits and precautions of the asanas and pranayamas.

Yoga helps in building purposeful life and
giving it a new direction.
–RJT

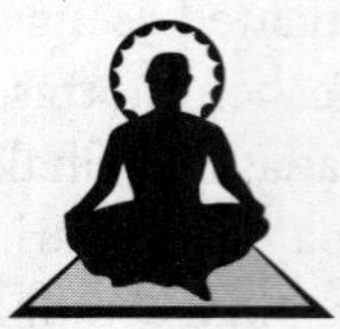

Which Asanas to Not Do and When

High blood pressure/giddiness/mental disorders/complicated heart diseases/chronic diseases related to the throat

Sheershasana, Halasana, Vipareetkarani, Dhanurasana, Sarvangasana (do not do it for a very long time), follow the precautions mentioned with each yogasana.

Pus formation in the ears/squinted eyes

Asanas with turning and rolling actions

Appendicitis/hernia

Pashchimottanasana, Yogmudrasana, asanas done by turning and bending backwards

Slip disc/sciatica/cervical pain

Asanas done by bending forward

During pregnancy

Do only those asanas which do not exert any pressure on the abdominal region. Consult an expert yoga teacher before doing the asanas

After pregnancy (delivery)

Do not do any asana till at least three months after the delivery. Afterwards, do light sookshma vyayama

For women

Never do any asana during menstruation, and asanas like Sarvangasana, Sheershasana should never be done.

Special note:

- Those who are suffering from high blood pressure, heart diseases or hernia and are unable to do the asanas properly should do them under the guidance of an expert yoga guru.
- After every asana, we have mentioned the diseases it can cure along with its other benefits. Please keep these in mind before doing the asana.
- All the asanas in yoga are beneficial, nevertheless, it is important for a person suffering from a particular disease to know which asana he/she should do and which he/she should not. Therefore, before doing yogabhyasa please read this book with concentration and wisdom.

Everyone must adopt yoga sadhana in his/her life.
However, it is preferential that a sadhaka first understands
all the facts about yogabhyasa and then puts it to practice.
This will give him/her more benefits.

–RJT

Exercise Schedule

(One Look)

It is not wise to prepare the same exercise schedule for everyone because everyone has a different built, age, body constitution, attitude and diseases. I have tried to make this book as complete as possible. Therefore, please read this book as many times as possible and prepare a list of asanas and pranayama suitable to you. To initiate you in to the schedule, I am categorising it under four headings:

Exercise for beginners: Under this category, those people are included who want to begin doing yoga, those who have a rigid body, or are suffering from some very complicated disease and therefore, cannot do asanas of the higher order. Pregnant women should also do simple exercises for the first 3-4 months, but they should also consult their doctor before starting the exercises.

First month, 1 hour: Yogic Sookshma Vyayama/asanas of the pavanmuktasana and energy-giving group (40 minutes). Anuloma-viloma pranayama (10 minutes); Shavasana/Hasya Yoga/Yoga Nidra (10 minutes)

Second month, 1 hour: Yogic Sookshma Vyayama/asanas of the Pavanmuktasana and energy-giving group (40 minutes); Anuloma-viloma/Ujjayi Pranayama (10 minutes); Makarasana, Shavasana, Yoga Nidra/Hasya Yoga (10 minutes)

Third month, 1 hour: Asanas of the Pavanmuktasana and energy-giving group (30 minutes); Vajrasana, Marjari Asana, Shavasana (15 minutes); Anuloma-viloma Pranayama, Ujjayi, Yoga Nidra, Hasya Yoga (15 minutes)

Medium level exercises

First month, 1 hour: Specific exercises of the pavanmuktasana and energy-giving group (15 minutes); Vajrasana, Marjari Asana, Vyaghrasana (first variation), Shashankasana, Bhujangasana,

Tadasana, Ardha Shalahasana (20 minutes); Anuloma-viloma, Ujjayi (15 minutes); Makarasana, Shavasana, Yoga Nidra, Hasya Yoga (10 minutes)

Second month, 1 hour or 80 minutes: Exercises of the Pavanmuktasana group (please choose according to your convenience), Surya Namaskara 2–3 rounds (15-20 minutes); Sukhasana, Ardha Padmasana, Vajrasana, Shashankasana, Bhujangasana, Tiryaka Bhujangasana, Shalabhasana, Tadasana, Trikonasana, Chakrasana, Dhanurasana, Hastpadasana, Shavasana, Ujjayi Pranayama, Bhramari Pranayama, Udgeetha Pranayama, Yoga Nidra, Hasya Yoga

Third month, 1 hour or 80 monutes: Surya Namaskara (2-3 rounds), Padmasana, Vajrasana, Supta Vajrasana, Shashankasana, Bhujangasana, Tiryaka Bhujangasana, Sarvangasana, Trikonasana, Chakrasana, Dhanurasana, Halasana, Matsyasana, Tadasana, Pashchimottanasana, Shavasana, Ujjayi, Kapala-bhati (slowly), Bhramari, Udgeetha Pranayama, Yoga Nidra, Hasya Yoga

Along with the exercises of the middle level, start some exercises of the higher level. The above mentioned exercise schedule has been prepared for an average person, it should be practiced under the guidance of a guru along with a lot of wisdom. The time limit for yoga is one to one and a half hours. This time must include asanas from all groups which will work together to cure various diseases.

We should do Sookshma Vyayama, Sthoola Vyayama, specific exercises and kriyas which provide energy, some kriyas from the Pavanmuktasana group, which the person feels are important, for about 10-15 minutes so that the body can be prepared for the next set of exercises. Then, start with Padmasana and related asanas of the group, followed by Tadasana and related asanas. However, one thing must be kept in mind, that whichever asana you do, you must also do the asanas of the opposite direction. By doing this, you can get rid of any complication which might have arise due to that particular asana. For example, if you do Sheershasana, then it should be followed by Tadasana; Dhanurasana should be followed by Pashchimottanasana, and if you sit in Padmasana with the left leg on the top, repeat it with the right leg on top. In this way, you should adopt yoga in your life by understanding all the processes thoroughly to gain total benefit.

Medium and higher level asanas: Prepare the list of medium level and higher level asanas according to your convenience.

Great yogis do not do different kriyas,
rather they do every kriya with a positive attitude.

–RJT

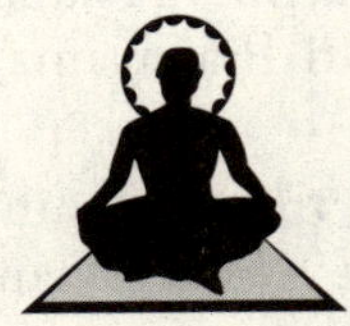

Asanas to be Done According to the Days of the Week

Monday: Kriyas to control the wind, Gatimaya Advasana, Gatimaya Gomukhasana, Makarasana, Gatimaya Makarasana, Sarpasana, Ardha Shalabhasana, Shalabhasana, Bhujangasana, Surya Namaskara, Anuloma-viloma Pranayama, Ujjayi Pranayama, Yoga Nidra; do Sookshma Vyayama for 10-15 minutes as per your convenience

Tuesday: Kriyas for the abdominal region, Tiryak Bhujangasana, Vipareet Naukasana, Pashchimottanasana, Gatimay Pashchimottanasana, Padmasana, Trilokasana, Gatimaya Trilokasana, Kati Vrittasana, Surya Namaskara, Anulom-viloma Pranayama, Ujjayi Pranayama, Yoga Nidra; do Sookshm Vyayam as per your convenience

Wednesday: Kriyas of Shaktibandha, Gomukhasana, Gatimaya Gomukhasana, Shalabhasana, Gatimaya Shalabhasana, Bhujangasana, Tiryaka Bhujangasana, Mendhaka Kooda, Murga Asanatmaka Kriya, Kati Vrittasana, Anuloma-viloma Pranayama, Udgeetha Pranayama, Kapala-bhati Pranayama, Yoga Nidra, do Sookshma Vyayama as per your convenience

Thursday: Kriyas to control the air, kriyas of Sookshma Vyayama as per your convenience, Padmasana,

Siddhasana, Vajrasana, Ananda Madirasana, Padadirasana, Marjari Asana, Tadasana, Trikonasana, Surya Namaskara, Ujjayi Pranayama, Kapala-bhati Pranayama, Bala Machalana Kriya, Yoga Nidra

Friday: Kriyas of the abdominal region, Padmasana, Muktasana, Shashankasana, Ushtrasana, Vyaghrasana (first variation), Tadasana, Trikonasana, Gatimaya Trikonasana, Padhastasana, Sarvangasana, Halasana, Pashchimottanasana, Udgeetha Pranayama, Ujjayi Pranayama, Kapala-bhati Pranayama, Yoga Nidra

Saturday: Kriyas of Shaktibandha, Tadasana, Tiryaka Tadasana, Kativrittasana, Padmasana, Baddha Padmasana, Pashchimottanasana, Sarvangasana, Halasana, Dhanurasana, Chakrasana, Marjari Asana, Vyaghrasana (first variation), Gomukhasana, Gatimaya Gomukhasana, Shashankasana, Mandookasana, Vajrasana, Surya Namaskara, Hasya Yoga, Ujjayi Pranayama, Bhastrika Pranayama, Kapala-bhati Pranayama, Yoga Nidra

Sunday: Kriyas of the Pavanmuktasana group (as per your convenience), energy-giving asanas, Padmasana, Baddha Padmasana, Vajrasana, Shashankasana, Mandookasana, Marjari Asana, Vyaghrasana (first variation), Pashchimottanasana, Gatimaya Pashchimottanasana, Sarvangasana, Halasana, Chakrasana, Dhanurasana, Bhujangasana, Tiryaka Bhujangasana, Tadasana, Tiryaka Tadasana, Bhastrika, Anuloma-viloma Pranayama, Yoga Nidra, Hasya Yoga

We have prepared this general list for an average person. You can consult a yoga teacher and practice the asanas according to your physical condition. Choose from the energy-giving exercises, asanas from the Pavanmuktasana group, Yogic Sookshma Vyayama and Sthoola Vyayama according to your condition and imply them in your life.

Yoga for Children

Whether it is an issue of physical development or the development of mental capacity of children, yoga is as important for them as sports or other activities.

Yoga should be made compulsory for the sake of their consistent development. Children can easily improve the flexibility and suppleness of their body by regular practice and eventually do the asanas of the higher level. By doing yogabhyasa everyday all the parts of their body start functioning effectively.

From the age of 8 years to 16 years, the life of a child is like soft wet clay. It can be molded in any shape. By teaching them Yama and Niyama in Ashtanga Yoga, we can make them well-cultured, thereby making their future brighter.

The best medium to fulfill physical and mental needs such as enhancing enhance the memory, increasing height, curing the disorders of the eye, is through complete yoga training. That is why children should adopt yoga in their lives.

We are presenting a short list of asanas for them: First and foremost, children should learn Yogic Sookshma Vyayama, followed by Yogic Sthoola Vyayama, kriyas of the Pavanmuktasana group and specific exercises and kriyas that provide energy for at least two to six months. This will make their bodies swift, provide freshness and firmness, and increase their interest in yoga.

Gradually light exercises, Anuloma-viloma Pranayama, Ujjayi, Bhramari, Udgeetha Pranayama and Yoga Nidra can be introduced. With regular practice, they will be able to awaken new self-confidence within themselves which would be nothing less than a great achievement for their future. Children can get a list of asanas prepared according to their interest and convenience and imbibe this skill in their lives.

Yoga for Women

Women are often worried about their health. Most women believe that they are suffering from some disease or the other. There are very few women who consider themselves healthy and fit. Nowadays, a woman's life is different as compared to the earlier times. Earlier women used to be engaged in household chores the entire day. And while doing them, they unknowingly did yogic kriyas. Getting up before sunrise, sweeping, cleaning, filling water, cleaning the grains, cooking food, grinding the grains on the mill, churning the curd, taking out butter and making ghee, etc. were some of the many jobs. They used to get tired at the end of the day, and as a result, get a good sound sleep. Nowadays, the environment has changed. Today's woman has started going out for work and is managing business too. Many have handed over the responsibility of the household to their servants. Most of the is being done through electronic gadgets. There are many other reasons due to which women have started becoming prone to various diseases like backache, obesity, hysteria, leukemia, headache, disorders of the wind, insomnia, white discharge, diabetes, heart diseases, constipation, arthritis and mental tension.

Yogabhyasa is the only medium which can provide total health and beauty to them. Therefore, it is very important for them to take out at least one hour for regular yogasana and pranayama. Read this book and choose your asana and pranayama according to your requirements. Women can do the following asanas and gain total good health.

Start with simple and easy asanas like Yogic Sookshma Vyayama, Yogic Sthoola Vyayama, asanas of the Pavanmuktasana group, asanas and kriyas which provide energy, Ardha Padmasana, Padmasana, Vajrasana, Shashankasana, Bhujangasana, Tiryaka Bhujangasana, Chakrasana, Shalabhasana, Makarasana, Gomukhasana, Ushtrasana, Tadasana, Tiryaka Tadasana, Padhastasana, Trikonasana, Hastottanasana, Pashchimottanasana, Mandookasana, Marjari Asana, Sarvangasana, Vipareetkarani, Shavasana, Yoga Nidra, etc. Women can do Nadi-shodhana Pranayama, Anuloma-viloma, Ujjayi, Bhastrika, Bhramari, Udgeetha and Kapala-bhati Pranayama and make themselves beautiful.

In this way women can become healthy and help their family members become healthy.

Yoga for Office Workers

People working in the office can bring a little change in their routine and gain health benefits. For example, as soon as you reach office, try to feel fresh mentally and sit joyfully on your chair. Keep your spine straight; close your eyes and chant *Om* or the name of your God. Inhale and exhale deeply, five times. Then, get ready for your work.

When you work on a desk, a lot of strain is exerted on the spine, neck, eyes and brain. So, you must change the way you sit on the chair. Keep your spine erect. When you work with a bent neck, disorders of the neck are bound to occur. Do Greeva Shakti Vikasaka Kriya for 2-5 minutes while sitting on your chair. Do not forget to do eye exercises, Yoga Nidra, Dhyana Yoga and Pranayama regularly for the development of the brain.

Spare 1 hour in the morning. Start with the easy exercises. Exercises of the Pavanmuktasana group, energy-giving exercises, Ardha Padmasana, Padmasana, Baddha Padmasana, Vajrasana, Shashankasana, Mandookasana, Bhujangasana, Tiryaka Bhujangasana, Chakrasana, Dhanurasana, Pashchimottanasana, Sarvangasana, Vipareetkarni, Tadasana, Tiryaka Tadasana and Anuloma-viloma, Ujjayi, Bhastrika, Kapala-bhati, Udgeetha, and Bhramari Pranayama should be incorporated in the routine. After these, do Yoga Nidra.

We have mentioned the above asanas and pranayamas in a simple manner. Please read the entire book and make a list of asanas and pranayamas according to your physical condition and diseases. Do these regularly with a happy disposition.

Contextual Text

Patanjal Yoga Pradeep, Gheranda Samhita, Vasishtha Samhita, Hatha Yoga Pradeepika, Maranyakantika, Skandapurana, Manusmriti, Shrimada Yoga Gita, Shrimada Bhagwata Gita, Yoga Tatvopnishada, Yoga Kundilyopnishada, Yoga Choodamani, Shandilyopnashishada, Koorma Purana Uttarardha, Gyanarnava, Samadhitantra, Lingapurana Poorvardha, Svara Vigyana, Vayu Purana, Markandeya Purana, Narada Purana, Agni Purana, Yoganka (Gita Press), Yogsaara, Yoga aur Ayurveda, Yoga Darshana, Shiva Samhita, Tantra Saar, Dhyana Bindu Upnishada, Amritasheeti – Shrimada Acharya Yogindu Deva, Yoga Vasishtha, Makundya Upanishada, Kalyana (Gita Press), Tantra Kriya aur Yoga Vidya – Swami Satyananda Sarawati, Shakti ka Jagarana aur Kundalini – M M P Gopinath Kaviraj, Savitri Kundalini Tantra – Shri Ram Sharma Acharya, American Yoga – Cary Schneider, Ayurvedic Chikitsa – Jha, Hatha Yoga Vidya – Swami Vigyananda Sarawati, Manava Shareera Rachna aur Shareera Kriya Vigyana – Vijay Kumar, Yogic Sookshma Vyayama – Dheerendra Bramhachari, Light on Yoga – B K S Iyengar, Food and Nutrition – Swaminathan, Nutrient Value of Indian Food – Rajgopalan, Anatomy and Physiology – Tora Tora, Prakritika Chikitsa: Siddhanta Evam Vyavahara – Dr P D Mishra, Yogasana – Swami Kuvalyananda, First step to Higher Yoga – Shri Yogeshwaranand Paramhans, Arogya Anka (Gita Press), Dhyana Vichara – Acharya Shri Vijay Kalapoorn Suriji, Statistics in Psychology and Education – Garret, Bharatiya Darshan – Radhakrishna, Foundation of Behaviours and Research – Kerrlinger, Samanya Manovigyan – Dr Arun Kumar, Patanjal Yoga Pradeep – Omanand Teerth, Office Yoga – Fred Burger, Theory of Personality – Swami Vidyanand Videh, Hatha Yoga Pradeepika – Svatmaram Yogi, Sadhanank (Gita Press), Svasthya Vritt – Ram Harsh Singh, Shiv Svarodaya – Tr HareKrishna Shastri, Yoga Saar Prabhoot – Acharya Amit Gati, Yoga Patha – Prabhuvad Swami, Yogshastra – Acharya Hemchandra, Moksha Pahuṇ – Acharya Shri Kund Kund Swami, Philosophy of Upanishad, Vasishth Samhita (Yoga Kanda) – Swami Digambarji, Yoga Darshan – Harikrishna Das, Yoga ke Siddhanta Evam Abhyasa – Dr Kalidas and Dr Ganesh Shankar, Kalyana Karaka – Ugradityacharya, Patanjal Yoga Evam Jain Yoga ka Tulanatmak Adhyayan – Aruna Anand, Yoga Darshana – Sampoornanad, Vivek Choodamani and Saundarya Lahri, Shandilya Upnishad – Jinendra Siddhant Khosh.

Conclusion

न धर्मस्य कर्ता न चार्थस्य हर्ता, न कामस्य भोक्ता न मोक्षस्य पाता।
नरो बुद्धिमान धीरसत्वोऽपि रोगी, यतस्तद्विनाशाद्भवेन्नैव मर्त्यः ।।

Kalyankarak

Shri Ugradityacharya maharaj

Meaning: A man might be intelligent and strong-willed but if he is sick, then he can neither do his duty (dharma) nor earn money (artha); he can neither enjoy the materialistic pleasures (kaama) nor attain salvation (moksha). In other words, he is unable to work towards the attainment of all the four goals of life. Such a person, even though he may have been born as a human being, is not worth being called one. The worth of being lies in his/her hard work.

These words of wisdom which were written thousands of years ago hold true and are applicable to people even today because the meaningfulness of a person's life will depend on being disease free. Through the above mentioned shloka, Shri Ugradityacharya Maharaj says that if you are ill, first get your disease treated and cured, and then work wisely towards the attainment of the four goals of life.

This book has been created to put the above mentioned ideology into practice. I have been practicing Ashtanga Yoga for the last 27 years, but have always felt the lack of such a book that would include all the aspects of Ashtanga Yoga, to be studied in totality. This very thought gradually took the shape of this book, by the grace of God.

The intricacies I have learnt in my 32 years of practicing of Yoga, I have tried to impart them to the readers through this book. Another important point is that I have tried to present the scientific reasons, tables of diseases, art of living as per today's scenario, and along with these, I have tried to enumerate topics such as 'what is yoga', 'how does it work', 'what are its benefits' for the reader's benefit. I feel that readers should read this book again and again and put the given techniques and theories to practice with a lot of wisdom.

My aim is to help you keep your body healthy and acquire beauty along with physical, mental, materialistic and spiritual happiness, peace, prosperity and absolute bliss.

May you always enjoy total health in your life, this is the wish and prayer of 'Trilok'.

Yogacharya Rajeev Jain 'Trilok'

rajeevjaintrilok@gmail.com

Yogabhyasa, simultaneously calms a person down and makes him/her more active.

– RJT

INDEX

B

D

E

H

R

V

Other titles by Author:

In Hindi

- ***Sampurn Yog Vidhya***
  (also in Gujarati and Marathi)
- ***Sampurn Yog Vigyan***
- ***Power Yoga***
- ***Sabhi Ke Liye Yogasan Aivam Pranayam***
- ***Khel Khel Mein Yog***
- ***Aao Yog Karen Hum***

In English

- ***Yoga for Children***
- ***Playing Yoga***